Cancer Pain Procedural Techniques

AF793114

ANESTHESIA ILLUSTRATED

Keith J. Ruskin, MD and Barbara K. Burian, PhD
Series Editors

Published and Forthcoming Titles:

Pediatric Anesthesia Procedures, edited by Anna Clebone and Barbara Burian

Ultrasound Guided Procedures and Radiologic Imaging for Pediatric Anesthesiologists, edited by Anna Clebone, Joshua Finkle, and Barbara Burian

Emergency Anesthesia Procedures, edited by Lauren C. Berkow

Cancer Pain Procedural Techniques, edited by Amitabh Gulati, Neal Rakesh, Grant Chen, Storm Horine, Ali Valimahomed, and Ehtesham Baig

Cancer Pain Procedural Techniques

EDITED BY

Amitabh Gulati
Neal Rakesh
Grant Chen
Storm Horine
Ali Valimahomed
Ehtesham Baig

OXFORD
UNIVERSITY PRESS

OXFORD
UNIVERSITY PRESS

Oxford University Press is a department of the University of Oxford. It furthers the University's objective of excellence in research, scholarship, and education by publishing worldwide. Oxford is a registered trade mark of Oxford University Press in the UK and certain other countries.

Published in the United States of America by Oxford University Press
198 Madison Avenue, New York, NY 10016, United States of America.

© Oxford University Press 2025

All rights reserved. No part of this publication may be reproduced, stored in a retrieval system, or transmitted, in any form or by any means, without the prior permission in writing of Oxford University Press, or as expressly permitted by law, by license, or under terms agreed with the appropriate reproduction rights organization. Inquiries concerning reproduction outside the scope of the above should be sent to the Rights Department, Oxford University Press, at the address above.

You must not circulate this work in any other form
and you must impose this same condition on any acquirer.

Library of Congress Cataloging-in-Publication Data
Names: Gulati, Amitabh [editor], Rakesh, Neal [editor],
Chen, Grant [editor], Horine, Storm [editor],
Valimahomed, Ali [editor], Baig, Ehtesham [editor]
Title: Cancer pain procedural techniques
Edited by Amitabh Gulati, Neal Rakesh, Grant Chen, Storm Horine,
Ali Valimahomed and Ehtesham Baig
Description: New York, NY, United States of America :
Oxford University Press, [2025] | Series: Anesthesia illustrated |
Includes bibliographical references and index.
Identifiers: LCCN 2024049642 | ISBN 9780190933524 epub |
ISBN 9780190933500 paperback | ISBN 9780190933517 | ISBN 9780190933531
Subjects: LCSH: Cancer pain—Treatment | Pain management—Technique
Classification: LCC RC262 .C359 2025 | DDC 616.99/40472—dc23/eng/20241205
LC record available at https://lccn.loc.gov/2024049642

This material is not intended to be, and should not be considered, a substitute for medical or other professional advice. Treatment for the conditions described in this material is highly dependent on the individual circumstances. And, while this material is designed to offer accurate information with respect to the subject matter covered and to be current as of the time it was written, research and knowledge about medical and health issues is constantly evolving and dose schedules for medications are being revised continually, with new side effects recognized and accounted for regularly. Readers must therefore always check the product information and clinical procedures with the most up-to-date published product information and data sheets provided by the manufacturers and the most recent codes of conduct and safety regulation. The publisher and the authors make no representations or warranties to readers, express or implied, as to the accuracy or completeness of this material. Without limiting the foregoing, the publisher and the authors make no representations or warranties as to the accuracy or efficacy of the drug dosages mentioned in the material. The authors and the publisher do not accept, and expressly disclaim, any responsibility for any liability, loss or risk that may be claimed or incurred as a consequence of the use and/ or application of any of the contents of this material.

DOI: 10.1093/med/9780190933500.001.0001

Printed by Integrated Books International, United States of America

MIX
Paper
FSC FSC® C183721

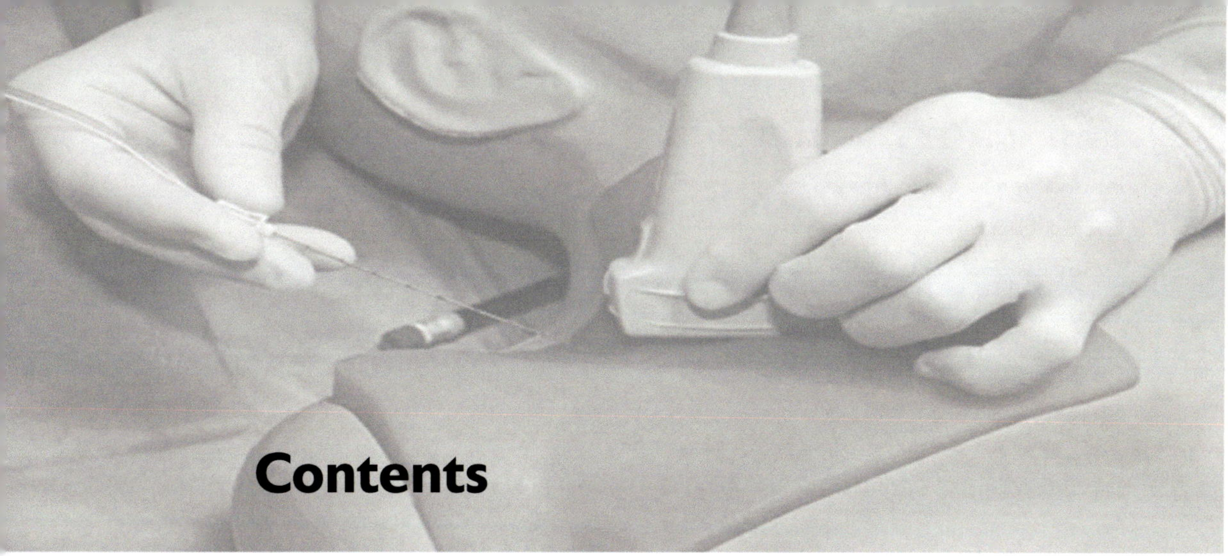

Contents

3. BREAST AND CHEST WALL SECTION

4. ABDOMINOPELVIC SECTION

5. NEUROAXIAL INTERVENTIONS

6. EXTRA-AXIAL SECTION

7. ADVANCED PROCEDURES SECTION

Contributors

Ehtesham Baig, BSc, MSc, MD, FRCPC, University Health Network—Toronto Western Hospital

Richard J. Batka, MD, Physician NYU Langone

Shane Brogan, MD, University of Utah School of Medicine—Huntsman Cancer Institute

A.C. Camargo, Cancer Center Professor Antonio Prudente—senior private health operator, A C Carmargo Cancer center

Erdong Chen, MD, Stanford Health Care

Grant Chen, MD, Attending at University of Texas at Houston Medical Center

Lucas First, MD, New York–Presbyterian Hospital Weill Cornell Medicine

Ale Ismael García-Cazares, MD, FIPP, National Cancer Institute, Mexico City—Clinica Alive

Akshat Gargya, MBBS, Physician at University of Vermont Medical Center

Priyanka Ghosh, MD, Physician San Mateo CA

Amitabh Gulati, MD, Attending Memorial Sloan Kettering Cancer Center

Rocío Guillén-Nuñez, MD, National Cancer Institute, Mexico City—Clinica Alive

Paul Ryan Haffey, DO, New York–Presbyterian Hospital Weill Cornell Medicine

B. Carolina Hernández-Porras, MD, MSc, FIPP, CIPS, National Cancer Institute, Mexico City—Centro Médico ABC

Lee Hingula, MD, Physician Santa Clara Valley Medical Center

Storm Horine, MD, Memorial Sloan Kettering Cancer Center

Angel Manuel Juárez-Lemus, MD, CIPS, ASRA-PMUC, National Cancer Institute, Mexico City—Clinica Alive

Olga Komargodski, MD, Department of Physical Medicine and Rehabilitation, Stony Brook University/St. Charles Rehabilitation

Franchesca König, MD, Memorial Sloan Kettering Cancer Center

Kelly Leap, MSN, AGACNP-BC, Memorial Sloan Kettering Cancer Center

Aron Legler, MD, Memorial Sloan Kettering Cancer Center

Dustin Liebling, MD, Physician Bay Shore Long Island, USA

Tiffany Lin, MD, New York–Presbyterian/Weill Cornell Medical Center

Ojas Mainkar, MD, New York–Presbyterian Hospital—Weill Cornell Medical Center

Anthony Mazzola, MD, Assistant professor, Mount Sinai Medical Center

Andrew Mendelson, DO, New York–Presbyterian Hospital—Weill Cornell Medicine

Daniel Chun-suk, Oh, MD, New York–Presbyterian, The University Hospital of Columbia and Cornell Department of Rehabilitation and Regenerative Medicine

Ankur A. Patel, DO, Physician Novant Health Pain Management NC, USA

Manuel Cifrian Perez, MD, PhD, La Fe University and Polytechnic Hospital

Ricardo Plancarte, MD, PhD, FIPP, National Cancer Institute, Mexico City—Centro Médico ABC

Neal Rakesh, MD, MSE, Memorial Sloan-Kettering Cancer Center

Marcela Sámano-García, MD, National Cancer Institute, Mexico City

Madeline Scanlon, MD, Physician Essentia Health Moose Lake Clinic MN, USA

Frank V. Schirripa, DO, Department of Physical Medicine and Rehabilitation, NewYork–Presbyterian, The University Hospital of Columbia and Cornell

Ido Straus, MD, PhD, Tel-Aviv Medical Center

Anthony Tran, MD, NewYork–Presbyterian Hospital—University Hospital of Columbia and Cornell

Cory Ullger, DO, Department of Physical Medicine and Rehabilitation, New York University Langone Health/Rusk Rehabilitation

Cameran Vakassi, MD, Memorial Sloan Kettering Cancer Center

Xiang Qian, MD, PhD, Stanford Health Care

Ajax Yang, MD, Weill Cornell Medicine

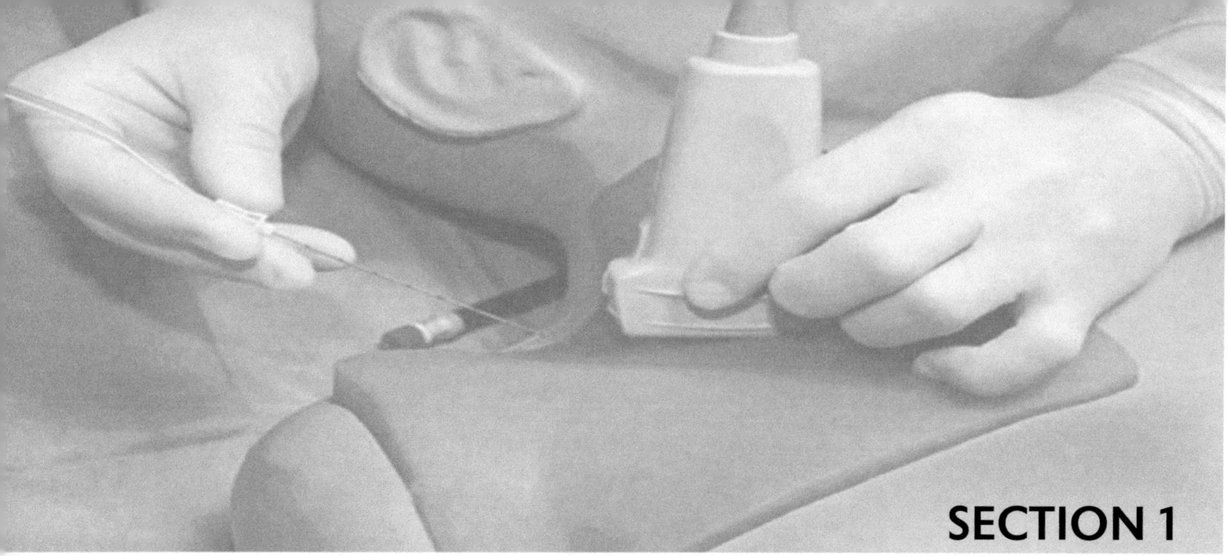

SECTION 1

INTRODUCTION

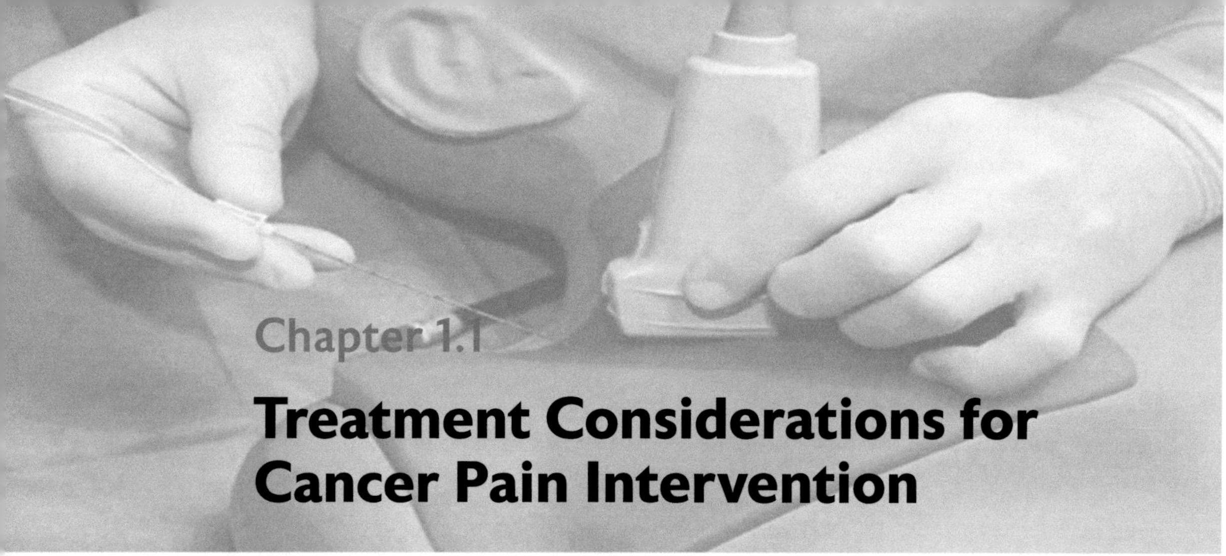

Chapter 1.1

Treatment Considerations for Cancer Pain Intervention

Kelly Leap and Grant Chen

Contents

Thrombocytopenia and Cancer Pain Population

Thrombocytopenia is defined as a platelet count of less than 150,000 platelets per microliter (μL) due to decreased platelet production, increased platelet consumption, or sequestration.[1] Thrombocytopenia is further broken down into mild (100,000–149,000 platelets per μL), moderate (50,000–99,000 platelets per μL), and severe (<50,000 platelets per μL).[1] Platelet counts less than 10,000 platelets per μL are associated with a very high risk for spontaneous bleeding.[1]

Thrombocytopenia in the oncologic population is often the result of bone marrow suppression from the tumor, chemotherapy, radiotherapy, or surgical trauma.[2,3] Bone marrow suppression is especially common in lymphoma, metastatic breast cancer, and metastatic lung cancer.[4] Nonmalignant causes of thrombocytopenia should also be considered in the oncologic population including infection, immune thrombocytopenia, disseminated intravascular coagulation, and drug-induced thrombocytopenia. Common triggers for drug-induced thrombocytopenia are heparin, vancomycin, linezolid, or ganciclovir.[4]

There is very limited evidence to guide perioperative management of patients with thrombocytopenia, and recommendations are mostly based on low-quality evidence and are, therefore, controversial.[1] According to a recent Cochrane review in 2018, the minimum recommended platelet counts for thrombocytopenic patients undergoing lumbar puncture or epidural anesthesia vary significantly across countries.[5] Although a consensus on a standard platelet count threshold has yet to be determined, current recommendations range from 20,000 to 50,000 platelets per μL for lumbar puncture and 50,000 to 80,000 platelets per μL for epidural anesthesia.[5] These recommendations vary from older and more conservative recommendations for 100,000 platelets per μL prior to epidural anesthesia.[6] Many studies, specifically in the obstetric setting, have supported these lower thresholds.[7–10] Although thrombocytopenia is a risk factor for epidural or spinal hematoma, great variability among recommendations exist due to the rarity of these complications, which are estimated to be 1:150,000 after epidural anesthesia and 1:220,000 after spinal anesthesia.[11,12] These inconsistencies in practice lead to provider uncertainty in safely performing pain management interventions.[5] Though these recommendations provide a basis for practice, the platelet threshold for performing neuraxial anesthesia should be individualized based on patient factors, the increased risk of bleeding in the oncological population,[13] the necessity of the intervention, and a risk versus benefit analysis.[8,11,14] Other weak or not graded recommendations include a platelet threshold of 100,000 platelets per μL for ophthalmic surgery and neurosurgery and 50,000 platelets per μL for major surgery or invasive procedures.[1,3,15,16] In nonemergent or elective procedures, a hematology consult may be beneficial in determining the cause of the patient's thrombocytopenia and the appropriate treatment plan, such as a platelet transfusion. Platelet transfusion comes with its own set of problems such fevers, rigors, urticaria, and a progressive decrease in platelet count as the number of transfusions increases.[17] Prior to performing the procedure, a thorough discussion of the risks of thrombocytopenia should occur between the provider and the patient.

Concurrent Chemotherapy/Radiation Therapy and Thrombocytopenia

Thrombocytopenia is considered an acute dose-limiting toxicity of chemotherapy and radiation therapy.[2,4] Chemotherapeutic agents differ in how they cause thrombocytopenia, but the most common causes include endothelial injury, reduced synthesis of coagulation factors in the liver, or platelet dysfunction.[2] Patients at highest risk for bleeding during chemotherapy include patients with prior episodes of bleeding, treatment with a drug affecting platelet function, bone marrow metastases, baseline platelet count less than 75,000, and genitourinary or gynecologic malignancy.[2] The highest rates of thrombocytopenia are associated with gemcitabine and platinum-based regimens[4] (Box 1.1.1). Another common offending agent is cabozantinib, which causes thrombocytopenia in approximately 34% of patients.[18] Contrarily, most standard nonmyeloablative therapies were developed to decrease the risk for thrombocytopenia and are, therefore, rarely complicated by low platelet count.[4]

Generally, after chemotherapy, the platelet count begins to drop by the 7th day, reaches its nadir by the 14th day, and then gradually returns to baseline by the 28th to 30th day.[4] After radiation, the platelet count begins to drop by the 7th to 10th day and may not return to baseline for 30 to 60 days.[4] Chemotherapy and radiation therapy dose reductions and platelet transfusions remain the mainstay treatment for related thrombocytopenia.[4,19] Prior to performing a high-risk procedure for a patient who is on chemotherapy or radiation, a provider should consider avoiding procedure around the anticipated time of platelet nadir or obtain a platelet count to ensure it is within normal limits. Collaboration with the oncologist may be beneficial in determining the safest and most ideal time for a patient on chemotherapy or radiation therapy to undergo a pain procedure.

BOX 1.1.1 Common Chemotherapy Regimens Associated with Thrombocytopenia (Adapted from Kuter[4] and Weycker et al.[19])

Common Chemotherapy Regimens Associated with Thrombocytopenia

Bortezomib
Carboplatin
Cisplatin
Cyclophosphamide
Docetaxel
Fluorouracil
Gemcitabine
Ibritumomab tiuxetan
Oxaliplatin
Temozolomide
Vincristine
Gemcitabine/Cisplatin
Gemcitabine/Oxaliplatin
Gemcitabine/Carboplatin
Pemetrexed/Cisplatin
Pemetrexed/Carboplatin
R-CHOP (Rituximab/Cyclophosphamide/Doxorubicin Hydrochloride/Vincristine/Prednisone)
ICE (Ifosfamide/Doxorubicin/Dacarbazine)
MAID (Mesna/Doxorubicin/Ifosfamide/Dacarbazine)
Fluorouracil/Doxorubicin/Cyclophosphamide
FOLFOX (Folinic Acid/Fluorouracil/Oxaliplatin)

Other Coagulation Disorders and Cancer Pain Population

Cancer patients are an especially vulnerable population, as they often have coagulation disorders. Cancer itself causes a hypercoagulable state, but patients are also often coagulopathic, either from disease affecting liver function or due to other sequelae of cancer like disseminated intravascular coagulation (DIC).[2,20] Providers should assess for bleeding risk factors in the patient's medical history and family history. Physical exam findings of easy bruising or petechiae can also help identify bleeding diathesis. Venous thromboembolism (VTE), which includes deep venous thrombosis and pulmonary embolism, is most commonly associated with acute myeloid leukemia, non-Hodgkin lymphoma, renal cell, ovarian, pancreatic, gastric, and lung cancers.[2] DIC is most commonly associated with the acute leukemias and prostate cancer.[2] Given the liver's significant role in blood coagulation, liver cancer or metastases to the liver can also cause coagulopathy.

These coagulation disorders are caused not only by the disease itself but also by the related treatments.[2,20] Radiation to the rectum, vagina, prostate, and bladder has been associated with an increased risk for bleeding.[2] Various surgeries and chemotherapy regimens have been associated with an increased risk for both thromboembolism and bleeding.[2] Many oncologic patients are also prescribed prophylactic or therapeutic anticoagulant or antiplatelet therapy, further exacerbating a cancer patient's risk for bleeding.

Antiplatelet/Anticoagulant Therapy and Cancer Pain Interventions

Prior to interrupting a patient's antiplatelet or anticoagulant regimen, one must weigh a patient's thromboembolic versus bleeding risk. Thromboembolic risk is estimated by first determining the reason for anticoagulation and, therefore, the risk of recurrent VTE.[20] Atrial fibrillation and previous thromboembolic events are common causes of VTE.[20] Bleeding risk is estimated by the type of the procedure and patients' comorbidities, such as renal impairment.[20] Recommended platelet cutoffs for invasive procedures are discussed in the section above. Societal recommendations for International normalized Ratio (INR) cutoffs exist for neuraxial anesthesia but vary slightly. The American Society of Regional Anesthesia and Pain Medicine (ASRA) recommends INR ≤1.4 in patients not on warfarin and ≤1.2 in patients who have discontinued warfarin for 5 days, while the European Society of Anesthesiology (ESA) and British guidelines recommend INR ≤1.4.[21,22]

The American Society of Regional Anesthesia and Pain Medicine (ASRA), European Society of Regional Anaesthesia and Pain Therapy, American Academy of Pain Medicine, International Neuromodulation Society, North American Neuromodulation Society, and World Institute of Pain created updated guidelines for nononcologic patients who are taking antiplatelet and anticoagulant medication and undergoing interventional spine and pain procedures (Tables 1.1.1 and 1.1.2).[22] No guidelines currently exist for the cancer pain population; thus, these guidelines are often applied to oncologic patients.

Table 1.1.1 Pain Procedures Classification Based on Potential Risk of Serious Bleeding (Adapted from Narouze et al.[22])

Low-Risk Procedures*	Intermediate-Risk Procedures*	High-Risk Procedures
- Peripheral nerve blocks - Peripheral joints and musculoskeletal injections - Trigger point injections including piriformis injection - Sacroiliac joint injection and sacral lateral branch blocks - Thoracic and lumbar facet MBNB and RFA - Peripheral nerve stimulation trial and implant - Pocket revision and implantable pulse generator - Intrathecal pump replacement	- Interlaminar ESIs (cervical, thoracic, lumbar, sacral) - Transforaminal ESIs (cervical, thoracic, lumbar, sacral) - Cervical facet MBNB and RFA - Intradiscal procedures (cervical, thoracic, lumbar) - Sympathetic blocks (stellate, thoracic, splanchnic, celiac, lumbar, hypogastric) - Trigeminal and sphenopalatine ganglia blocks - Peripheral nerve stimulation trial and implant	- Spinal cord stimulation trial and implant - Dorsal root ganglion stimulation trial and implant - Intrathecal catheter and pump implant - Vertebral augmentation (vertebroplasty and kyphoplasty) - Percutaneous decompression laminotomy - Epiduroscopy and epidural decompression

*Patients with high risk for bleeding (old age, history of bleeding tendency, concurrent uses of other anticoagulants/antiplatelets, liver cirrhosis/advanced liver disease, and advanced renal disease) undergoing low- or intermediate-risk procedures should be treated as intermediate or high risk, respectively.

Table 1.1.2 Preprocedural/Postprocedural Anticoagulation Guidelines (Adapted from Narouze et al.[22])

Medication	Discontinuation Prior to Procedure	Resumption Post-Procedure
Aspirin (ASA)	LOW: N/A INTERMEDIATE: Per assessment/ risk stratification HIGH: 6 days (primary prophylaxis); Per assessment/risk stratification (secondary prophylaxis)	24 hours
Diclofenac, Ketorolac, Ibuprofen	LOW: N/A INTERMEDIATE: N/A HIGH: 24 hours	24 hours
Etodolac, Indomethacin	LOW: N/A INTERMEDIATE: N/A HIGH: 2 days	24 hours
Naproxen, Meloxicam	LOW: N/A INTERMEDIATE: N/A HIGH: 4 days	24 hours
Nabumetone	LOW: N/A INTERMEDIATE: N/A HIGH: 6 days	24 hours
Oxaprozin, Piroxicam	LOW: N/A INTERMEDIATE: N/A HIGH: 10 days	24 hours
Coumadin	LOW: Per assessment/risk stratification INTERMEDIATE: 5 days; Normal INR HIGH: 5 days; Normal INR	6 hours
Subcutaneous heparin (BID, TID)	LOW: 6 hours INTERMEDIATE: 6 hours HIGH: 24 hours	LOW: 2 hours INTERMEDIATE/HIGH- 6–8 hours
IV heparin	LOW: 6 hours INTERMEDIATE: 6 hours HIGH: 6 hours	2 hours
Enoxaparin (prophylactic)	LOW: 12 hours INTERMEDIATE: 12 hours HIGH: 12 hours	LOW: 4 hours INTERMEDIATE/HIGH: 12–24 hours
Enoxaparin (therapeutic)	LOW:24 hours INTERMEDIATE: 24 hours HIGH: 24 hours	LOW: 4 hours INTERMEDIATE/HIGH: 12–24 hours
Dalteparin	LOW: 24 hours INTERMEDIATE: 24 hours HIGH: 24 hours	LOW: 4 hours INTERMEDIATE/HIGH: 12–24 hours
Rivaroxaban, Apixaban, Edoxaban	LOW: Per assessment/risk stratification INTERMEDIATE: 3 days HIGH: 3 days	24 hours

(*continued*)

Table 1.1.2 Continued

Medication	Discontinuation Prior to Procedure	Resumption Post-Procedure
Fondaparinux	LOW: Per assessment/risk stratification INTERMEDIATE: 4 days HIGH: 4 days	LOW: 6 hours INTERMEDIATE/HIGH: 24 hours
Cangrelor	LOW: Per assessment/risk stratification INTERMEDIATE: 3 hours HIGH: 3 hours	24 hours
Ticagrelor	LOW: Per assessment/risk stratification INTERMEDIATE: 5 days HIGH: 5 days	24 hours
Dabigatran	LOW: Per assessment/risk stratification INTERMEDIATE: 4 days; 5–6 days (impaired renal function) HIGH: 4 days; 5–6 days (impaired renal function)	24 hours
Clopidogrel	LOW: Per assessment/risk stratification INTERMEDIATE: 7 days HIGH: 7 days	12-24 hours
Prasugrel	LOW: Per assessment/risk stratification INTERMEDIATE: 7–10 days HIGH: 7–10 days	24 hours

Leukocytosis and Leukopenia in the Cancer Pain Population

Leukocytosis is defined as a white blood cell count greater than 11,000 per mm^3. Neutrophilia is the most common form of leukocytosis and is defined as an absolute number of mature neutrophils greater than 7,000 per mm.[3,23] Common causes of neutrophilia include stress, infection, chronic inflammation, and medications. Of the medications that may induce neutrophilia, corticosteroids are a common offending agent and are of special concern in the cancer pain setting.[23] Corticosteroid-induced leukocytosis can be differentiated from bacterial infection, as corticosteroids typically do not cause the same degree of a left shift.[24] The main mechanism of action behind corticosteroid-induced leukocytosis is the release of granulocytes from the bone marrow and the inhibition of neutrophil apoptosis.[25,26] The most common infection in the interventional pain management setting is an epidural abscess, and the most common pathogen is *Staphylococcus aureus*.[27]

The evidence that corticosteroid-induced leukocytosis is caused by steroid injections is lacking. Studies have associated corticosteroid-induced leukocytosis with chronic systemic steroid administration, raising the concern that steroid injections may pose similar risks.[28] Controversy exists when there is a correlation between the systemic corticosteroid dose and the degree of leukocytosis; however, one study found earlier leukocytosis with higher doses.[24] Corticosteroid-induced leukocytosis can begin within hours of steroid administration and typically decreases on discontinuation of the steroid.[25]

Leukopenia, on the other hand, is defined as white blood count below 4,000 per mm^3. Leukopenia in the cancer patient can result from leukemia and other cancers, chemotherapy, radiation treatment, immunosuppression therapy, or bone marrow transplant. Neutropenia is a specific type of leukopenia defined as low numbers of neutrophils (usually under 1,500 neutrophils per mm^3). Both leukopenic and neutropenic patients are prone to infection, so while there are no preprocedural guidelines, the recommended standard of care is to assess the risks and benefits for each patient individually along with their severity of leukopenia and current cancer stage.

Concurrent Immunotherapy and Cancer Pain Interventions

Given corticosteroids' immunosuppressive properties, prudent use is recommended prior to the start of immunotherapy as they can decrease the efficacy of immunotherapy. A study by Arbour and colleagues found that the use of systemic adrenal glucocorticoids prior to the start of immunotherapy in patients with non-small-cell lung cancer was associated with poorer outcomes.[29] In congruence with these findings, most immunotherapy clinical trial protocols exclude patients who take prednisone doses greater than or equal to 10 mg per day.[29]

References

1. Nagrebetsky A, Al-Samkari H, Davis NM, Kuter DJ, Wiener-Kronish JP. Perioperative thrombocytopenia: evidence, evaluation, and emerging therapies. Br J Anaesth. 2019;122(1):19–31. doi:10.1016/j.bja.2018.09.010
2. Kvolik S, Jukic M, Matijevic M, Marjanovic K, Glavas-Obrovac L. An overview of coagulation disorders in cancer patients. Surg Oncol. 2010;19(1):e33–e46. doi:10.1016/j.suronc.2009.03.008
3. Gauer RL, Braun MM. Thrombocytopenia. Am Fam Physician. 2012;85(6):612–622.
4. Kuter DJ. Managing thrombocytopenia associated with cancer chemotherapy. Oncology (Williston Park). 2015;29(4):282–294.
5. Estcourt LJ, Malouf R, Hopewell S, Doree C, Van Veen J. Use of platelet transfusions prior to lumbar punctures or epidural anaesthesia for the prevention of complications in people with thrombocytopenia. Cochrane Database Syst Rev. 2018;4(4):CD011980. doi:10.1002/14651858.CD011980.pub3
6. Rolbin SH, Abbott D, Musclow E, Papsin F, Lie LM, Freedman J. Epidural anesthesia in pregnant patients with low platelet counts. Obstet Gynecol. 1988;71(6 Pt 1):918–920.
7. Tanaka M, Balki M, McLeod A, Carvalho JC. Regional anesthesia and non-preeclamptic thrombocytopenia: time to re-think the safe platelet count. Rev Bras Anestesiol. 2009;59(2):142–153. doi:10.1590/s0034-70942009000200002
8. Douglas MJ. Platelets, the parturient and regional anesthesia. Int J Obstet Anesth. 2001;10:113–120.
9. Goodier CG, Lu JT, Hebbar L, Segal BS, Goetzl L. Neuraxial anesthesia in parturients with thrombocytopenia: a multisite retrospective cohort study. Anesth Analg. 2015;121(4):988–991. doi:10.1213/ANE.0000000000000882
10. Beilin Y, Zahn J, Comerford M. Safe epidural analgesia in thirty parturients with platelet counts between 69,000 and 98,000 mm(-3). Anesth Analg. 1997;85(2):385–388. doi:10.1097/00000539-199708000-00025
11. Grant GJ. Adverse effects of neuraxial analgesia and anesthesia for obstetrics. In: Post T, ed. UpToDate. Waltham, Mass.: UpToDate; 2021. www.uptodate.com. Accessed March 9, 2021.
12. Vandermeulen EP, Van Aken H, Vermylen J. Anticoagulants and spinal-epidural anesthesia. Anesth Analg. 1994;79(6):1165–1177. doi:10.1213/00000539-199412000-00024
13. Al-Samkari H, Connors JM. Managing the competing risks of thrombosis, bleeding, and anticoagulation in patients with malignancy. Blood Adv. 2019;3(22):3770–3779.
14. Frenk V, Camann W, Shankar KB. Regional anesthesia in parturients with low platelet counts. Can J Anaesth. 2005;52(1):114. doi:10.1007/BF03018594
15. Liumbruno GM, Bennardello F, Lattanzio A, Piccoli P, Rossetti G; Italian Society of Transfusion Medicine and Immunohaematology (SIMTI) Working Party. Recommendations for the transfusion management of patients in the peri-operative period. I. The pre-operative period. Blood Transfus. 2011;9(1):19–40. doi:10.2450/2010.0074-10

16. Yuan S, Goldfinger D. Clinical and laboratory aspects of platelet transfusion therapy. In: Post T, ed. UpToDate. Waltham, Mass.: UpToDate; 2021. www.uptodate.com. Accessed February 15, 2021.
17. Slichter SJ, Davis K, Enright H, Braine H, Gernsheimer T, Kao KJ, et al. Factors affecting posttransfusion platelet increments, platelet refractoriness, and platelet transfusion intervals in thrombocytopenic patients. Blood. 2005;105:4106–4114.
18. Cabozantinib (Rx). Medscape. https://reference.medscape.com/drug/cometriq-cabometyx-cabozantinib-999791#4. Accessed May 25, 2021.
19. Weycker D, Hatfield M, Grossman A, et al. Risk and consequences of chemotherapy-induced thrombocytopenia in US clinical practice. BMC Cancer. 2019;19:151.
20. Douketis JD, Lip GYH. Perioperative management of patients receiving anticoagulants. In: Post T, ed. UpToDate. Waltham, Mass.: UpToDate; 2021. www.uptodate.com. Accessed February 15, 2021.
21. Horlocker TT, Vandermeuelen E, Kopp SL, Gogarten W, Leffert LR, Benzon HT. Regional anesthesia in the patient receiving antithrombotic or thrombolytic therapy: American Society of Regional Anesthesia and Pain Medicine evidence-based guidelines (fourth edition). Reg Anesth Pain Med. 2018;43(3):263–309.
22. Narouze S, Benzon HT, Provenzano D, et al. Interventional spine and pain procedures in patients on antiplatelet and anticoagulant medications (second edition): Guidelines from the American Society of Regional Anesthesia and Pain Medicine, the European Society of Regional Anaesthesia and Pain Therapy, the American Academy of Pain Medicine, the International Neuromodulation Society, the North American Neuromodulation Society, and the World Institute of Pain. Reg Anesth Pain Med. 2018;43(3):225–262. doi:10.1097/AAP.0000000000000700
23. Riley LK, Rupert J. Evaluation of patients with leukocytosis. Am Fam Physician. 2015;92(11):1004–1011.
24. Shoenfeld Y, Gurewich Y, Gallant LA, Pinkhas J. Prednisone-induced leukocytosis: influence of dosage, method and duration of administration on the degree of leukocytosis. Am J Med. 1981;71(5):773–778. doi:10.1016/0002-9343(81)90363-6
25. Coates TD. Approach to the patient with neutrophilia. In: Post T, ed. UpToDate. Waltham, Mass.: UpToDate; 2021. www.uptodate.com. Accessed February 17, 2021.
26. Ronchetti S, Ricci E, Migliorati G, Gentili M, Riccardi C. How glucocorticoids affect the neutrophil life. Int J Mol Sci. 2018;19(12):4090. doi:10.3390/ijms19124090
27. Weng M, Sun Z, Miao C. Corticosteroid induce leukocytosis during the pain management. Pain Med. 2014;15(9):1645–1646. doi:10.1111/pme.12510
28. Frenkel A, Kachko E, Cohen K, Novack V, Maimon N. Estimations of a degree of steroid induced leukocytosis in patients with acute infections. Am J Emerg Med. 2018;36(5):749–753. doi:10.1016/j.ajem.2017.10.003
29. Arbour KC, Mezquita L, Long N, et al. Impact of baseline steroids on efficacy of programmed cell death-1 and programmed death-ligand 1 blockade in patients with non-small-cell lung cancer. J Clin Oncol. 2018;36(28):2872–2878. doi:10.1200/JCO.2018.79.0006

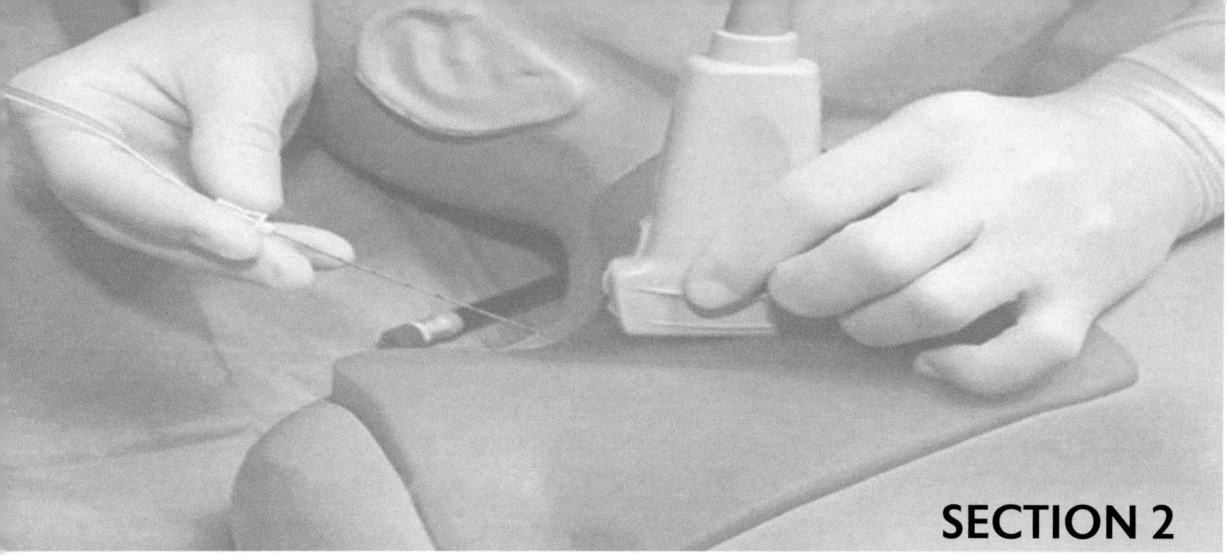

HEAD AND NECK INTERVENTIONS

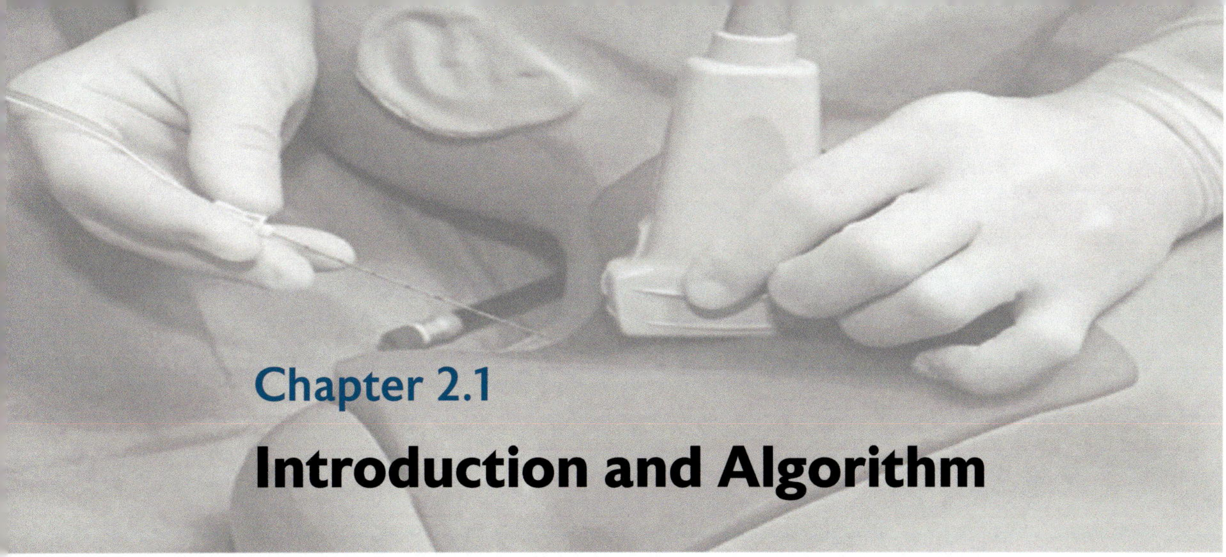

Chapter 2.1

Introduction and Algorithm

Ethesham Baig and Amitabh Gulati

Contents

Introduction

Cancers of the head and neck were the seventh most common cancer worldwide in 2018 (890,000 new cases and 450,000 deaths),[1] accounting for 3% of all cancers (51,540 new cases) and just over 1.5% of all cancer deaths (10,030 deaths) in the United States.[2] Within a cohort of head and neck cancer patients, the incidence of pain was 50%, 81%, and 70%, before, during and after oncologic treatments, respectively. Six months postcurative treatment, 36% of patients continued to report pain symptoms with 30% reporting higher severity of pain compared to the pretreatment period.[3]

The most frequent risk factors associated with head and neck cancer include smoking, alcohol consumption, human papillomavirus (HPV) infection (especially for oropharyngeal cancers), and Epstein-Barr virus (EBV) infection (especially for nasopharyngeal cancers in Asia).[4] There has been a steady decline globally of head and neck cancer associated with tobacco and alcohol use; however, HPV-associated oropharyngeal cancer cases have been increasing reflecting a latency of 10 to 30 years after oral-sex exposure.[5] The American Joint Committee on Cancer (AJCC) along with the Union for International Cancer Control (UICC) have therefore revised the classification system to include HPV status as part of diagnosis and staging.[6]

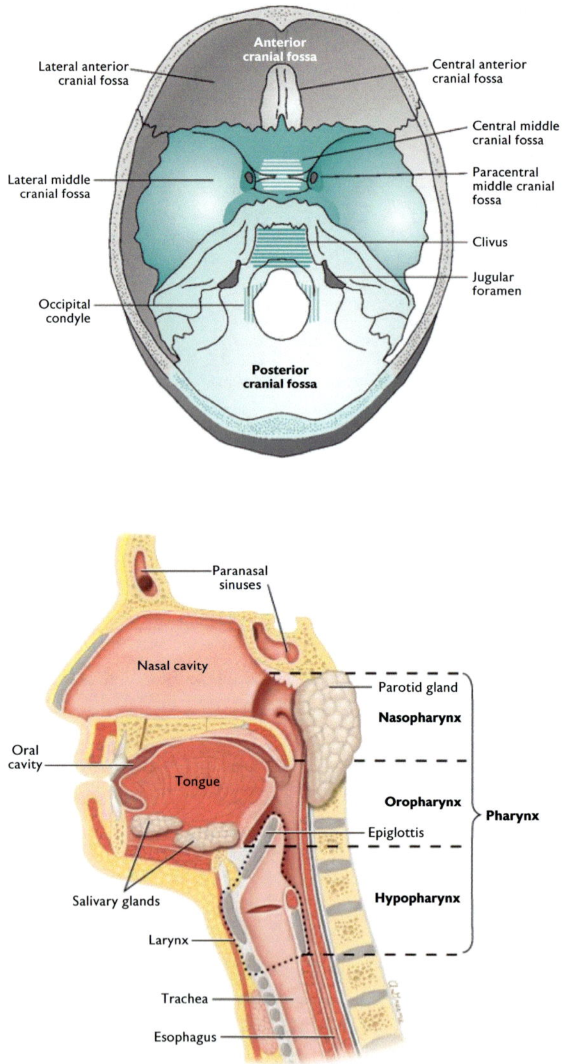

Figure 2.1.1 **a,** Anatomy of the skull base. **b,** Anatomy of the head and neck region (UpToDate: Overview of the diagnosis and staging of head and neck cancer)

For the purposes of this textbook, head and neck cancers include the following cancer sites: skull base, oral cavity, pharynx, larynx, the nasal cavity and paranasal sinuses, the major and minor salivary glands, and the thyroid gland (Figure 2.1.1).[7]

Mechanisms of Pain in the Head and Neck Region

Head and neck tumors produce pain through several mechanisms, including stimulation of nerve endings in mucous membranes, compression or invasion of sensory nerves, ulceration and infection, and bony invasion and destruction.[8] Nociceptive pain can be a direct effect of the tumor from expansion, inflammation, compression, ischemia, and destruction of surrounding tissue.[9] Bone invasion by tumor does not initially produce pain, but as the tumor grows, or becomes infected, it causes the periosteum to expand, which stimulates the nociceptive afferents that innervate the periosteum. Neuropathic pain may be due to direct tumor involvement of nerves such as the trigeminal nerve (CN V) and its branches, the facial nerve (CN VII), and the glossopharyngeal nerve (CN IX), as well as any sensory nerves in the face, skull, neck, or shoulder.[10] Patients with tumors located in the skull base or metastatic lesions to the brain may present with headaches.

Oral mucositis is a side effect of chemotherapy or radiation to the head and neck. It affects up to 80% of patients and is the most frequently reported pain syndrome in head and neck cancer.[11,12] Radiation to the head and neck can cause damage from fibrosis, necrosis, tissue atrophy, and vascular damage. Specific regional syndromes due to radiation of the head and neck region include trismus, dysphagia, dysgeusia, and chronic pain.[13] Metastatic disease to the lymph nodes within the neck may cause mass effect and related pain syndromes. Surgical resection via radical neck dissection is associated with long-term musculoskeletal impairments. Neck and shoulder pain is prevalent in many patients who have undergone lymph node dissection. Injury to the spinal accessory nerve (CN XI) can lead to shoulder disability and glenohumeral stiffness from scapulohumeral girdle muscle weakness. Various studies have shown that sparing the accessory nerve during neck dissection significantly decreases both acute and chronic postoperative shoulder pain and improves functional status.[14–15] Mandibular resection, maxillectomy, and other surgical resections also cause damage to vital structures resulting in chronic pain post-surgery.

Head and Neck Cancer Pain Syndromes

Major pain syndromes associated with head and neck oncology include headaches, facial pain, and neck pain (Table 2.1.1). The initial interventional approach usually involves nerve blocks targeting central and peripheral nerves for diagnostic purposes. These can be followed by longer-acting therapeutic interventions including radiofrequency ablation and chemical or electrical neurolysis. Neural structures that can be treated include sympathetic ganglia and somatic nerves of the head and neck region. Advanced techniques including spinal cord stimulation, intrathecal drug delivery, and neurosurgical procedures may be utilized if pain remains refractory to pharmacologic management and percutaneous interventional modalities. Figures 2.1.2a–c outline the interventional treatment algorithm for each of the three main head and neck pain symptom clusters.

Table 2.1.1 Head and Neck Pain Syndrome Etiologies

• Tumor-related • Myofascial pain syndrome • Boney metastasis • Cervical radiculopathy • Facet arthropathy • Spinal stenosis • Leptomeningeal disease • Cranial nerve compression • Complex regional pain syndrome • Hormonal therapy induced • Arthralgias • Postsurgical pain	• Radiation dermatitis • Chemotherapy or radiation-induced mucositis • Radiation-induced fibrosis • Dropped head syndrome • Mandibular osteonecrosis • Anxiety/depression • Lymphedema • Polyneuropathy • Mononeuropathy • Contractures • Fibromyalgia

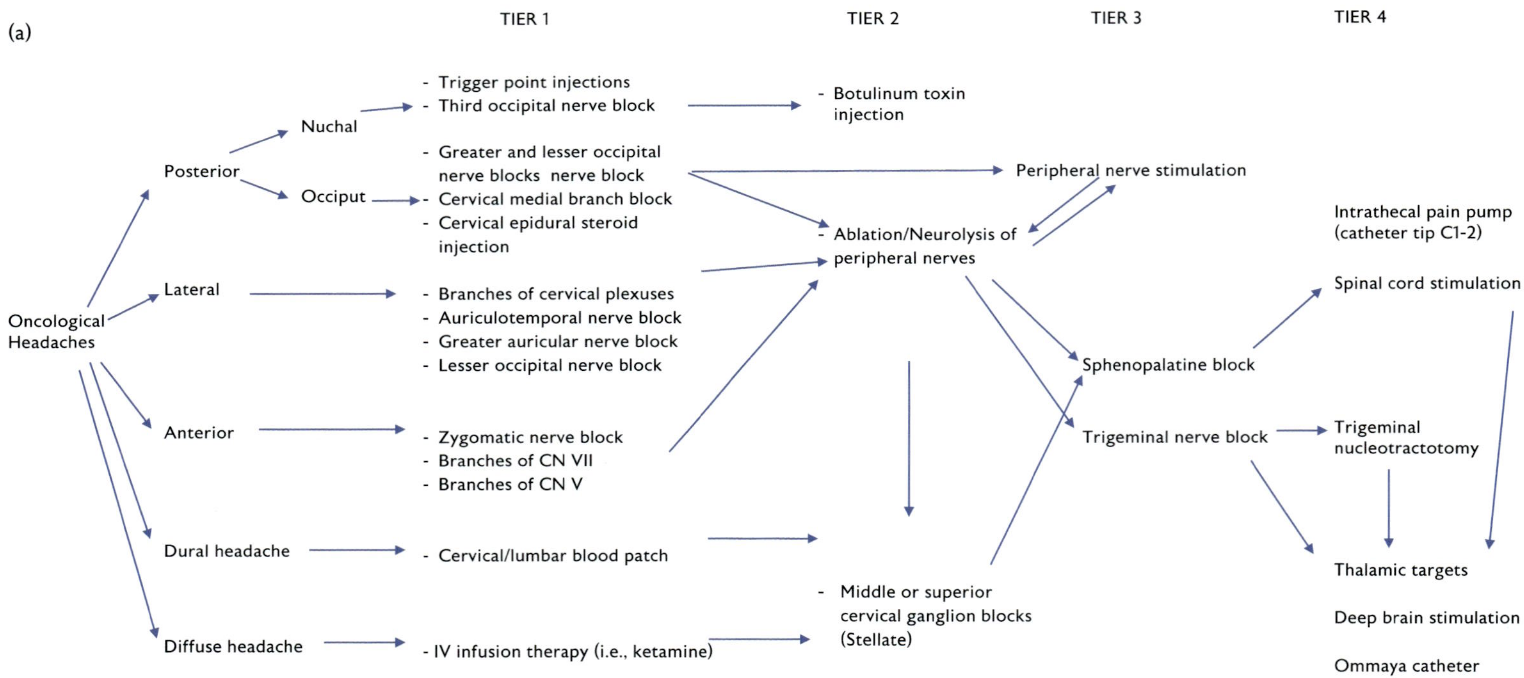

Figure 2.1.2 a–c. Interventional treatment algorithm for head and neck pain. **a,** Headaches.

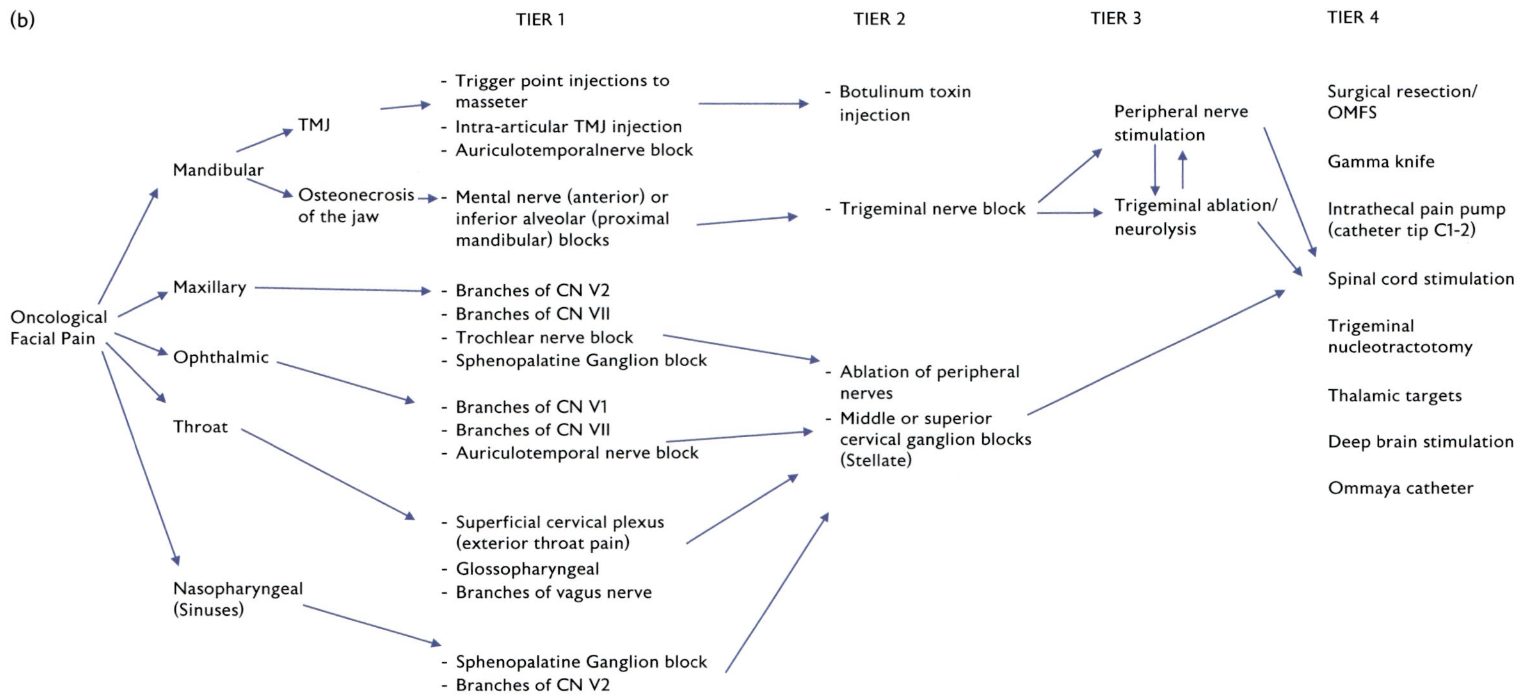

Figure 2.1.2 b. Facial pain.

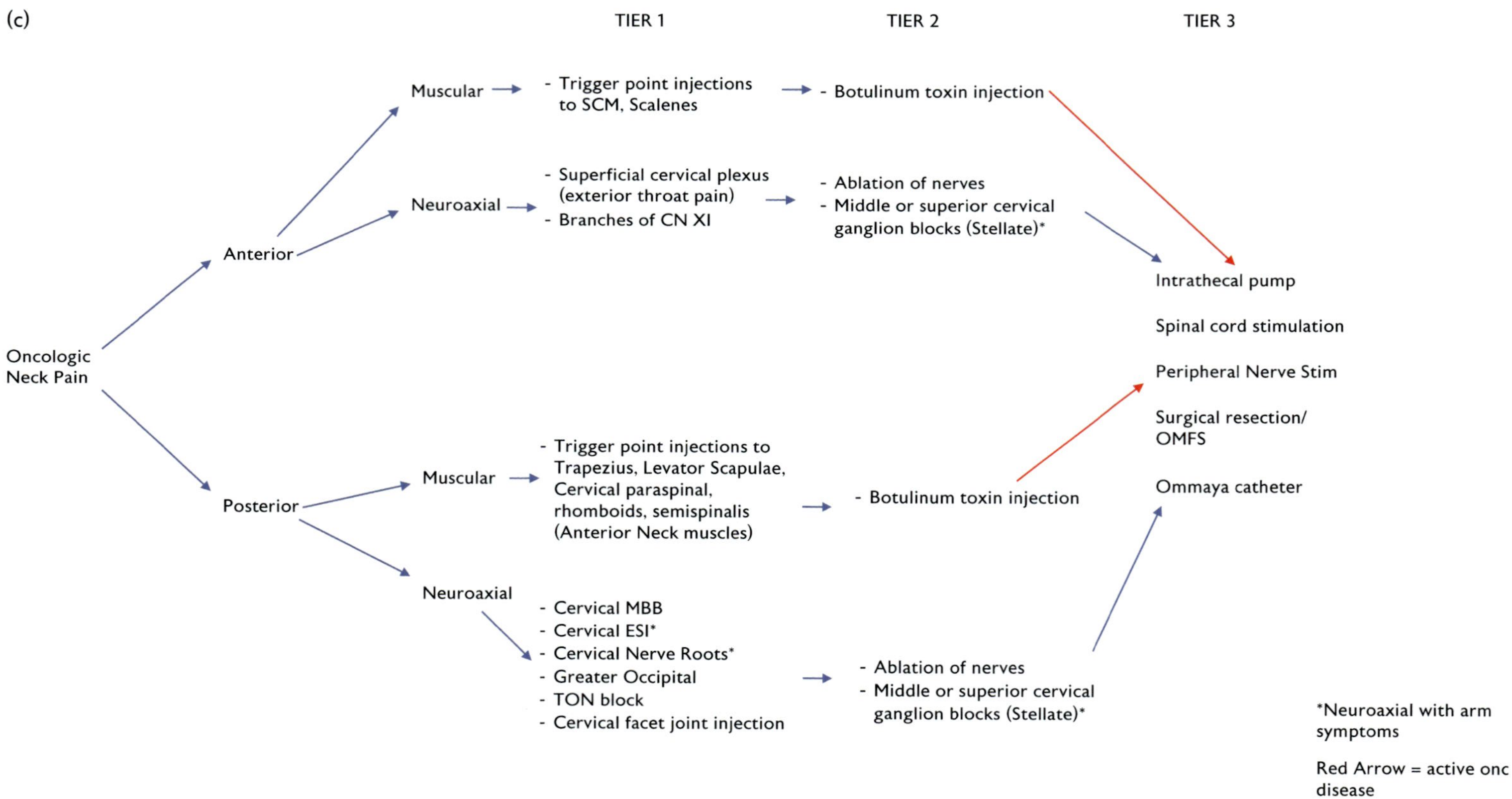

Figure 2.1.2 c. Neck pain.

Table 2.1.2 Contraindications to Head and Neck Interventions

Contraindications	Related-Types
Absolute	Refusal for the procedure Localized or systemic infection Severe coagulopathy
Relative	Thrombocytopenia Anticoagulation Immunocompromised patients Distorted anatomy Prior nerve injury or damage Allergy to anesthetics Implanted pacemaker Recent myocardial infarction Recent pulmonary embolism Cardiac conduction block (type 2 or higher A-V block) Severe emphysema Allodynia Glaucoma Mass preventing access to target location Inability to consent the procedure

Interventional Treatment Contraindications

The absolute contraindications to head and neck interventions are patient refusal for the procedure, localized or systemic infection, and severe coagulopathy.

Relative contraindications include thrombocytopenia, anticoagulation, immunocompromised state, distorted anatomy, prior nerve injury or damage, allergy to anesthetics, and inability to consent to the procedure. Table 2.1.2 outlines the contraindications and recommended treatment intervention to mitigate overall risk to the patient.

Conclusions

Head and neck cancer is associated with a high prevalence of pain syndromes due to underlying pathology and treatment regimens. Individualized analgesic plans, involving medical and interventional options, are necessary to address the pain symptoms that patients suffer. A recommended treatment approach includes local anesthetic blockade for diagnostic purposes and then ablative techniques utilizing chemical or thermal techniques. Depending on patient response, invasive strategies such as intrathecal drug delivery, dorsal column or peripheral nerve stimulation, and neurosurgical ablative techniques can be utilized.

References

1. Bray F et al. Global cancer statistics 2018: GLOBOCAN estimates of incidence and mortality worldwide for 36 cancers in 185 countries. CA Cancer J Clin. 2018; 68: 394–424.
2. Siegel R et al. Cancer statistics, 2018. CA Cancer J Clin. 2018; 68: 7–30.
3. Epstein JB et al. A systematic review of orofacial pain in patients receiving cancer therapy. Support Care Cancer. 2010; 18(8): 1023–1031.
4. Sankaranarayanan R et al. Head and neck cancer: a global perspective on epidemiology and prognosis. Anticancer Res. 1998; 18(6B): 4779–4786.

5. Global Burden of Disease Cancer Collaboration. Global, regional, and national cancer incidence, mortality, years of life lost, years lived with disability, and dis- ability-adjusted life-years for 32 cancer groups, 1990 to 2015: a systematic analysis for the global burden of disease study. JAMA Oncol. 2017; 3: 524–548.
6. Amin MB et al. The eighth edition AJCC cancer staging manual: continuing to build a bridge from a population-based to a more "personalized" approach to cancer staging. CA Cancer J Clin. 2017; 67: 93–99.
7. Mechtler L. Chapter 5: Pain due to tumors of the skull base. In: Cancer Pain: Pharmacologic, Interventional, and Palliative Approaches, 1st ed., edited by deLeon-Cassasola OA. Saunders First Edition, Philadelphia, PA: USA; 2000.
8. Datta S et al. Interventional approaches to management of pain of oral cancer. Oral Maxillofac Surg Clin North Am. 2006; 18(4): 627–641.
9. Binczak M et al. Management of somatic pain induced by head-and-neck cancer treatment: definition and assessment. Guidelines of the French Oto-Rhino-Laryngology- Head and Neck Surgery Society. Eur Ann Otorhinolaryngol Head Neck Dis. 2014; 131(4): 243–247.
10. Mehio AK et al. Alleviating head and neck pain. Otolaryngol Clin North Am. 2009; 42(1): 143–159.
11. Riley P et al. Interventions for preventing oral mucositis in patients with cancer receiving treatment: oral cryotherapy. Cochrane Database of Systematic Reviews 2015; 12.
12. Pandya JA et al. Post-radiation changes in oral tissues: an analysis of cancer irradiation cases. South Asian J Cancer. 2014; 3(3): 159–162.
13. Straub JM et al. Radiation-induced fibrosis: mechanisms and implications for therapy. J Cancer Res Clin Oncol. 2015; 141(11): 1985–1994.
14. Chan JY et al. Shoulder dysfunction after selective neck dissection in recurrent nasopharyngeal carcinoma. Otolaryngol Head Neck Surg. 2015; 153(3): 379–384.
15. Terrell JE et al. Pain, quality of life, and spinal accessory nerve status after neck dissection. Laryngoscope. 2000;110(4): 620–626.

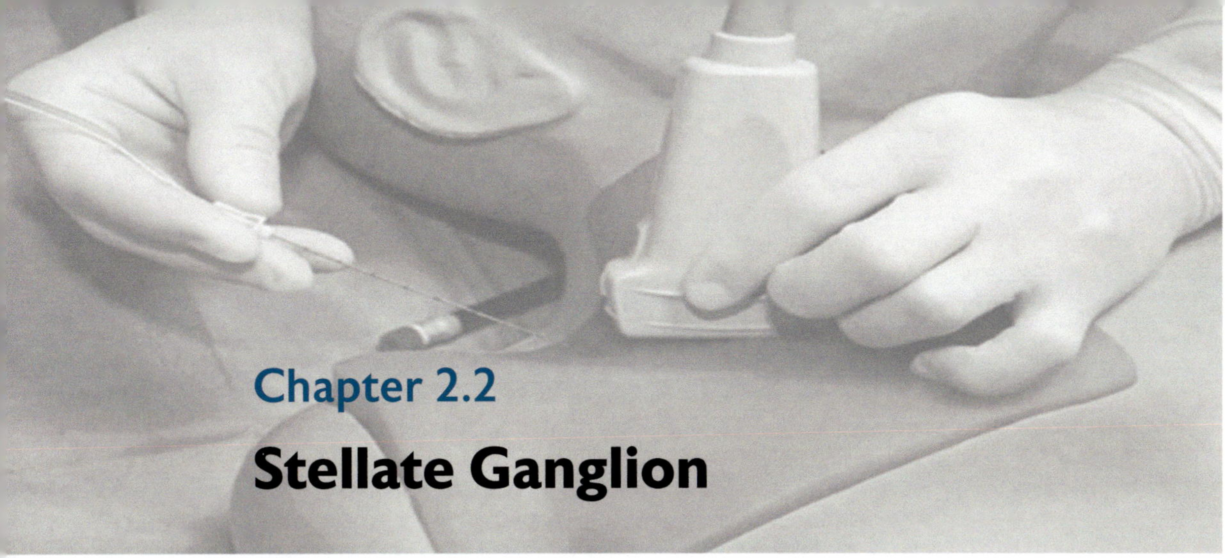

Chapter 2.2

Stellate Ganglion

Akshat Gargya

Contents

Introduction

The stellate ganglion block (SGB) is a common interventional procedure performed in cancer patients to manage ipsilateral upper extremity, neck, and facial pain. It is a safe procedure that can be performed in outpatient settings. Gunduz et al. proposed that stellate ganglion block inhibits the sympathetic/adrenergic hypersensitivity and central hyperexcitability.[1] It has also been demonstrated that sympathetic inhibition of upper extremity, neck, and head causes vasodilation that contributes to analgesia.[2]

Indications

An SGB is useful for pain in the upper extremity, face, and head in the oncologic population. Acute and chronic pain syndromes can occur due to direct tumor involvement or as sequelae of treatments from radiation, chemotherapy, or surgery. It can also be done as a diagnostic tool to confirm sympathetic mediated pain. Other indications for SGB include pain arising from intractable angina, phantom limb, postherpetic neuralgia, Raynaud's disease, thalamic pain syndrome, hyperhidrosis, peripheral vascular disease, and intractable cardiac arrythmias.[3–7]

Critical Anatomy

The stellate ganglion is formed by fusion of inferior cervical (C7, C8) and upper thoracic (T1, T2) sympathetic ganglia.[1,8,9] In up to 80% of the population, it lies anterior to the neck of the first rib and anterolateral to the C7 vertebral body (Figure 2.2.1). At the level of C7, the stellate ganglion is located anterior to the vertebral artery, posteromedial medial to the common carotid artery and internal jugular vein, and lateral to the thyroid, esophagus, and trachea. The suprapleural membrane lies just inferior to the ganglion. The stellate ganglion itself is enclosed beneath the prevertebral fascia over the longus colli muscle.[9] Blocking the stellate ganglion is usually performed at the level of C6 vertebrae. This level is easily recognized by its prominent anterior tubercle and tends to be the safest point to target the sympathetic fibers.[10] The anterior tubercle should reduce incidence of inadvertent injection into the vertebral artery. At C7 and T1, the vertebral artery is located anterior to the ganglion (Figure 2.2.2). This location may better target the true sympathetic ganglion and more effectively capture fibers to the distal arm. On the other hand, injecting medication at C6 level also minimizes the risk of pneumothorax due to the ganglion's proximity to the apex of the lung at C7.[8] Additionally, targeting the sympathetic chain at C6 and above may preferentially target fibers to the high cervical nerve roots and ipsilateral face and head. The shape and size of stellate ganglion are variable with average dimensions in literature approximated to 25 × 10 × 5 mm.[10,11]

Equipment and Patient Preparation

1. Monitors and Sterility
   a. No specific monitors are needed for this procedure, but emergency resuscitation equipment should be available immediately. This includes adult cardiac life support (ACLS) drugs, supplemental oxygen, airway adjuncts, and suction.
   b. Strict antiseptic technique should be observed including sterile probe cover, ultrasound gel, and sterile gloves. Chlorhexidine or other skin prep agent should be used to clean the skin prior to commencing the procedure.
   c. Peripheral IV should be placed for this procedure in case of emergency, and IV intralipid should be available immediately.
2. Equipment
   a. Probe: High-frequency linear array transducer (8–12 MHz)
   b. Needle type: 25-gauge, 1.5- to 2-inch needle
   c. Local anesthetic (2–4 mL): Lidocaine 1%–2%; ropivacaine 0.2%–0.5%; bupivacaine 0.25%–0.5%
   d. Adjuvant (0.5–1 mL): Nonparticulate (recommended) or particulate steroid

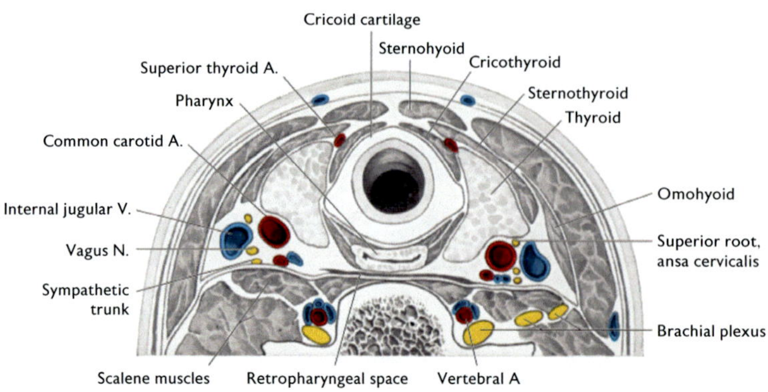

Figure 2.2.1 Schematic drawing of transverse section of the neck at the level of the cricoid cartilage and C7 illustrating the location of the sympathetic trunk/Stellate ganglion. (Reprinted with permission from Cunningham's Manual of Practical Anatomy: Head, Neck and Brain, 16th Edition)

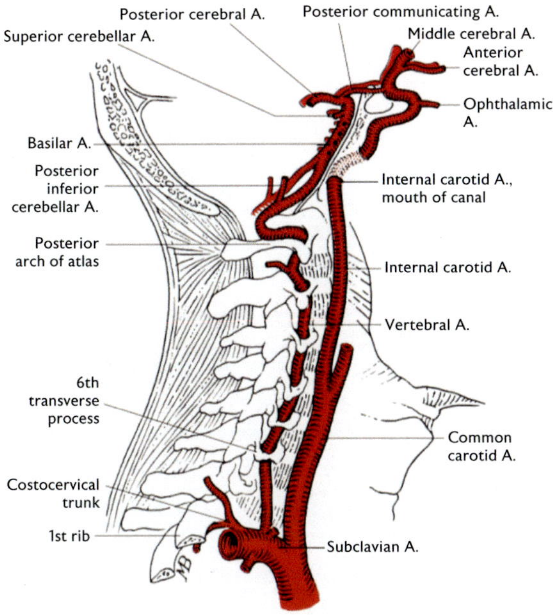

Figure 2.2.2 The course and communications of the internal carotid and vertebral arteries. (Reprinted with permission from Cunningham's Manual of Practical Anatomy: Head, Neck and Brain, 16th Edition)

3. Position
   a. Supine with head in contralateral rotation and extension

Procedure Technique

1. **Prepare equipment and supplies, position the patient supine with the head turned away from the procedural side, and clean the skin around the area of the block with antiseptic solution.** Palpate the cricoid cartilage, which is a surface marker to locate C6 level (Figure 2.2.3).
2. **Place the ultrasound probe in a transverse orientation on the neck to identify critical structures including the trachea, thyroid, esophagus, carotid artery, and internal jugular vein.**
3. **Scan cephalad and caudad to identify the C6 and C7 cervical levels.** The C6 level can be identified by its prominent anterior tubercle, which is called Chassaignac's or the Carotid tubercle. The C7 level can be identified by the absence of an anterior tubercle (Figure 2.2.4).
4. **Identify smaller adjacent vascular structures to avoid vascular injury, hematoma, and intravascular injection.** The vertebral artery is typically exposed at the C7 level and should be protected within the transverse foramen at C6. The inferior thyroid artery can often be visualized medially to the stellate ganglion at C6 or C7.
5. **Move the US probe to C6.** Identify the stellate ganglion below the carotid artery and above the longus colli muscle. Use doppler to confirm the procedural path does not involve vasculature.
6. **Insert the procedural needle using an in-plane approach with continuous ultrasound visualization.** Direct the needle between the carotid artery and longus colli muscle.
7. **After negative aspiration, deposit medication.** The stellate ganglion should be surrounded by the injectate.

Tips

- Use doppler to search for and identify cervical radicular arteries near the target area to avoid during procedures.
- If the cervical nerve roots are difficult to visualize, instead identify the neural foramen at a desired level based on anterior and posterior tubercles of the transverse processes.

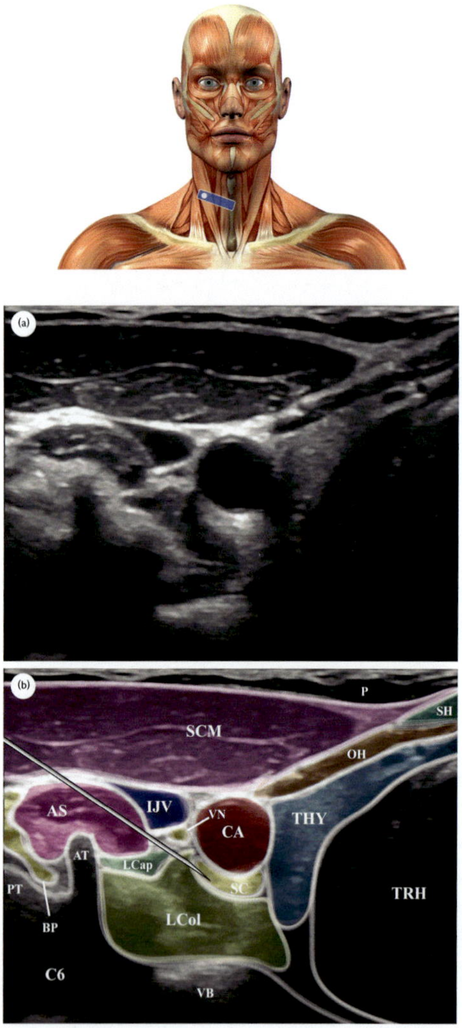

Figure 2.2.3 **a,** Ultrasound image of the anterolateral neck in an axial oblique plane at the C6 level. **b,** Labeled ultrasound image of in-plane needle placement within the subfascial plane for the location of the sympathetic chain with spread to the stellate ganglion in short-axis. *P* platysma, *SCM* sternocleidomastoid, *OH* omohyoid muscle, *SH* sternohyoid muscle, *BP* brachial plexus, *AS* anterior scalene, *IJV* internal jugular vein, *VN* vagus nerve, *CA* carotid artery, *THY* thyroid, *TRH* trachea, *C6 VB* vertebral body & *AT* anterior tubercle & *PT* posterior tubercle, *LCap* longus capitus, *SC* location of sympathetic chain, *LCol* longus colli.

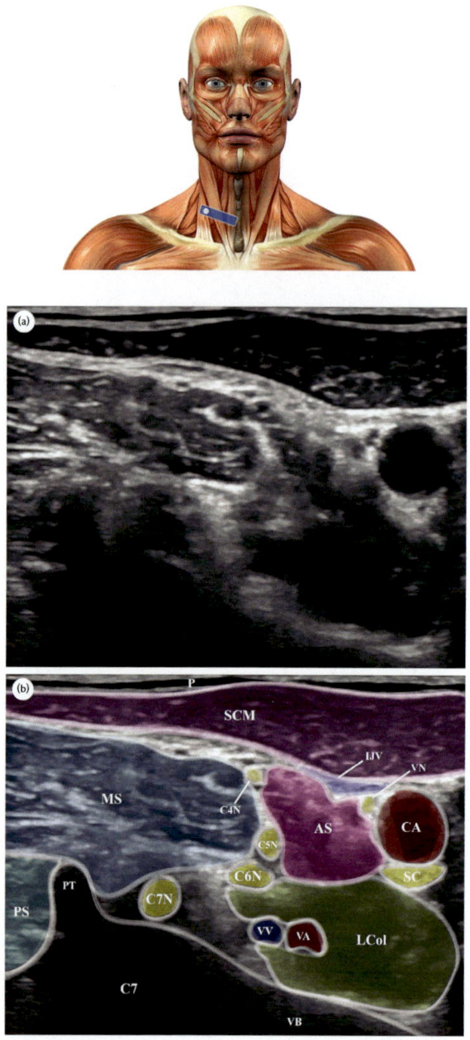

Figure 2.2.4 **a,** Unlabeled and **b,** labeled ultrasound image of the anterolateral neck in an axial oblique plane at the C7 level. *P* platysma, *SCM* sternocleidomastoid, *MS* middle scalene, C4N C4 nerve root, C5N C5 nerve root, C6N C6 nerve root, *AS* anterior scalene, *IJV* internal jugular vein, *VN* vagus nerve, *CA* carotid artery, *PS* posterior scalene, *C7 VB* vertebral body & *PT* posterior tubercle, C7N C7 nerve root, *SC* location of sympathetic chain, *VV* vertebral vein, *VA* vertebral artery, *LCol* longus colli.

Safety Considerations

- Avoid aiming anteriorly to puncture the carotid artery/internal jugular, vagus, and spinal nerves. However, sometimes a transinternal jugular venous approach is necessary to avoid the other structures by compressing the vein with pressure of the ultrasound probe.
- Avoid large volume injections (greater than 5 mL) to reduce the chance of spread to the recurrent laryngeal nerve causing dysphagia and hoarseness.

Postprocedure Management

Expected postprocedural considerations include Horner's syndrome, hoarseness of the voice, and ipsilateral phrenic nerve block with associated transient diaphragmatic paralysis. Horner's syndrome presents with drooping of the eyelid and pupil size changes that could be misinterpreted as signs of stroke or transient ischemic attack. Horner's syndrome is usually evidence of successful sympathetic block; however, it does not indicate complete sympathectomy. Patients should be educated about these temporary side effects and other signs of sympathectomy like conjunctival hyperemia, flushing of face, nasal stuffiness, and increased lacrimation. Hoarseness of the voice is due to blockade of the recurrent laryngeal nerve and is also temporary. Transient phrenic nerve block can present as shortness of breath that is typically positional and improved with sitting upright. Other potential complications include paratracheal hematoma formation, local anesthetic systemic toxicity from intravascular injection, pneumothorax, epidural or subarachnoid injection, and esophageal or tracheal perforation, which the patient should be monitored for. Postprocedurally, patients should be assessed for level of pain and a repeat neurological examination should be done.

References

1. Gunduz O, Kenis Coskun O. Ganglion blocks as a treatment of pain: current perspectives. Journal of Pain Research. 2017;10:2815–2826.
2. Song R. Effects of stellate ganglion block on cerebrovascular vasodilation in elderly patients and patients with subarachnoid hemorrhage. British Journal of Anaesthesia. 2016;117:el_13711.
3. Mekhail N, Kapural L. Complex regional pain syndrome type I in cancer patients. Current Review of Pain. 2000;4(3):227–233.
4. Michaels R, Sorber J. Reflex sympathetic dystrophy as a probable paraneoplastic syndrome: case report and literature review. Arthritis and Rheumatism. 1984;27(10):1183–1185.
5. Medsger TA, Dixon JA, Garwood VF. Palmar fasciitis and polyarthritis associated with ovarian carcinoma. Ann Intern Med. 1982;96:424–431.
6. Piraccini E, Chang KV. Stellate ganglion blocks. [Updated 2019 Jun 18]. In: StatPearls [Internet]. Treasure Island (FL): StatPearls Publishing; 2019 Jan. Available from: https://www.ncbi.nlm.nih.gov/books/NBK507798/
7. Duong S, Bravo D, Todd K, Finlayson R, Tran D. Treatment of complex regional pain syndrome: an updated systematic review and narrative synthesis. Canadian Journal of Anesthesia/Journal canadien d'anesthésie. 2018;65(6):658–684.
8. Marcer N, Bergmann M, Klie A, Moor B, Djonov V. An anatomical investigation of the cervicothoracic ganglion. Clinical Anatomy. 2011;25(4):444–451.
9. Ghai A, Kaushik T, Wadhera R, Wadhera S. Stellate ganglion blockade-techniques and modalities. Acta Anesthesiology Belgium. 2016;67(1):1–5.
10. Drake LD, Vogl W, Michel AW. Head and neck. In: Gray's anatomy for students, 1st ed., edited by Henry Gray. New York: Churchill Livingstone, 2005, 933.
11. Elias M1. Cervical sympathetic and stellate ganglion blocks. Pain Physician. 2000;3(3):294–304.

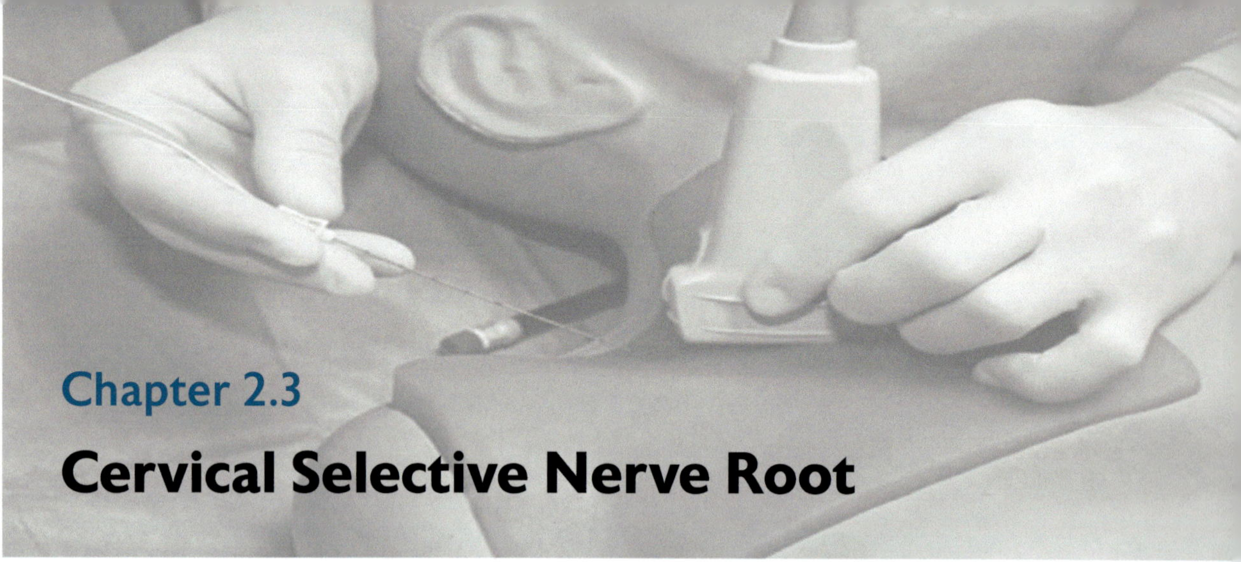

Chapter 2.3

Cervical Selective Nerve Root

Ajax Yang and Anthony Mazzola

Contents

Introduction

Cervical spinal nerve injuries that result from direct compression from a tumor, ischemia, radiation-induced or chemotherapy-induced neuritis, surgical manipulation, or chemical irritation (from tumor release of proinflammatory peptides, degenerative disc disease, etc.) can result in cervical radiculopathy and radicular pain.[1] However, it is important to note that radicular pain and radiculopathy are not synonymous. Studies show that compression of a spinal nerve alone does not cause pain except when dorsal root ganglion is involved.[2] Noninflammatory lesions such as malignancy, cysts, disc herniation, and osteophytes may cause direct mechanical compression, while leaking intradiscal exudates can result in chemical irritation. Radiation may also alter the nerve root as well as the surrounding anatomy. Cervical radicular pain is typically lancinating, deep, and experienced in the upper extremities.[3] Cervical radiculopathy, specifically, is a neurologic condition characterized by nerve conduction block that results in sensory or motor loss, or impaired reflexes, or a combination of these neurological deficits in a segmental or dermatomal distribution.[2]

Indications

Macnab and colleagues first described the selective nerve root block in 1971 as a method to evaluate patients with signs and symptoms of nerve root irritation but with incongruent image findings.[4] Since then, selective nerve root blocks have been used as diagnostic and treatment modalities when the etiology of pain is uncertain, such as:

1. Neck and upper extremity radicular pain of unspecified origin, resistant to conservative medical management. This is especially true after oncologic injury as described above.
2. Nonspecific neck and upper extremity pain with imaging showing pathology affecting multiple levels of spinal nerves.
3. Neck and upper extremity pain without clear radiologic pathology.
4. Neck and upper extremity pain with diagnostic imaging obscured by hardware artifact.

Traditionally fluoroscopic guidance has been the predominant method to target the cervical nerve roots.[5] More recently, ultrasound guidance techniques have been developed. Ultrasound-guided selective nerve block for the treatment C6 and C7 radicular pain was demonstrated in randomized clinical trials and retrospective studies to be as effective as a fluoroscopy-guided transforaminal block for cervical radicular pain.[6] Ultrasound-guided cervical nerve blocks have also been shown to have comparable outcomes to fluoroscopy-guided cervical epidural injections in regard to functional improvement when treating radicular pain of the lower cervical spine.[7,8] In the oncologic population, common indications to target cervical nerve roots include compressive tumors, such as Pancoast tumor, and radiation neuritis.

Critical Anatomy

The osseous structures of the seven cervical vertebrae are traditionally divided into the upper (C1 and C2) and lower (C3–C7) cervical spine with neurovascular elements exiting above each corresponding vertebral body.[9] C1 (atlas) is made up of two enlarged lateral masses. The lateral masses of C1 articulate with the occipital condyles to form the atlanto-occipital (AO) joint. Immediately behind the anterior arch of C1 is the vertically projecting odontoid process (axis) of the C2 vertebral body. The lower cervical vertebral bodies are similar in shape. Each vertebra consists of a pair of pedicles connecting the vertebral body to the lamina and bifid spinal process forming the spinal canal. Intervertebral foramina are bordered by the superior notch of the vertebra below, inferior notch of the vertebra above, vertebral body, and the facet joint. There are eight pairs of cervical nerve roots separated by seven vertebral bodies. Spinal neurovascular structures such as spinal nerves, dorsal root ganglia, sinuvertebral nerves, spinal arteries, and communicating veins are found inside the intervertebral foramina. Adjacent to the pedicles of C1–C6 are anterior and posterior tubercles, which combine to form the transverse foramina. The vertebral artery is usually encased in the transverse foramina from C1 to C6 and exposed from C7 caudally (Figure 2.3.1). The bony congruence is further enhanced by uncovertebral joints formed by the uncinate processes of adjacent vertebral bodies. The confluence of spinal nerves C1–C4, spinal accessory (CN XI), hypoglossal (CN XII) nerve, and sympathetic trunk form the cervical plexus. Spinal nerves C5–T1 form the brachial plexus to innervate the upper extremities (Figures 2.3.2 and 2.3.3). Uncovertebral osteophytes and protruding discs can cause stenosis and nerve root impingement anteriorly, while facet joint arthropathy and ligamentum flavum hypertrophy can cause posterior nerve root compression and radiculopathy.[9–10]

Anatomical studies demonstrated that cervical spine degenerative changes often alter the position of the vertebral artery and increase the risk of vascular compromise as the artery begins to more completely cover the nerve root in the lateral part of the foramen.[11,12] In patients with prior surgical debulking or facet degeneration, ultrasound may be particularly useful to discover atypical locations of the cervical vessels. While fluoroscopic digital subtraction may detect active

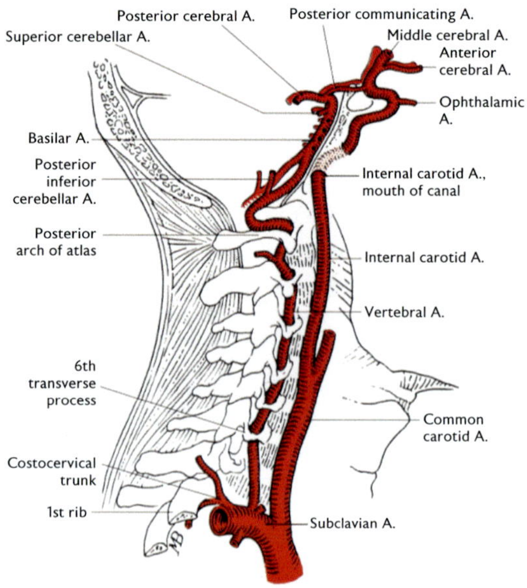

Figure 2.3.1 The course and communications of the internal carotid and vertebral arteries. (Reprinted with permission from Cunningham's Manual of Practical Anatomy: Head, Neck and Brain, 16th Edition)

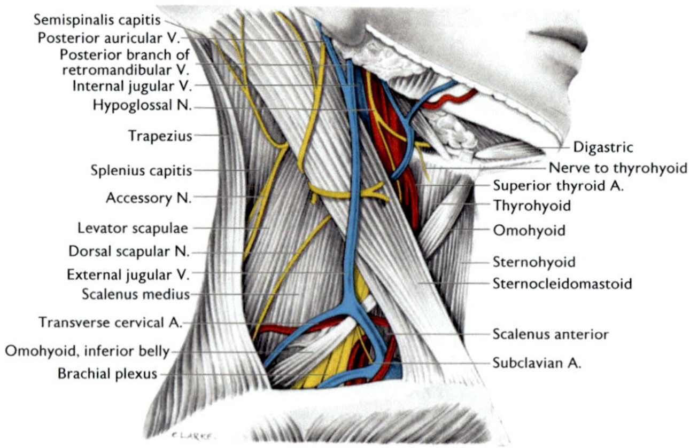

Figure 2.3.2 Lateral view of the superficial structures in the neck. (Reprinted with permission from Cunningham's Manual of Practical Anatomy: Head, Neck and Brain, 16th Edition)

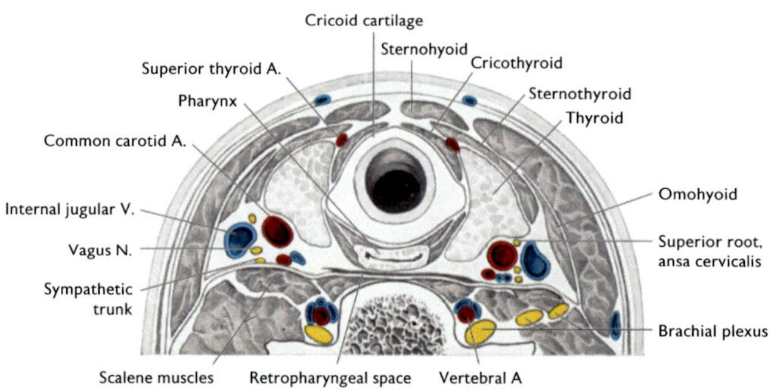

Figure 2.3.3 Schematic drawing of transverse section of the neck at the level of the cricoid cartilage and C7 illustrating the location of the brachial plexus. (Reprinted with permission from Cunningham's Manual of Practical Anatomy: Head, Neck and Brain, 16th Edition)

intravascular injections of contrast at the expense of significant radiation exposure,[13] ultrasound visualization offers the advantage of detecting blood vessels prior to performing any intravascular injection. Caution must be used, as current ultrasound technology is not completely sensitive in detecting minuscule vessels in which injection or spasm could still produce devastating neurologic deficits.[14] Furthermore, radiation may alter anatomy around the nerve root, and even the nerve root itself. In these cases, ultrasound will help identify neuromuscular changes.

Equipment and Patient Preparation

1. Monitors and Sterility
   a. No specific monitors are needed for this procedure, but emergency resuscitation equipment should be available immediately. This includes adult cardiac life support (ACLS) drugs, supplemental oxygen, airway adjuncts, and suction.
   b. Strict antiseptic technique should be observed including sterile probe cover, ultrasound gel, and sterile gloves. Chlorhexidine or other skin prep agent should be used to clean the skin prior to commencing the procedure.
2. Equipment
   a. Probe: High-frequency linear array transducer (8–12 MHz)
   b. Needle type: 22- or 25-gauge, 1.5- to 2-inch needle
   c. Local anesthetic (1–2 mL): Lidocaine 15%–2%; ropivacaine 0.2%–0.5%; bupivacaine 0.25%–0.5%
   d. Adjuvant (0.5–1 mL): Nonparticulate steroid
3. Position
   a. Supine (preferred) or lateral decubitus

Step-by-Step Technique

Selective Nerve Root Block (C4–C7)

1. **Prepare equipment and supplies, position the patient in the lateral decubitus position with the procedural side up, and clean the skin around the area of the block with antiseptic solution.** Alternative positioning is supine with the head rotated away from the procedural side.
2. Place the ultrasound probe in a transverse orientation to identify critical structures including the trachea, thyroid, esophagus, carotid artery, and internal jugular vein.
3. **Scan cephalad-caudad to identify cervical spine anatomy in the short-axis view.** C5 is notable for anterior and posterior tubercles of similar size (Figure 2.3.4). C6 has a more prominent anterior tubercle, which is known as the Carotid Tubercle or Chassaignac's Tubercle (Figure 2.3.5). C7 has a rudimentary or absent anterior tubercle and a large posterior tubercle (Figure 2.3.6).
4. **Identify the exposed vertebral artery.** This is typically found at C7 as it becomes encased within the transverse foramen by C6. Rule out atypical anatomy that could increase the risk of intravascular injection.
5. **Identify the nerve root at the desired cervical level.** Nerve roots have a characteristic circular, hypoechoic appearance and emerge from between the anterior and posterior tubercles at each level.
6. **Insert the needle at a 30- to 45-degree angle with an in-plane approach using a posterior-to-anterior direction (Figures 2.3.4–6).** The target portion of the cervical spine nerve is immediately distal to its exit from the anterior and posterior tubercles.
7. **Aspirate to rule out intravascular or intradural injection and inject 1–2 mL of local anesthetic and 0.25–0.5 mL of nonparticulate steroid.** Remove the needle and apply a dressing.

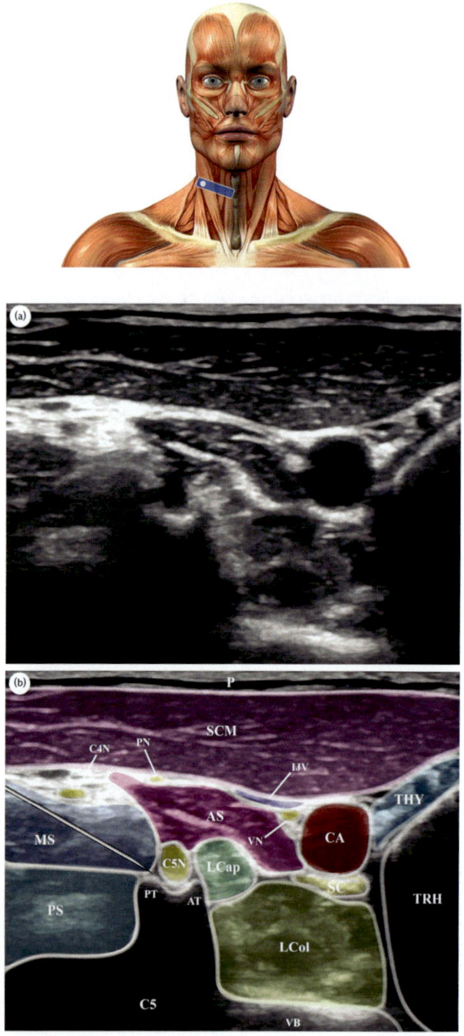

Figure 2.3.4 a, Ultrasound image of the anterolateral neck in an axial oblique plane at the C5 level. **b,** Labeled ultrasound image of in-plane needle placement of the C5 nerve root for a selective nerve root block in short-axis. *P* platysma, *SCM* sternocleidomastoid, *MS* middle scalene, *C4N* C4 nerve root, *AS* anterior scalene, *IJV* internal jugular vein, *PN* phrenic nerve, *VN* vagus nerve, *CA* carotid artery, *PS* posterior scalene, *C5N* C5 nerve root, *C5 VB* vertebral body & *PT* posterior tubercle, *SC* location of sympathetic chain, *LCap* longus capitus, *SC* location of sympathetic chain, *LCol* longus colli.

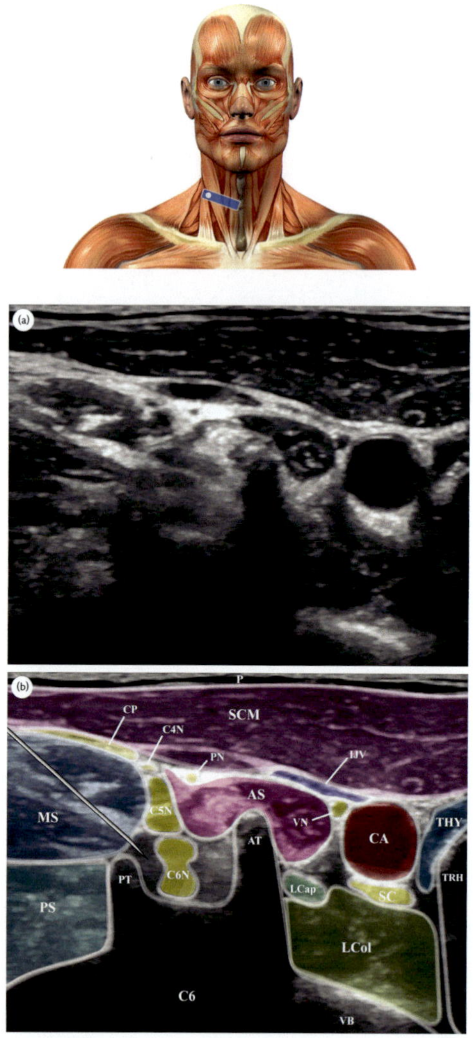

Figure 2.3.5 a, Ultrasound image of the anterolateral neck in an axial oblique plane at the C6 level. **b,** Labeled ultrasound image of in-plane needle placement of the C6 nerve root for a selective nerve root block in short-axis. *P* platysma, *SCM* sternocleidomastoid, *PN* phrenic nerve, *IJV* internal jugular vein, *MS* middle scalene, *CP* cervical plexus, *C4N* C4 nerve root, *C5N* C5 nerve root, *AS* anterior scalene, *VN* vagus nerve, *CA* carotid artery, *THY* thyroid, *TRH* trachea, *PS* posterior scalene, *C6 VB* vertebral body & *AT* anterior tubercle & *PT* posterior tubercle, *C6N* C6 nerve root, *LCap* longus capitus, *SC* location of sympathetic chain, *LCol* longus colli.

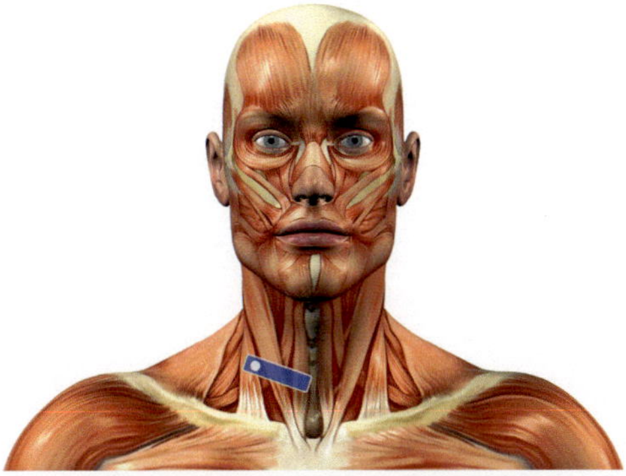

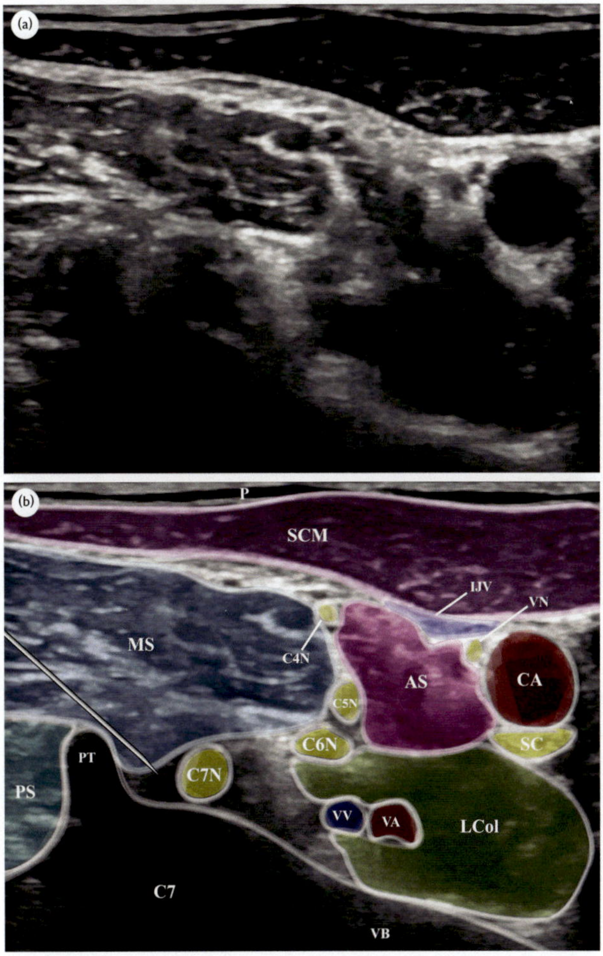

Figure 2.3.6 a, Ultrasound image of the anterolateral neck in an axial oblique plane at the C7 level. **b,** Labeled ultrasound image of in-plane needle placement of the C7 nerve root for a selective nerve root block in short-axis. *P* platysma, *SCM* sternocleidomastoid, *MS* middle scalene, *C4N* C4 nerve root, *C5N* C5 nerve root, *C6N* C6 nerve root, *AS* anterior scalene, *IJV* internal jugular vein, *VN* vagus nerve, *CA* carotid artery, *PS* posterior scalene, *C7 VB* vertebral body & *PT* posterior tubercle, *C7N* C7 nerve root, *SC* location of sympathetic chain, *VV* vertebral vein, *VA* vertebral artery, *LCol* longus colli.

Tips

- Use doppler to search for and identify cervical radicular arteries near the target area to avoid during procedures.
- If you are having difficulty visualizing the cervical roots, scan cephalad to visualize the corresponding nerve roots as they enter the neural foramina between the anterior and posterior tubercles.
- Consider combining ultrasound with fluoroscopy when first mastering this technique.

Safety Considerations

- Avoid aiming anteriorly to puncture the carotid artery/internal jugular and spinal nerves.

Postprocedure Management

It is recommended to perform a thorough upper extremity neurological and cranial exam before discharging the patient. Written instructions should be given to the patient to monitor any signs and symptoms of infection, epidural hematoma, intravascular and neurological compromises. In situations where selective nerve injection is performed for the diagnostic purpose as part of preoperative planning, the patients should be educated to monitor the duration and degree of pain relief in relation to the type of local anesthetic used.

Further Reading

- Narouze SN. Ultrasound-guided cervical nerve root block. 2018. In: Narouze S (ed), Atlas of Ultrasound-Guided Procedures in Interventional Pain Management. Springer, New York.
- Jankovic D, Peng P. Regional nerve blocks in anesthesia and pain therapy. In: Peng P (ed), Pulsed Radiofrequency Treatment Adjacent of the Cervical Dorsal Root Ganglion. Textbook, Springer 4th edition, Switzerland; 2015:239–245. doi:10.1007/978-3-319-05131-4
- Korbe S, Udoji EN, Ness TJ, Udoji MA. Ultrasound-guided interventional procedures for chronic pain management. *Pain Manag*. 2015;5(6):465–482. doi:10.2217/pmt.15.46
- Asenjo JF, Jackson J. 2019. Atlas of ultrasound-guided procedures in interventional pain management, 2nd ed. *Anesthesia and Analgesia.* 129(2):e56.

References

1. Iyer S, Kim HJ. Cervical radiculopathy. *Curr Rev Musculoskelet Med*. 2016;9(3):272–280.
2. Eloqayli H. Clinical decision-making in chronic spine pain: dilemma of image-based diagnosis of degenerative spine and generation mechanisms for nociceptive, radicular, and referred pain. *BioMed Research International*. 2018;2018:1–6. doi:10.1155/2018/8793843
3. Murphy DR, Hurwitz EL, Gerrard JK, Clary R. Pain patterns and descriptions in patients with radicular pain: does the pain necessarily follow a specific dermatome? *Chiropr Osteopat*. 2009;17:9.
4. Macnab I. Negative disc exploration: an analysis of the causes of nerve-root involvement in sixty-eight patients. *J Bone Joint Surg Am*. 1971;53(5):891–903.
5. Rathmell JP, Aprill C, Bogduk N. Cervical transforaminal injection of steroids. *Anesthesiology*. 2004;100(6):1595–1600.
6. Jee H, Lee JH, Kim J, Park KD, Lee WY, Park Y. Ultrasound-guided selective nerve root block versus fluoroscopy-guided transforaminal block for the treatment of radicular pain in the lower cervical spine: a randomized, blinded, controlled study. *Skeletal Radiology*. 2013;42(1):69–78. doi:10.1007/s00256-012-1434-1
7. Park Y, Ahn JK, Sohn Y, et al. Treatment effects of ultrasound guide selective nerve root block for lower cervical radicular pain: a retrospective study of 1-year follow-up. *Ann Rehabil Med*. 2013;37(5):658–667.

8. Park KD, Lee WY, Nam SH, Kim M, Park Y. Ultrasound-guided selective nerve root block versus fluoroscopy-guided interlaminar epidural block for the treatment of radicular pain in the lower cervical spine: a retrospective comparative study. *Journal of Ultrasound*. 2019;22(2):167–177. doi:10.1007/s40477-018-0344-z
9. Tanaka N, Fujimoto Y, An HS, Ikuta Y, Yasuda M. The anatomic relation among the nerve roots, intervertebral foramina, and intervertebral discs of the cervical spine. *Spine*. 2000;25(3):286–291.
10. Kushchayev SV, Glushko T, Jarraya M, et al. ABCs of the degenerative spine. *Insights Imaging*. 2018;9(2):253–274.
11. Lee HH, Park D, Oh Y, Ryu JS. Ultrasonography evaluation of vulnerable vessels around cervical nerve roots during selective cervical nerve root block. *Ann Rehabil Med*. 2017;41(1):66–71.
12. Fitzgerald RT, Bartynski WS, Collins HR. Vertebral artery position in the setting of cervical degenerative disease: implications for selective cervical transforaminal epidural injections. *Interv Neuroradiol*. 2013;19(4):425–431.
13. Park SK, Choi YS. Advantages of digital subtraction angiography during nerve block. *Anesthesiology and Pain Medicine*. 2014;4(5):E19927. doi:10.5812/aapm.19927
14. Ter Haar G. Ultrasonic imaging: safety considerations. *Interface Focus*. 2011;1(4):686–697.

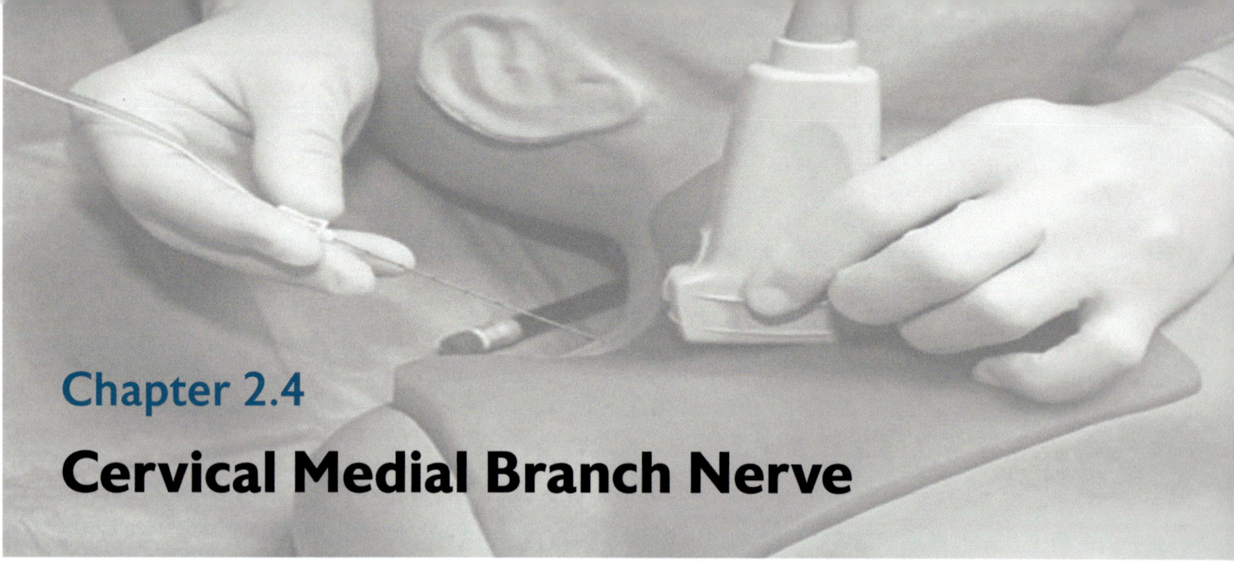

Chapter 2.4
Cervical Medial Branch Nerve

Ajax Yang and Anthony Mazzola

Contents

Introduction

Cervical facet mediated neck pain accounts for 33%–65% (atraumatic: 25%–65%; traumatic 50%–60%) of the total reported chronic neck pain cases, with disease occurring most frequently at the mid- and low-cervical levels (C4–C7).[1,2] Although injecting local anesthetic into the facet joint or next to the medial branch are both reliable methods of identifying and addressing the underlying neck pain generator, cervical facet injection poses a considerably higher risk. Given the neck is a densely vascularized region, patient positioning and imaging optimization will maximize patient comfort and procedural safety.[3] In this chapter, we will discuss the clinical, anatomical, and technical considerations relating to performing ultrasound- (US-) guided cervical medial branch blocks in the oncologic population.

Cervical medial branch blocks have conventionally been performed under fluoroscopic guidance, utilizing an anatomical landmark approach.[4] However, there is increasing evidence to support the use of ultrasound guidance in order to minimize radiation exposure to the patient and allow for the dynamic visualization of vessels and nerves, leading to a safer procedure.[5,6] When comparing ultrasound-guided cervical medial branch injections to conventional fluoroscopic guidance, both methods resulted in similar improvement in verbal numeric pain scale and neck disability index.[7] However, ultrasound image guidance offers the advantage of faster procedure times with fewer needle passes compared to fluoroscopy.[7] In addition, cancer patients often have significant changes to their muscular and vascular anatomy due to surgical and radiation treatment with subsequent revascularization of the region.

Indications

While modern imaging modalities are valuable in detecting structural pathologies, imaging alone is unable to delineate which spinal segment is symptomatic. This is especially true in the setting of multilevel spinal spondylosis or facet arthropathy where the source of axial spine pain is often multifactorial. Patients with cervical facetogenic pain typically present with uni- or bilateral axial neck pain with or without radiation into their shoulders or interscapular region.[4] In the authors' experience, common causes of neck pain syndromes in the oncologic population include surgical debulking/decompression and fusion of the cervical spine, radiation to the posterior vertebral and muscular components of the neck (head and neck and neuroaxial tumors), inflammatory response to oncologic treatments (immunotherapy and hormonal treatments), postural stresses due to tumor-related changes, and deconditioning after treatment.

Each facet joint has a typical pain pattern. The C2/3 joint often presents with pain over the posterior neck and head, while the C6/7 joint often presents with lower cervical pain over the upper back and scapular region.[4] Lateral flexion and rotation range of motion deficits are typically present without neurological compromise. Radiological findings cannot predictably identify painful facet joints, and imaging is primarily used to exclude other etiologies of axial spine pain.[8–9] Baseline pain scores should be recorded at rest and with cervical facet loading. Patients are then instructed to quantify neck pain relief after diagnostic medial branch blocks. Following successful blocks, radiofrequency ablation of the medial branches can provide prolonged pain relief. Falsely positive diagnostic medial branch blocks are minimized by using small volumes of injectate (0.2–0.5 cc) at each level and repeating the procedure to verify pain relief.[10]

Diagnostic blocks followed by therapeutic injections is a time-consuming process. Leeway may be given for expediting definitive pain treatment in the oncologic patient population and especially for those with terminal cancer. In these circumstances, corticosteroids are often added to diagnostic blocks for therapeutic effect.

Cervical medial branch blocks are indicated in patients with somatic or nonradicular neck pain without evidence of either disc herniation, radiculopathy, or discogenic pain.[8] Additionally, medial branch blocks can be considered in the following situations:[11,12]

1. Severely arthritic, obliterated, or fused facet joints
2. Treatment-resistant chronic (>6 months) axial neck pain
3. Radiologic and clinical evidence is insufficient to locate the symptomatic facet joint
4. Prior to rhizotomy, cryoablation, or radiofrequency ablation
5. Osseous facet destruction or medial branch compression from:
    a. Local tumor invasion
        i. Metastatic spine tumors
        ii. Primary bone tumor, extradural
            1. Benign (osteochondroma, chondroma, chondromyxoid fibroma, osteoid osteoma, giant cell tumor, benign osteoblastoma, fibroma, hemangioma, lipoma)
            2. Malignant (myeloma, chondrosarcoma, osteosarcoma, malignant giant cell tumor, Ewing's tumor, chordoma, hemangioendothelioma, hemangiopericytoma)
    b. Medial branch neuritis (radiation-induced, tumor-induced release of inflammatory neuropeptides).

Critical Anatomy

The facet joints are synovial joints formed between the superior articular process and the inferior articular process of two adjacent vertebrae. These joints allow for flexion, extension, and rotation. Each cervical facet joint is innervated by the medial branch from its respective spinal level and the one below. The C2–3 facet joint is innervated by the C2 dorsal ramus and the C3 superficial branch of the medial branch, also known as the third occipital nerve.[4] Dorsal rami of C3–8 spinal nerves give medial branches, which travel dorsolaterally wrapping around the articular pillars to innervate their respective cervical facet joints resulting in each facet joint innervated by the medial branch from above and below. Cervical medial branches also supply deep segmental muscular stabilizing muscles such as multifidus, semispinalis capitis, and semispinalis cervicis.

The C7 vertebra can be identified by its single prominent posterior tubercle and small anterior tubercle on ultrasound. The C6 vertebra can be identified where the vertebral artery enters the foramen transversalis of the transverse processes. The articular pillar of C2 can be identified just caudad to the mastoid. By identifying these structures, the other levels can be counted. The mountain peaks of the articular pillars are the facet joints, whereas the valleys correspond with the location of the medial branches. On ultrasound imaging, these valleys are the waist of the articular pillars as seen on fluoroscopy.

Several studies have acknowledged the increased vasculature concerns regarding interventional procedures at the cervical level.[13–15] One such study examined 1,005 cervical levels of 102 patients and identified 363 incidental vessels, of which 238 were arteries. These small periforaminal arteries are prevalent along the lateral aspect of the cervical spine including the articular pillars of C6 and C7 where 19% and 16% of vessels were shown, respectively. Increased changes in vascularity are also likely after radiation to the neck. Doppler should be used to identify vasculature near injection sites to mitigate the risks of vascular injury or injection.[14]

Equipment and Patient Preparation

1. **Monitors and Sterility**
    a. No specific monitors are needed for this procedure but emergency resuscitation equipment should be available immediately. This includes adult cardiac life support (ACLS) drugs, supplemental oxygen, airway adjuncts, and suction.
    b. Strict antiseptic technique should be observed including sterile probe cover, ultrasound gel, and sterile gloves. Chlorhexidine or other skin prep agent should be used to clean the skin prior to commencing the procedure.
2. **Equipment**
    a. Probe: High-frequency linear array transducer (8–12 MHz)
    b. Needle type: 22- or 25-gauge, 1.5- to 2-inch needle
    c. Local anesthetic (0.1–0.5 mL per medial branch): Lidocaine 1%–2%; ropivacaine 0.2%–0.5%; bupivacaine 0.25%–0.5%
    d. Adjuvant (0.1–0.5 mL per medial branch): Particulate or non-particulate steroid
3. **Position**
    a. Lateral decubitus (preferred) or prone

Step-by-Step Technique

Cervical Medial Branch Block—Ultrasound Approach

1. **Prepare equipment and supplies, position the patient in the prone position, and clean the skin around the area of the block with antiseptic solution**
2. **Place the probe to view the cervical spine coronally.** Identify the ipsilateral mastoid process with the caudal cervical articular pillars (Figure 2.4.1). The vertebral artery will be in view as it enters the C2 foramen. Immediately posterior to the C2 foramen lies the C2/3 facet articulation and, possibly, the third occipital nerve, which lies on the superior portion on the C3 articular pillar and can be targeted here in-plane (Figure 2.4.1).
3. **Move the transducer caudally in a coronal view so facet joints and articular pillars appear as peaks and valleys (Figure 2.4.2).** Each divot in the peak denotes a joint line. The medial branch will appear as hypoechoic structures except for C7, where the view to the medial branch is commonly obscured by the surrounding soft tissue.

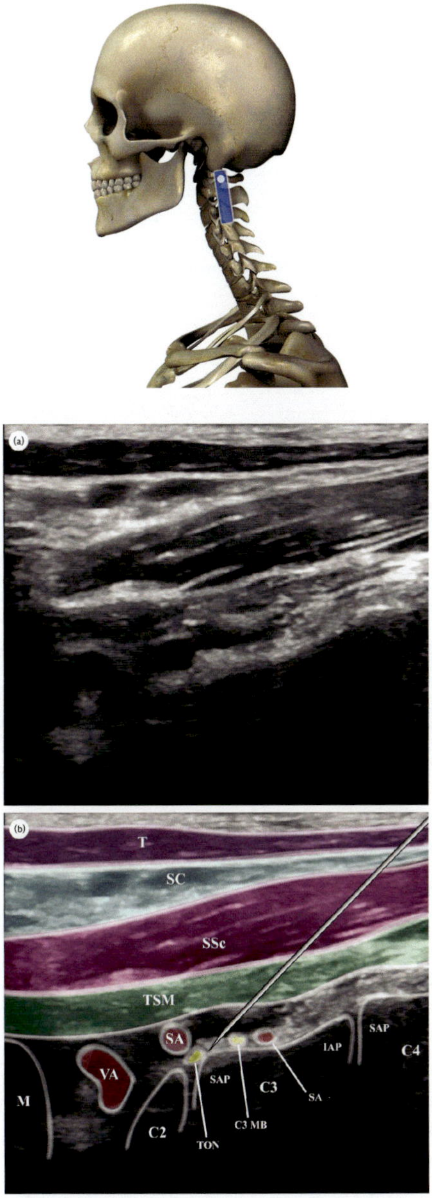

Figure 2.4.1 a, Ultrasound image of the lateral neck at the mastoid and upper cervical spine level in a coronal oblique plane. **b,** Labeled ultrasound image of in-plane needle placement for a third occipital nerve (TON) or superficial branch of the C3 medial branch in short-axis. *T* trapezius muscle, *SC* splenius capitus muscle, *SSc* semispinalis capitus muscles, *TSM* transversospinalis muscles, *M* mastoid, *VA* vertebral artery, *SA* satellite artery, *TON* third occipital nerve, *C3 MB* deep branch of C3 medial branch, *C2* C2 articular pillar, *C3* C3 articular pillar with superior articular process (*SAP*) and inferior articular process (*IAP*), *C4* C4 articular pillar with superior articular process (*SAP*).

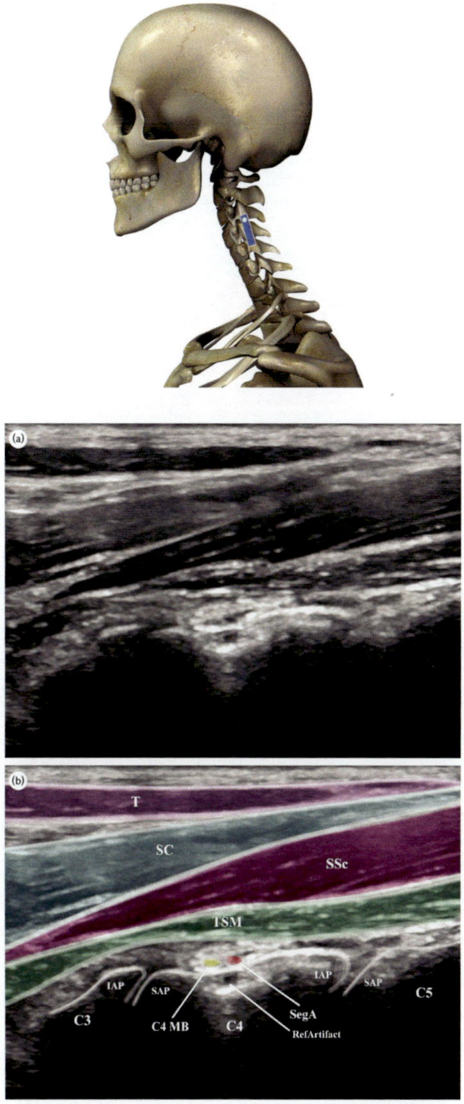

Figure 2.4.2 a, Ultrasound image of the lateral neck at the mid-cervical-spine level in a coronal oblique plane. **b,** Labeled ultrasound image of an out-of-plane needle placement for the C4 medial branch in short-axis. *T* trapezius muscle, *SC* splenius capitus muscle, *SSc* semispinalis capitus muscles, *TSM* transversospinalis muscles, *C4 MB* C4 medial branch, ***SegA*** segmental artery, *C3* C3 articular pillar with inferior articular process (*IAP*), *C4* C4 articular pillar with superior articular process (*SAP*) and inferior articular process (*IAP*), ***RefArtifact*** refractive artifact from segmental artery, *C5* C5 articular pillar with superior articular process (*SAP*).

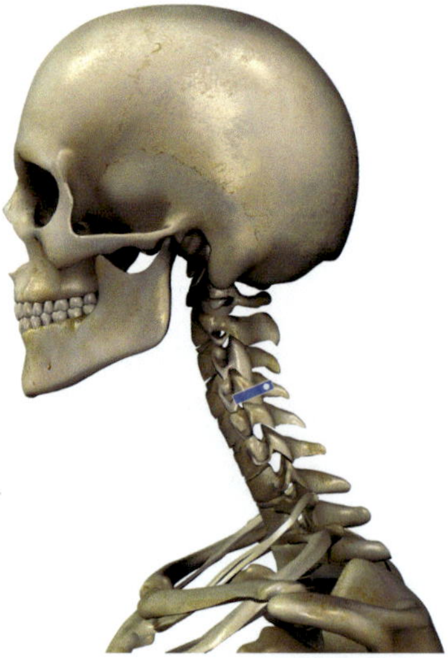

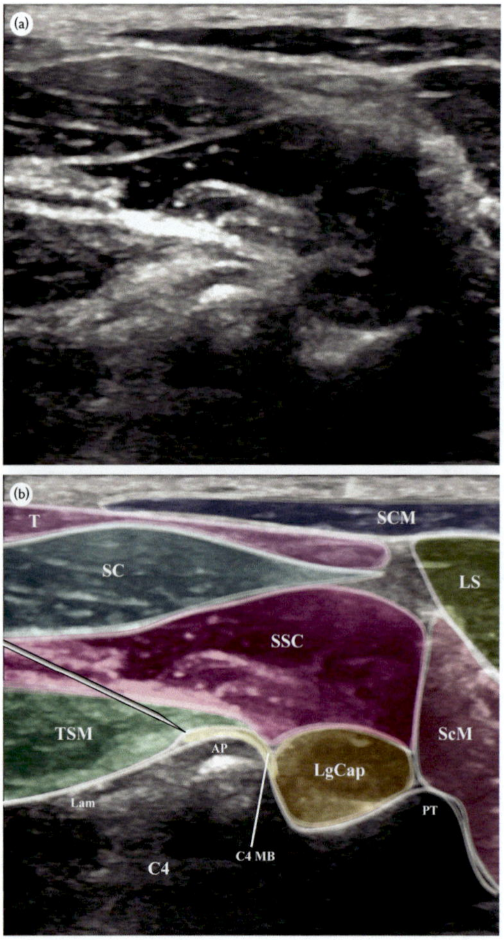

Figure 2.4.3 a, Ultrasound image of the lateral neck at the C4 level in an axial oblique plane. **b,** Labeled ultrasound image of in-plane needle placement for the C4 medial branch in long-axis. *SCM* sternocleidomastoid muscle, *T* trapezius muscle, *SC* splenius capitus muscle, *LS* levator scapulae muscle, *SSC* semispinalis capitus muscles, *ScM* scalene muscles, *TSM* transversospinalis muscles, *C4 MB* C4 medial branch, *LgCap* longissimus capitus muscle, *C4* C4 articular pillar (*AP*) with lamina (*Lam*) and posterior tubercle (*PT*).

4. **Insert the needle in an out-of-plane (Figure 2.4.2) or in-plane (Figure 2.4.3) approach to the articular pillar.** Inject 0.2–1 mL of injectate to each targeted medial branch. It is important to avoid intravascular and neuroforaminal injections. Note if the needle is too anterior the injectate can spread into the transforaminal space.

Tips

- Use doppler to visualize and avoid cervical radicular arteries near the target area.

Safety Considerations

- Avoid aiming too far anteriorly on the articular pillar, which increases the risk of injury to the vertebral artery and spinal nerves.
- Avoid anterior spread of injectate, which may enter the foraminal space and potentially anesthetize the corresponding nerve root.
- Be aware of muscular changes or scarring secondary to radiation effects.

Postprocedure Management

The patient should be evaluated for postprocedural dizziness and nausea, especially after the bilateral cervical medial branch block. It is recommended that the patient should not operate vehicles or drive themselves home immediately following the injection. Rare complications include hemorrhage, dural puncture, intra-arterial or intravenous injection, paralysis from spinal cord trauma, infection, and hematoma.

Further Reading

- Gellhorn AC. Cervical facet-mediated pain. *Physical Medicine and Rehabilitation Clinics of North America*. 2011;22(3):447–458. doi:10.1016/j.pmr.2011.02.006
- Gofeld M. Ultrasonography in pain medicine: a critical review. *Pain Pract*. 2008;8(4):226–240.
- Hadzic A. *Hadzic's Textbook of Regional Anesthesia and Acute Pain Management*. McGraw Hill Professional; 2017.
- Siegenthaler A, Eichenberger U. Ultrasound-guided third occipital nerve and cervical medial branch nerve blocks. In: Narouze SN, ed. *Atlas of Ultrasound-Guided Procedures in Interventional Pain Management*. New York, NY: Springer New York; 2011:107–117.
- Siegenthaler A, Schliessbach J, Curatolo M, Eichenberger U. Ultrasound anatomy of the nerves supplying the cervical zygapophyseal joints, an exploratory study. Reg Anesth Pain Med. 2011;36:606–10.
- Thonnagith A, Elgueta MF. Ultrasound-guided cervical medial branch blocks: a technical review. *International Journal of Physical Medicine & and Rehabilitation*. 2016;4(2). doi:10.4172/2329-9096.1000329
- Waldman S. *Comprehensive Atlas of Ultrasound-Guided Pain Management Injection Techniques*. Lippincott Williams & Wilkins; 2014.

References

1. Fejer R, Kyvik KO, Hartvigsen J. The prevalence of neck pain in the world population: a systematic critical review of the literature. *Eur Spine J*. 2006;15(6):834–848.
2. Binder AI. Neck pain. *BMJ Clin Evid*. 2008;2008:1103. https://www.ncbi.nlm.nih.gov/pubmed/19445809.
3. Martinoli C, Bianchi S, M'hamed D, Pugliese F, Bianchi-Zamorani M, Valle M. Ultrasound of tendons and nerves. *European Radiology*. 2002;12(1):44–55. doi:10.1007/s00330-001-1161-9

4. Bogduk N. *Practice Guidelines for Spinal Diagnostic and Treatment Procedures*. International Spine Intervention Society; 2013.
5. Siegenthaler A, Mlekusch S, Trelle S, Schliessbach J, Curatolo M, Eichenberger U. Accuracy of ultrasound-guided nerve blocks of the cervical zygapophysial joints. *Anesthesiology*. 2012;117(2):347–352.
6. Finlayson RJ, Etheridge J-PB, Tiyaprasertkul W, Nelems B, Tran DQH. A prospective validation of biplanar ultrasound imaging for C5–C6 cervical medial branch blocks. *Regional Anesthesia and Pain Medicine*. 2014;39(2):160–163. doi:10.1097/aap.0000000000000043
7. Park KD, Lim D-J, Lee WY, Ahn J, Park Y. Ultrasound versus fluoroscopy-guided cervical medial branch block for the treatment of chronic cervical facet joint pain: a retrospective comparative study. *Skeletal Radiol*. 2017;46(1):81–91.
8. Manchikanti L, Singh V, Falco FJE, Cash KM, Fellows B. Cervical medial branch blocks for chronic cervical facet joint pain: a randomized, double-blind, controlled trial with one-year follow-up. *Spine*. 2008;33(17):1813–1820.
9. Speldewinde GC, Bashford GM, Davidson IR. Diagnostic cervical zygapophyseal joint blocks for chronic cervical pain. *Med J Aust*. 2001;174(4):174–176.
10. Curatolo M, Bogduk N. Diagnostic blocks for chronic pain. *Scandinavian Journal of Pain*. 2010;1(4):186–192. doi:10.1016/j.sjpain.2010.07.001
11. Manchikanti L, Abdi S, Atluri S, et al. An update of comprehensive evidence-based guidelines for interventional techniques in chronic spinal pain. Part II: Guidance and recommendations. *Pain Physician*. 2013;16(2 Suppl):S49–S283.
12. MacVicar J, Borowczyk JM, MacVicar AM, Loughnan BM, Bogduk N. Cervical medial branch radiofrequency neurotomy in New Zealand. *Pain Medicine*. 2012;13(5):647–654. doi:10.1111/j.1526-4637.2012.01351
13. Curatolo M, Bogduk N. Diagnostic and therapeutic nerve blocks. In *Bonica's Management of Pain*, edited by Fishman SM, Ballantyne JC, Rathmell JP. Lippincott Williams and Wilkins: Philadelphia PA; 2010:723–753.
14. Finlayson RJ, Etheridge J-PB, Chalermkitpanit P, et al. Real-time detection of periforaminal vessels in the cervical spine. *Regional Anesthesia and Pain Medicine*. 2016;41(2):130–134. doi:10.1097/aap.0000000000000363
15. Kettler A, Werner K, Wilke H-J. Morphological changes of cervical facet joints in elderly individuals. *Eur Spine J*. 2007;16(7):987–992.

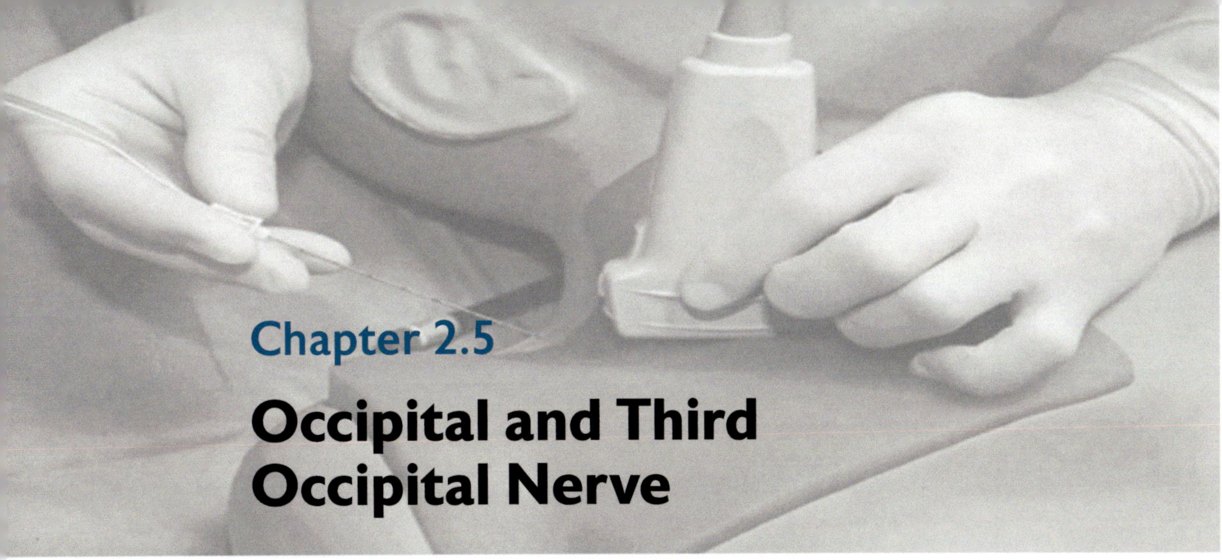

Chapter 2.5

Occipital and Third Occipital Nerve

Tiffany Lin

Contents

Introduction

Headaches are among the most common nervous system disorders, with a prevalence of more than 48% in the general population.[1] Headaches can be classified into primary, secondary, or other painful cranial neuropathies according to International Classification of Headache Disorders (ICHD).[2] In the oncologic patient, posterior skull-based headaches and posterior and lateral scalp pain may arise from multiple sources:

- Skull-based tumors and soft tissue tumors of the scalp
- Postsurgical pain from craniotomies
- Postradiation injury

Though difficult to treat, primary tumors of the brain may present as headaches and other neurologic sequelae. In many instances despite a plethora of treatment modalities, some forms of these headaches and somatic pain may remain resistant to conservative therapies. Interventional treatment options, such occipital nerve blocks, can be useful in diagnosis and treatment. These interventions should be considered in patients whose pain is not controlled by conservative therapies.

Critical Anatomy

The greater occipital nerve (GON) arises from the dorsal ramus of C2 with occasional contribution from C3.[3] It exits between the atlas (C1) and the axis (C2) and travels between the inferior obliquus capitis and semispinalis capitis muscles. It then penetrates the aponeurosis of the trapezius muscle inferior to the superior nuchal crest and medial to the occipital artery.[3,4] The GON innervates the medial portion of the posterior scalp up to the vertex of the head.[4]

The lesser occipital nerve (LON) is a branch of the superficial cervical plexus arising from the dorsal rami of C2 and C3.[3] It emerges along the posterior aspect of the sternocleidomastoid muscle and innervates the lateral portion of the posterior scalp and the cephalad surface of the pinna of the ear.[4]

The third occipital nerve (TON) is a superficial branch arising from the dorsal ramus of C3.[1,4] It curves dorsally and medially around the superior articular pillar of the C3 vertebral body and crosses the C2–C3 zygapophyseal joint either at the level of the joint or just below.[4] It then courses medially and superiorly to penetrate the semispinalis capitis muscle, running along the GON.[1,4] The TON is the only medial branch that innervates the C2–C3 facet joint.[4] See Figure 2.5.1 for illustration of the courses of the GON, LON, and TON.

Indications

Occipital nerve blocks are commonly performed to diagnose and treat cervicogenic headache (CGH), a secondary headache disorder due to pain etiologies in the areas innervated by the C1–C3 spinal nerves.[1] Cervicogenic pain is thought to arise from the convergence of upper cervical and trigeminal sensory pathways within the brainstem to the head and face.[1] Nociceptive stimuli from the interspinal muscles, facet joints, intervertebral discs, and trigeminal cervical complex can lead to referred pain in the scapular region extending through the occipital area, causing symptoms of headache.[1] Headache pain can also be related to osteoarthritis of the facet joints or trauma from whiplash injuries.[5] The Cervicogenic Headache International Study Group defines CGH as (1) pain with neck movement or sustained awkward positioning, (2) pain with applied pressure over the upper cervical or occipital region, (3) a positive response to anesthetic blockade of the cervical spine nerves, and (4) unilateral pain and restriction in neck range of motion.[1,6–8]

Greater, lesser, and third occipital neuralgia or cervicogenic headaches occur frequently in the oncological population. In our practice, we see pathology frequently in those patients who have undergone craniotomy or burr holes for surgical treatment of brain cancer, which can result in sacrifice of a nerve or neuritis. Head and neck cancer may result in occipital neuralgia from compressive forces due to tumor burden, inflammatory changes due to tumor, surgical lesioning of the nerves, or postsurgical swelling. Radiation therapy is known to cause fibrosis of the neck muscles, which may result in entrapment of the GON, LON, and TON at various locations throughout their course. Common locations for entrapment of the GON include[9–13]:

- Between the atlas and the axis
- Between the inferior obliquus capitis (IOC) and semispinalis capitis (SSC) muscles
- Exit point of the trapezius muscle
- Tendinous insertion of the trapezius muscle

Equipment and Patient Preparation

1. Monitors and Sterility
   a. No specific monitors are needed for this procedure, but emergency resuscitation equipment should be available immediately. This includes ACLS drugs, supplemental oxygen, airway adjuncts, and suction.
   b. Strict antiseptic technique should be observed including sterile probe cover, ultrasound gel, and sterile gloves. Chlorhexidine or other skin prep agent should be used to clean the skin prior to commencing the procedure.

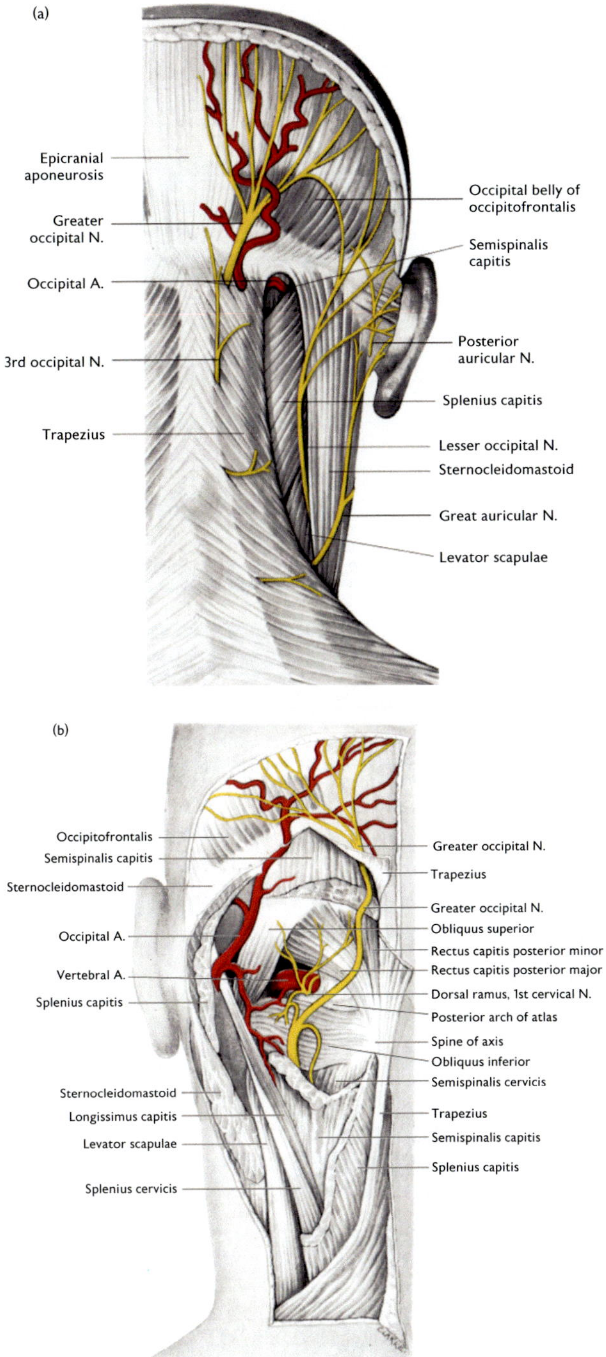

Figure 2.5.1 a, Cutaneous nerves and vessels of the posterior part of the scalp. **b,** The suboccipital region and deep structures of the back of the neck. (Reprinted with permission from Cunningham's Manual of Practical Anatomy: Head, Neck and Brain, 16th Edition)

2. Equipment
   a. Probe: High-frequency linear array transducer (8-12 MHz)
   b. Needle type: 25- or 30-gauge, 1- to 2-inch needle
   c. Local anesthetic (0.5 mL): Lidocaine 1%–2%; ropivacaine 0.2%–0.5%; bupivacaine 0.25%–0.5%
   d. Adjuvant (0.5 mL): Particulate or nonparticulate steroid
3. Position
   a. Seated (preferred) or prone

Procedure Technique

Distal Greater Occipital Nerve Approach

1. **Prepare equipment and supplies, position the patient in the prone position, and clean the procedural area with antiseptic solution.** Alternative positioning is seated with the head flexed inferiorly.
2. **Palpate the occipital protuberance** and visualize the occipital artery with the ultrasound probe in an oblique transverse orientation. The artery should be located at the level of the occiput.
3. **Identify the desired nerves based on anatomy position to the occipital artery.** The distal greater occipital nerve is usually 1 cm medial to the artery, while the lesser occipital nerve is usually 1 cm lateral to the artery.
4. **Introduce the procedural needle in an in-plane or out-of-plane approach to deposit medication as in Figure 2.5.2**. Remove the needle and apply a bandage.

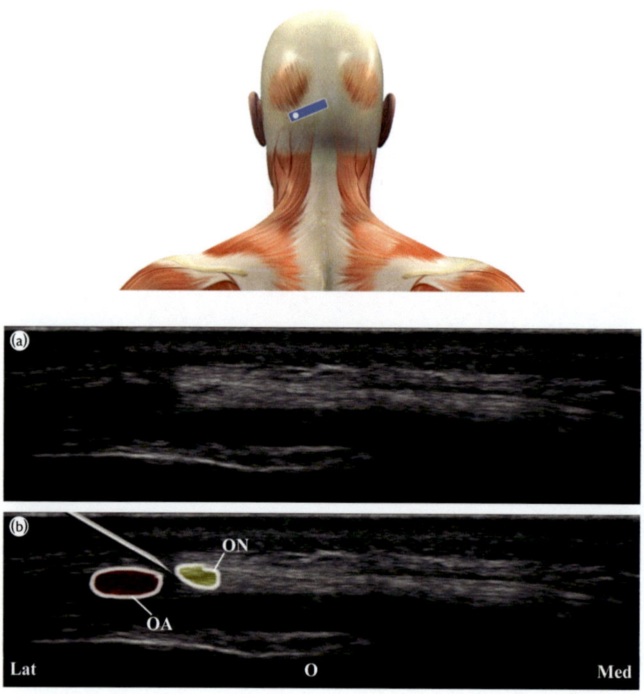

Figure 2.5.2 **a,** Ultrasound image of the posterior head near the nuchal line in an axial oblique plane. **b,** Labeled ultrasound image of in-plane needle placement for a distal greater occipital nerve block in short-axis. *GON* greater occipital nerve, *OA* occipital artery, *Lat* lateral, *O* occiput, *Med* medial.

Safety Considerations

- Avoid intravascular injection of the occipital artery by identifying on color or power doppler.
- Ensure that the needle tip is superficial to the nuchal ridge to avoid compromise of deeper neurovascular structures not seen under ultrasound.

Proximal Greater Occipital Nerve Approach

1. **Prepare equipment and supplies, position the patient in the seated position with neck in forward flexion, and clean the procedural area with antiseptic solution.**
2. **Palpate the occipital protuberance and place the ultrasound probe in the transverse plane at this position.** Translate the probe caudad until the bifid spinous process of C2 is identified (Figure 2.5.3).
3. **Translate the ultrasound probe laterally to the affected side to identify critical anatomic structures.** Identify the obliquus capitis inferior (OCI) muscle laying on top of the C2 lamina. Next, slowly translate the lateral aspect of the probe cephalad to obtain a parallel view of the OCI muscle spanning from the spinous process of C2 to the transverse process of C1 (Figure 2.5.3).
4. **The greater occipital nerve (GON) is found in the fascial plane superior to the OCI muscle and inferior to the semispinalis capitis (SSC)/trapezius muscles.**
5. **Introduce the procedural needle in an in-plane approach, from lateral to medial, toward the GON and deposit the medication as in Figure 2.5.3.** Remove the needle and apply a bandage.

Tips

- If the GON is not directly visualized, simply inject into the fascial plane in-between the OCI and the SSC/trapezius muscles.
- Inject around the nerve, which helps to decompress the nerve.
- Visual confirmation of a successful block is depicted as a "bull's eye" sign of medication deposited circumferentially around the nerve or as a separation of the muscle planes of the OCI and SSC/trapezius.
- Blocking the nerve at this proximal site will help with pain at all distal sites.
- The TON is cephalad and medial to the GON at this location and a larger volume may also inadvertently block the TON.

Safety Considerations

- Avoid injecting medial to laterally, as the vertebral artery is lateral and deep to the GON at this location and might be unprotected.
- Use doppler US and aspirate prior to injecting to avoid vascular injection to the suboccipital artery, which may run adjacent to the nerve at this level.
- Consider blocking only one side at a time. The GON and surrounding nerves (medial branches) help to contribute to proprioception and bilateral blockade may lead to temporary dizziness and decreased balance.
- Consider continuous heart rate monitor and initial test dose of lidocaine, as inadvertent vascular injection may result in rapid cardiac arrhythmia and seizure

Third Occipital Nerve Approach

1. **Prepare equipment and supplies, position the patient in the prone position, and clean the procedural area with antiseptic solution**
2. **Place the ultrasound probe in a parasagittal orientation lateral to the cervical spine. The mastoid process should be visible on the cephalad portion of the image, as shown in** Figure 2.5.4. **Adjust the probe so that the articular pillars are aligned.** The hyperechoic peaks are articular processes and joints, whereas the hyperechoic valleys are where the medial branches lie.

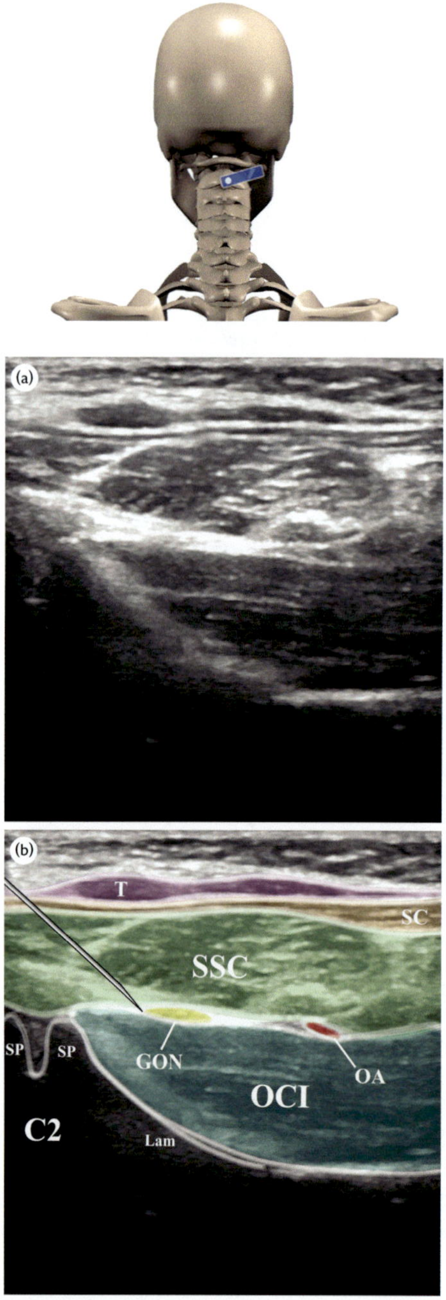

Figure 2.5.3 a, Ultrasound image of the posterior neck at the C2 level in an axial oblique plane. **b,** Labeled ultrasound image of in-plane needle placement for a proximal greater occipital nerve block in short-axis. *T* trapezius, *SC* splenius capitis, *SSC* semispinalis capitis, *GON* greater occipital nerve, *OA* occipital artery, *C2 SP* C2 bifid spinous process & *Lam* lamina, *OCI* obliquus capitis inferior.

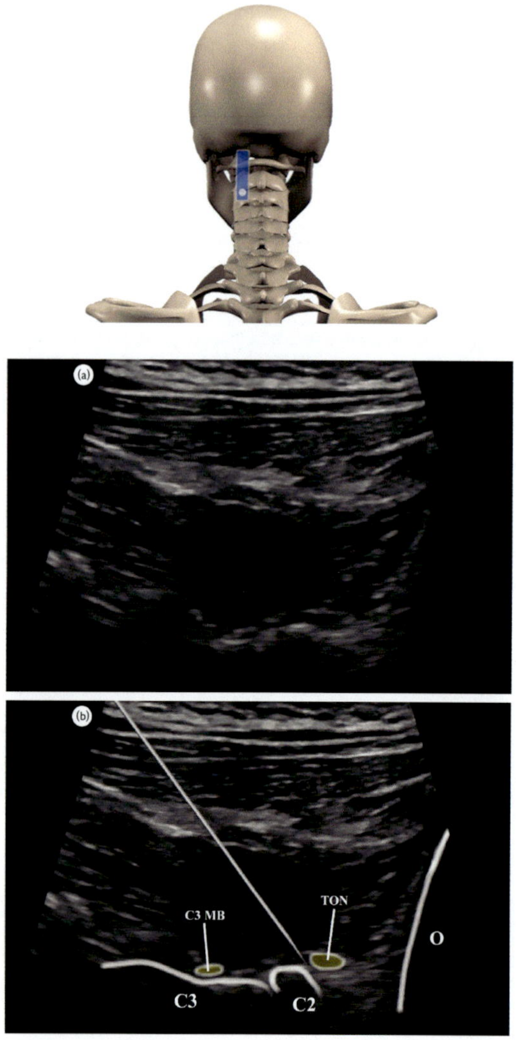

Figure 2.5.4 a, Ultrasound image of the posterior neck at the C2–3 level in a sagittal plane. **b,** Labeled ultrasound image of in-plane needle placement for a third occipital nerve block in short-axis. *C3 MB* C3 medial branch, *TON* third occipital nerve, *C3* C3 articular pillar, *C2* C2 articular pillar, *O* occiput.

3. **Visualize the C2–C3 articulation.** Follow the cervical spine caudally to the C2–C3 articulation, where a “break” is visualized as shown in Figure 2.5.4.
4. **Introduce the procedural needle in an in-plane or out-of-plane approach to deposit medication at the C2–3 articulation.** Remove the needle and apply a bandage.

Tips

- Use doppler to search for and identify cervical radicular arteries near the target area to avoid during procedures.

Safety Considerations

- Avoid aiming anteriorly past the articular pillar, which can puncture the vertebral artery and spinal nerves.
- Avoid anterior spread of injectate, which may enter the foraminal space and potentially anesthetizes the corresponding nerve root.

Postprocedure Management

There are no special postprocedure management considerations associated with this procedure. It is generally a safe and well-tolerated procedure. Most common adverse effects include pain at the injection site, numbness, lightheadedness, and syncope.[14] Others can include local infection, abscess or hematoma, steroid-related complications, and local anesthetic-related complications. There are two case reports of coma in patients with cranial bone defects after occipital nerve block.[14]

References

1. Gupta R, Fisher K, Pyati S. Chronic headache: a review of interventional treatment strategies in headache management. Current Pain and Headache Reports. 2019;23:68.
2. The International Classification of Headache Disorders, 3rd edition. Cephalalgia. 2018;38(1):1–211.
3. Lasaosa SS, Perez C, Peral G, et al. Consensus recommendations for anaesthetic peripheral nerve block. Neurologia. 2017;32(5):316–30.
4. Candido KD, Day M. Nerve Blocks of the Head and Neck. In: Practical Management of Pain, 5th ed., edited by Honorio Benzon, James P. Rathmell, Christopher L. Wu, Dennis C. Turk, Charles E. Argoff, Robert W. Hurley. Philadelphia: Mosby (Elsevier); 2014: 697–715.
5. Hurdle MB. Ultrasound-guided spinal procedures for pain. Phys Med Rehabil Clin N Am. 2016;27:673–686.
6. Curatolo M. Regional anesthesia in pain management. Curr Opin Anesthesiol. 2016;29:614–19.
7. Levin M. Nerve blocks in the treatment of headache. Neurotherapeutics. 2010;7(2):197–203.
8. Tobin J, Flitman S. Occipital nerve blocks: when and what to inject? Headache. 2009;1521–33.
9. Loukas M, El-Sedfy A, Tubbs RS, et al. Identification of greater occipital nerve landmarks for the treatment of occipital neuralgia. Folia Morphol (Warsz). 2006;65:299–304.
10. Natsis K, Baraliakos X, Appell HJ, et al. The course of the greater occipital nerve in the suboccipital region: a proposal for setting landmarks for local anesthesia in patients with occipital neuralgia. Clin Anat. 2006;19:332–36.
11. Hunter CR, Mayfield FH. Role of the upper cervical roots in the production of pain in the head. Am J Surg. 1949;48:743–52.
12. Bogduk N. Then anatomy of occipital neuralgia. Clin Exp Neurol. 1980;17:167–84.
13. Stechison MT, Mullin BB. Surgical treatment of greater occipital neuralgia: an appraisal of strategies. Acta Neurochir (Wien). 1994;131:236–40.
14. Blumenfeld A, Ashkenazi A, Evans RW. Occipital and trigeminal nerve blocks for migraine. Headache. 2015;55(5):682–89.

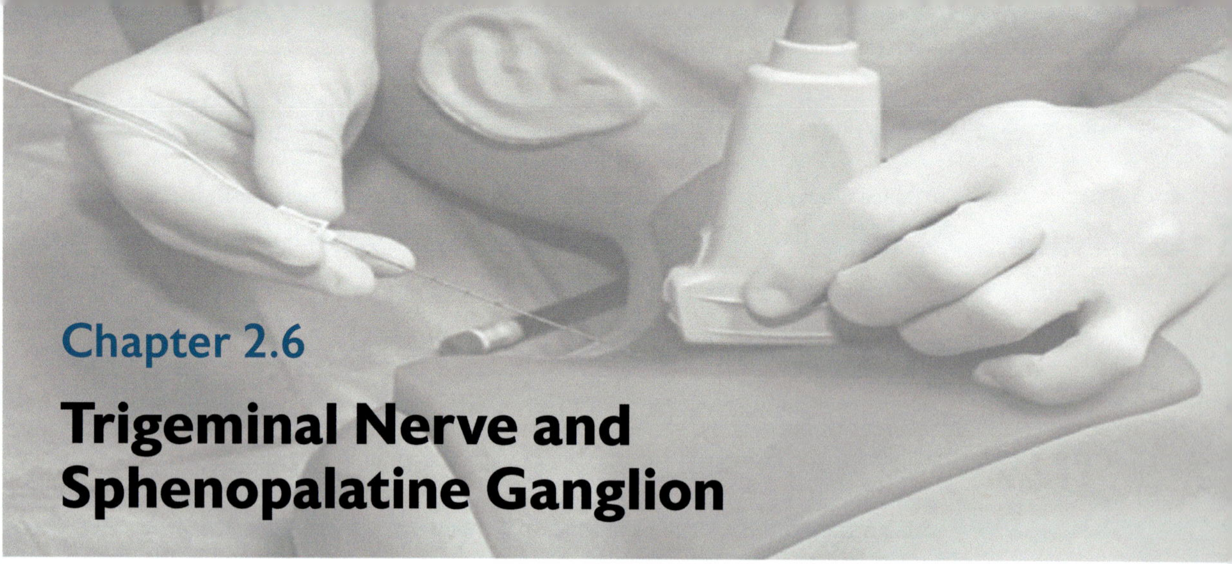

Chapter 2.6

Trigeminal Nerve and Sphenopalatine Ganglion

Tiffany Lin, Erdong Chen, and Xiang Qian

Contents

Introduction

The trigeminal nerve is the fifth cranial nerve (CN V) and supplies sensory innervation to the face via the ophthalmic (V1), maxillary (V2), and mandibular (V3) branches. Blockade of the trigeminal nerve is commonly used to treat facial pain from surgery or radiation, headaches, postherpetic neuralgia, and treatment-related complications such as osteonecrosis of the jaw. Typically, pain refractory to conventional pharmacologic therapy may be targeted with these interventions.[1] The trigeminal sensory nerves can be blocked either as they exit the cranium or as they exit through the facial bones. Similarly, the sphenopalatine ganglion (SPG), which is composed of sympathetic and parasympathetic innervation, may be targeted for pain syndromes that manifest as facial and headache type pain.

In cancer pain management, facial pain due to tumor invasion often necessitates more proximal blockade of the nerves. Fluoroscopy and ultrasound provide visualization of relevant anatomy and radiographic landmarks, which are often altered in the oncologic population and complicate blind landmark-based techniques.[2] When considering these blocks for postsurgical pain, surgical technique and evaluation of anatomy is needed for procedural planning.

Critical Anatomy

The trigeminal nerve sensory root arises from the pons and forms the trigeminal ganglion within Meckel's cave in the middle cranial fossa. Here, it is also referred to as the Gasserian ganglion. It then divides peripherally into the ophthalmic V1, maxillary V2, and mandibular V3 branches, as shown in Figure 2.6.1. The ophthalmic V1 division becomes the frontal nerve as it enters the superior orbital fissure. The frontal nerve then divides into the supraorbital and supratrochlear branches to provide sensory innervation to the forehead, medial upper eyelid, frontal portion of the cranium, and base of the nose. The maxillary V2 division exits the middle cranial fossa via the foramen rotundum, crosses the pterygopalatine fossa (PPF), and enters the orbit through the inferior orbital fissure.[1] Branches of the maxillary nerve include the infraorbital, superior alveolar, palatine, and zygomatic nerves. The branches provide sensory innervation to the maxilla, nasal cavity, palate, nasopharynx, and meninges of the anterior and middle cranial fossa.[1]

The mandibular V3 division exits through the foramen ovale and divides into the buccal, lingual, inferior alveolar, and auriculotemporal nerves.[1] These nerves carry sensory input from the buccal region, lateral head and scalp, inferior mandible, teeth, gums, anterior two-thirds of the tongue, chin, and inferior lip.[1] The motor component of V3 innervates the masseter, temporal, and medial and lateral pterygoid muscles.[1]

The SPG, also known as the pterygopalatine ganglion, is located in the PPF as shown in Figure 2.6.2. It is bordered anteriorly by the maxillary sinus, posteriorly by the medial pterygoid plate, medially by the palatine bone, and superiorly by the sphenoid sinus.[1] The fossa is in direct communication with the foramen rotundum superolaterally and the pterygoid canal inferomedially.[1] The maxillary artery resides in the fossa, while a large venous plexus overlies the fossa.[1] The SPG serves as a relay point for sensory pathways from the head and neck via the maxillary nerve, postganglionic sympathetics from the superior cervical ganglion, and parasympathetics via the greater and deep petrosal nerve.[2–4] Sensory fibers from the maxillary nerve pass through the SPG to the greater and lesser palatine nerves.[1,3] The greater palatine nerve supplies sensation to the bony palate, gingiva, and mucosa of the buccal cavity. The lesser palatine nerve supplies sensation to the uvula, tonsils, and soft palate.[3]

The SPG's sympathetic fibers arise from the superior cervical ganglion, which then forms the carotid sympathetic plexus as it travels toward the pterygoid canal. It then merges with the deep

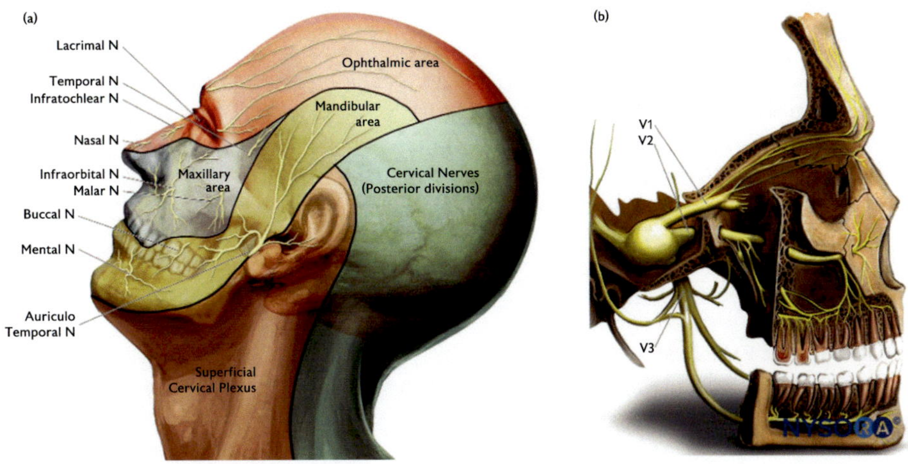

Figure 2.6.1 Distribution of the trigeminal nerves. (NYSORA)

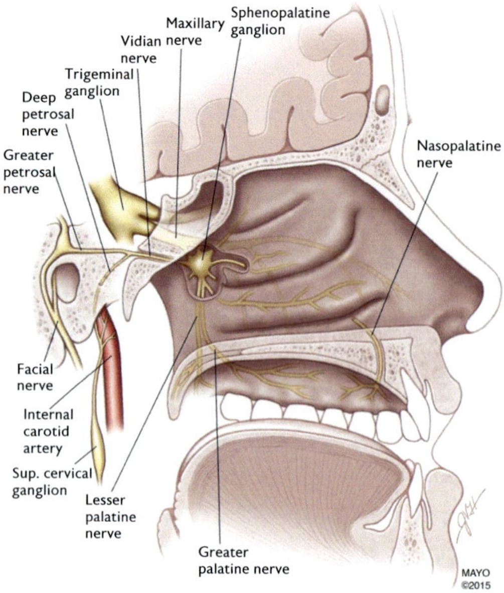

Figure 2.6.2 The sphenopalatine ganglion and its direct connections. (Obtained from Robbins MS, Robertson CE, Kaplan E, et al. The Sphenopalatine Ganglion: Anatomy, Pathophysiology, and Therapeutic Targeting in Headache. Headache. 2016;56(2):240–258.)

petrosal nerve. The deep petrosal nerve joins the greater petrosal nerve within the pterygoid canal to form the Vidian nerve, and then travels into the PPF.[3] These sympathetic fibers are predominantly distributed to the nasopharyngeal mucosa with some fibers reaching the lacrimal gland. Parasympathetic fibers from the superior salivatory nucleus in the brainstem travel through the geniculate ganglion to form the greater petrosal nerve, which eventually synapses in the SPG by way of the Vidian nerve.[3] These SPG postganglionic fibers travel with trigeminal nerve branches and provide secretomotor function to the mucous membrane of the nose, soft palate, tonsils, uvula, roof of the mouth, upper lip/gums, upper pharynx, lacrimal gland, and meningeal vessels.[3]

Clinical Applications

Maxillary V2 and mandibular V3 nerve blocks have demonstrated efficacy in treating pain syndromes attributed to trigeminal nerve involvement. They have also been utilized for surgical analgesia for procedures involving the maxilla or mandible. Mandibular V3 blocks have also been used in combination with cervical plexus blocks for analgesia for carotid endarterectomy.[1] Branches of the mandibular V3 nerve may be targeted for the treatment of pain from osteonecrosis of the jaw.

The SPG has long been implicated in the pathogenesis of headaches, and thus represents a therapeutic site for intervention.[3] Stimulation of the parasympathetic neurons of SPG has been shown to release acetylcholine, vasoactive intestinal peptide (VIP), and nitric oxide in dural blood vessels, leading to cerebral vasodilation and triggering headache.[3] Blocking the SPG, therefore, is thought to prevent that pathogenesis of headaches and it has been demonstrated to effectively treat cluster headache.[4] Cluster headache is the most prevalent subtype of the trigeminal autonomic cephalgias, which are a group of headaches characterized by short duration, strict unilaterality, and association with autonomic manifestations such as rhinorrhea, lacrimation, ptosis, and conjunctival injection.[1] Sphenopalatine ganglion block has also been used to treat acute migraine headache, chronic migraine headache, posttraumatic headache, and other facial neuralgias.[3,5,6] Though uncommon, we have also targeted the sphenopalatine fossa for atypical facial pain associated with radiation-induced pain of the nasal cavity.

Image Guidance Consideration

Fluoroscopy and ultrasound remain the predominant method of image guidance for percutaneous procedures. However, the complexity of skull base anatomy makes fluoroscopic and ultrasound guidance difficult, especially when anatomy is changed by cancer.

The percutaneous infrazygomatic SPG approach has the benefit of direct administration of medication to the ganglion, as opposed to the passive diffusion of local anesthetic through the mucosal walls.

When intervention is desired on individual trigeminal branches, manipulation of the needle within Meckel's cave can be very painful to the patient and technically challenging, which can necessitate general anesthesia and prolonged fluoroscopy times. With recent technological advances, the trigeminal nerve can be blocked with aid of needle guidance software and flat-panel C-arm CT. These advances allow interventions on V2 via a foramen rotundum approach and V3 via a foramen ovale approach.

Equipment and Patient Preparation

1. **Monitors and Sterility**
   a. No special monitors are needed for this procedure in an otherwise healthy patient.
   b. For patients with cardiac concerns, consider monitored anesthesia care in case of bradycardia and hypotension, which may result from activation of the trigeminal cardiac reflex.
   c. Emergency resuscitation equipment, supplemental oxygen, AMBU bag, suction, ACLS drugs, and intralipid should be available immediately.
   d. Peripheral IV should be placed.
2. **Equipment**
   a. Imaging:
      i. Fluoroscopy/CT-guided intervention: Fluoroscopy with C-arm CT capability and 3D navigation software such as Syngo Iguide
      ii. Ultrasound-guided block: High-frequency (7–12 MHz) linear array ultrasound probe
   b. Needle type:
      i. Fluoroscopy/CT-guided intervention:
         1. SPG block
            a. 22- or 25-gauge 3.5-inch spinal needle for SPG block
         2. V2/V3 Approach
            a. 5 mm tip 21-gauge radiofrequency needle for V2/V3 pulsed radiofrequency
      ii. Ultrasound-guided block: 22- or 25-gauge, 1.5- to 3.5-inch needle
   c. Local anesthetic (1–2 mL): Lidocaine 1%–2%; ropivacaine 0.2%–0.5%; bupivacaine 0.25%–0.5%
   d. Adjuvant (0.5–1 mL): Particulate or nonparticulate steroid
3. **Position**
   a. Fluoroscopy/CT-guided intervention: supine with neck mildly extended and head gently secured with a soft strap
   b. Ultrasound-guided approach: supine with a thin pillow under the head

Procedure Technique

Supraorbital and Supratrochlear Ophthalmic V1 Branch of Trigeminal Nerve Block

Landmark Approach

1. **Prepare equipment and supplies, position the patient supine, and clean the skin around the area of the block with antiseptic solution.**

2. **Identify the supraorbital and supratrochlear foramina (Figure 2.6.3).** The supraorbital foramen can be palpated along the supraorbital rim, typically same longitudinal plane as the pupil, which is where the supraorbital branch of the trigeminal nerve resides. The supratrochlear foramen can be palpated at the junction of the supraorbital rim and nasal spine, medial to the supraorbital foramen, and contained the supratrochlear branch of the trigeminal nerve.
3. **Insert the procedural needle inferior to the eyebrow from lateral to medial.** Direct the needle medially and cephalad.
4. **After negative aspiration, inject into the area.** Flush and remove the needle. Apply a bandage.

Tips

- Avoid crossing the eye of the patient with the needle, as it can often be discomforting to the patient during the procedure to see the needle cross the eye.

Safety Considerations

- Do not penetrate the foramen, which can cause uncontrolled spread of the medication into the eye.

Maxillary V2 and Mandibular V3 Nerve

Infraorbital Maxillary V2 Branch of Trigeminal Nerve Block—Landmark Approach

1. **Prepare equipment and supplies, position the patient supine, and clean the skin around the area of the block with antiseptic solution.**
2. **Identify the infraorbital foramen (Figure 2.6.3).** It can be palpated along the infraorbital rim, typically same longitudinal plane the patient's pupil.
3. **Insert the procedural needle from lateral to medial.** Direct the needle medially and caudad until bony contact.
4. **After negative aspiration, inject into the area.** Flush and remove the needle. Apply a bandage.

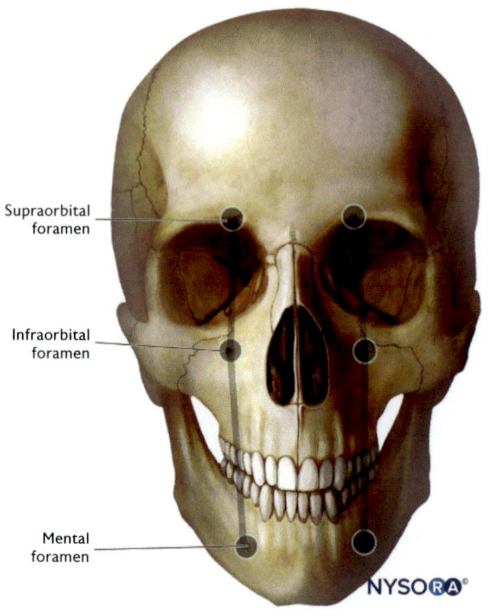

Figure 2.6.3 Anatomy of the supraorbital, infraorbital, and mental foramen where the terminal sensory branch of the trigeminal nerve exits the facial bone. (NYSORA)

Tips

- When palpating, the infraorbital foramen is often located in the same sagittal plane as the pupil.
- Avoid crossing the eye of the patient with the needle, as it can often be discomforting to the patient during the procedure to see the needle cross the eye.

Safety Considerations

- Do not penetrate the foramen, which can cause uncontrolled spread of the medication into the eye.

Mental Mandibular V3 Branch of Trigeminal Nerve Block—Landmark Approach

1. **Prepare equipment and supplies, position the patient supine, and clean the skin around the area of the block with antiseptic solution.**

2. **Identify the mental foramen (Figure 2.6.3).** It can be palpated along the mental process of the mandible, typically same longitudinal plane as the pupil.
3. **Insert the procedural needle in the lateral to medial direction.** Direct the needle medially until bony contact.
4. **After negative aspiration, inject into the area.** Flush and remove the needle. Apply a bandage.

Tips

- When palpating, the mental foramen is often located in the same sagittal plane as the pupil on the mandible.

Safety Considerations

- Do not penetrate the foramen, which could lead to uncontrolled spread of the medication into the mouth

V2/V3—Ultrasound Approach

1. **Prepare equipment and supplies, position the patient supine with the head turned away from the procedural side, and clean the skin around the area of the block with antiseptic solution.**
2. **Place the ultrasound probe in a transverse orientation to be parallel to and below the zygomatic arch**. Scan caudally to visualize the mandibular coronoid process anteriorly and the condylar process posteriorly. The lateral pterygoid plate can be seen at a depth of about 3–4 cm in this view with the pulsating maxillary artery superficial to it (as shown in Figure 2.6.4).
3. **Identify the desired nerve target based on position of the maxillary artery.** The maxillary V2 branch is captured anterior to the artery (Figure 2.6.4b), while the mandibular V3 branch is captured posterior to the artery (Figure 2.6.4c).
4. **Insert the procedural needle using an in-plane approach between the coronoid and condylar processes of the mandible to target the desired nerve.** After negative aspiration, inject into the region. Flush and remove the needle. Apply a bandage.

Tips

- Contact the lateral pterygoid plate with the needle first and then walk off anteriorly to reach the maxillary V2 nerve or posteriorly to reach the mandibular V3 nerve in the PPF.

Safety Considerations

- Use doppler to search for and identify the maxillary artery near the target area to avoid intravascular injection.

V2/3 Block and Radiofrequency Treatment—Combined Fluoroscopic/CT Approach

1. **Prepare equipment and supplies, position the patient in the supine position, and clean the procedural area with antiseptic solution.**
2. **Determine location of initial needle insertion.** Place a radiopaque BB marker on the skin (Figure 2.6.5a). Measure target depth from the skin on processed CT images and mark needle to this depth (Figure 2.6.5b). The initial needle skin entry point for the maxillary V2 branch is in the region of the intersection point of a vertical line drawn 1 cm lateral to the outer canthus and the horizontal line of the base of the nose. Skin entry for the mandibular V3 branch is approximately 2 cm lateral to the corner of the mouth.

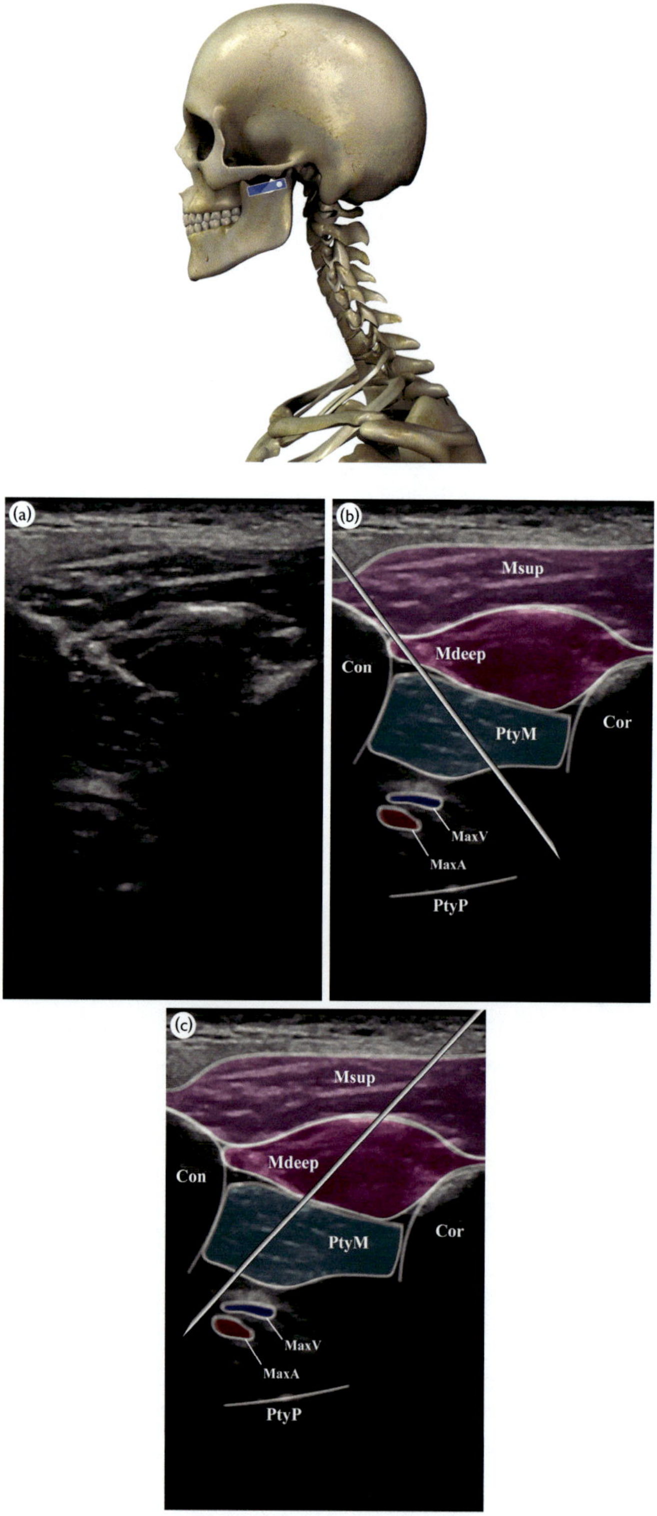

Figure 2.6.4 a, Ultrasound image of the lateral face with probe in an axial oblique plane. **b,** Labeled ultrasound image of in-plane needle placement for a maxillary V2 branch nerve block. **c,** Labeled ultrasound image of in-plane needle placement for a mandibular V3 branch nerve block. *Msup* superficial masseter muscle, *Mdeep* deep masseter muscle, *Con* condylar process of the mandible, *PtyM* pterygoid muscle, *Cor* coronoid process of the mandible, *MaxV* maxillary vein, *MaxA* maxillary artery, *PtyP* pterygoid plate

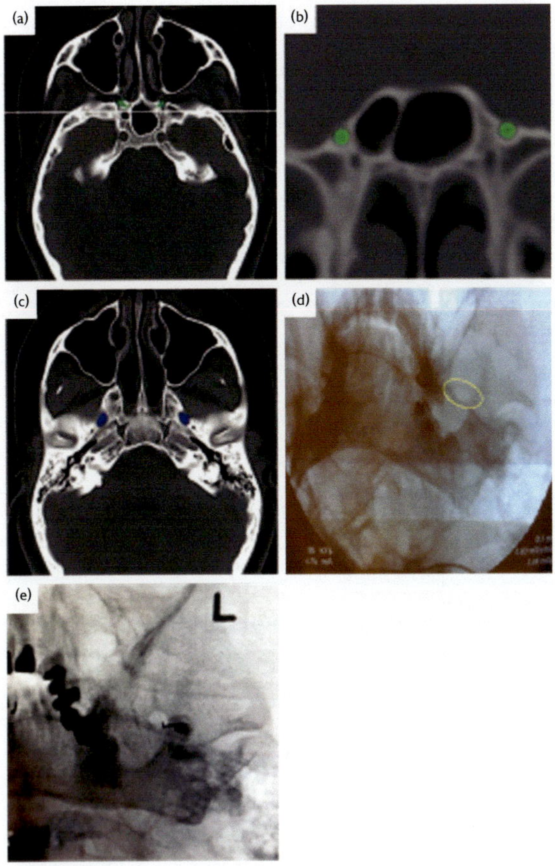

Figure 2.6.5 Normal anatomy of the foramen rotundum and ovale. **a,** The outlet of the foramen rotundum (green) lies within the pterygopalatine fossa, as depicted on an axial computerized tomography (CT) image. CT image through the coronal plane depicted in the line drawn. **b,** Demonstrates to better effect the anterior–posterior course of the foramen rotundum from Meckel's cave to the pterygopalatine fossa. **c,** The foramen ovale (blue) is easily identified in the axial plane anteromedial to the foramen spinosum, giving the appearance of a high- heeled shoe print. **d,** The foramen ovale can be visualized on fluoroscopy with ~20°–30° caudocephalic tilting of the C-arm and ~10°–20° head rotation to ipsilateral side (yellow circle) with the needle tip shown in (e). (Figure adapted from Telischak et al., Pain Medicine. January 2018, Pages 130–141 and Stanford Pain Clinic)

3. **Plan the procedural approach.**
   a. For maxillary V2 nerve blocks, the foramen rotundum can be approached from below the zygomatic arch to enter the PPF through the pterygomaxillary fissure (Figure 2.6.5, Figure 2.6.6).
   b. For mandibular V3 nerve blocks, the foramen ovale is recognized in the axial plane of a CT image, where it lies anterior and medial to the foramen spinosum. The two foramina together form the imprint of a high-heeled shoe (Figure 2.6.7c). The foramen ovale can also be visualized on fluoroscopy with 20–30 degree caudocephalic tilting of the C-arm and head rotation to 10–20 degrees ipsilateral side (Figure 2.6.7d). The V3 branch of the trigeminal nerve exits through the foramen ovale and may be selectively targeted with a skin entry point below the zygomatic arch and a straight-line needle trajectory reaching the foramen that can be visualized on fluoroscopy (Figures 2.6.7e, and 2.6.8a–d)
4. **Raise subcutaneous skin wheal with 1–2 cc 1% lidocaine at needle entry point.**
5. **Position the fluoroscopic C-arm so that a coaxial "bull's eye" approach can be taken to advance the needle to the desired target.**
6. **Perform postpositioning CT to confirm the needle location prior to treatment (Figures 2.6.5c–d and 2.6.8c–d).**
7. **With the needle in an appropriate position, replace the stylet with an RFA probe and perform electrostimulation to confirm the target.**

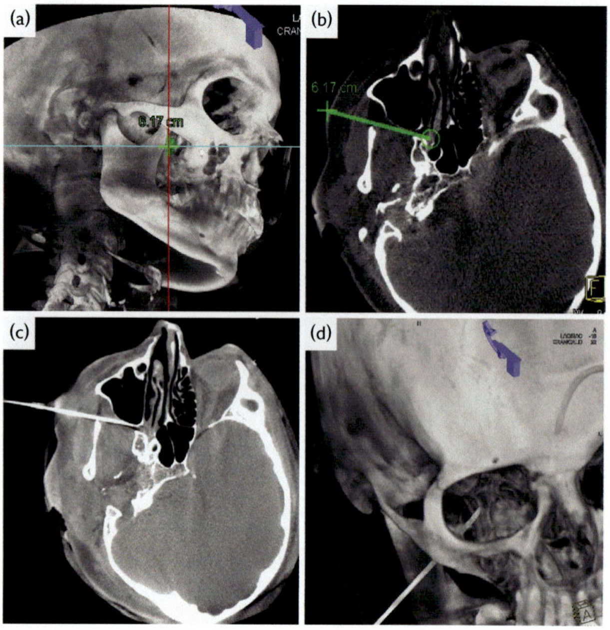

Figure 2.6.6 CT Guided Approach to maxillary V2 branch. **a & b,** A flat panel C-arm computerized tomography (CT) is performed. The C-arm CT is then used to select a needle path to the foramen rotundum using needle guidance software, and a lesion depth is calculated. **c,** The needle is then positioned in a bull's eye approach targeting the selected depth, with a post-positioning CT performed to confirm the needle location prior to treatment, as depicted on this multiplanar reformatted CT image. **d,** A 3D reconstructed image displays the needle in position within the foramen rotundum. (Figure adapted from Telischak, et. al, Pain Medicine. January 2018, Pages 130–141)

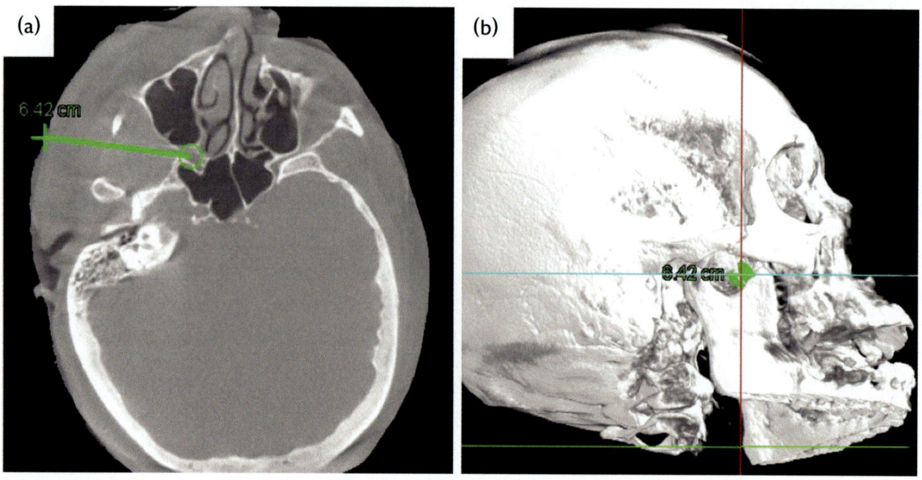

Figure 2.6.7 An illustration of the lateral supramandibular approach to the foramen rotundum. **a,** Axial computerized tomography (CT) image demonstrating the planned approach and target depth. **b,** 3D reconstructed CT image demonstrates the relationship with the mandibular condyle and coronoid process. (Figure adapted from Telischak, et. al, Pain Medicine. January 2018, Pages 130–141)

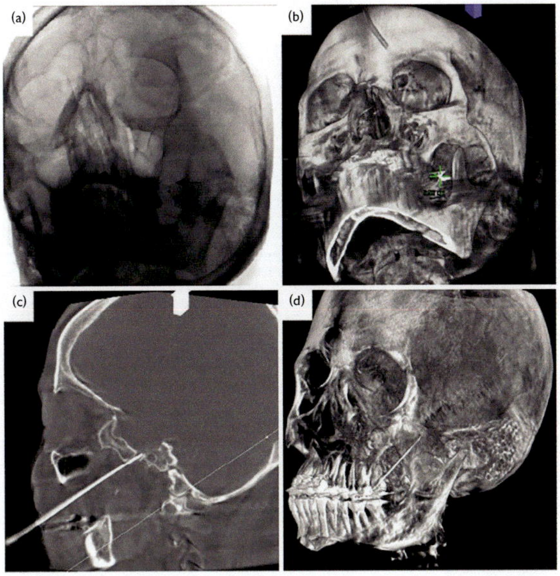

Figure 2.6.8 CT-guided approach to mandibular V3 branch. **a,** A BB marker is placed on the skin overlying the foramen ovale (black arrow) and a flat panel C-arm computerized tomography (CT) is performed. **b,** The C-arm CT is then used to select a needle path to the foramen ovale using needle guidance software, and a lesion depth is calculated. **c,** The needle is then positioned in a bull's eye approach targeting the selected depth, with a post-positioning CT performed to confirm the needle location prior to treatment, as depicted on this multiplanar reformatted CT image. **d,** A 3D reconstructed image displays the needle in position within the foramen ovale. (Figure adapted from Telischak et al., Pain Medicine. January 2018, Pages 130–141)

8. Nerve stimulation is performed, with the voltage slowly increased until stimulation can be confirmed. A voltage of less than 0.2–0.3 volts confirms adequate proximity to the nerve for successful treatment.
9. **Inject 0.5 to 1 mL 1% lidocaine to the target to achieve a dense sensory block,** in the corresponding dermatomal distribution, confirming the correct position of needle.
10. Once positioning is confirmed, perform continuous. **Perform radiofrequency ablation for 60 seconds at 60°C–80°C, twice, with the needle tip turned 180° between cycles.** Needle turning is performed to take advantage of the needle curvature to increase the treatment area volume by creating overlapping lesion spheres, increasing the likelihood of delivering a successful treatment to the target nerve.
11. **After negative aspiration, inject 2 mL mixture of 1 mL bupivacaine 0.25% and 1 mL methylprednisolone 10 mg to reduce the risk of postprocedural neuritis.**
12. **Flush needle with 1% lidocaine and withdraw the needle**. Apply a bandage.

Sphenopalatine Ganglion Block

Intranasal Approach

There are many documented techniques for SPG blocks, including infrazygomatic, intranasal, and transnasal approaches.[7] The intranasal approach is performed with a cotton-tipped applicator soaked in local anesthetic. It can also be done via SphenoCath or Tx360 nasal applicators.

1. **Prepare equipment and supplies, position the patient supine, and clean the skin around the area of the block with antiseptic solution.**
2. **Measure the approximate distance from the opening of the nare to the mandibular notch below the zygoma.**
3. **Insert a cotton-tipped applicator soaked in 4% lidocaine into the nare.** Slowly advance with the tip angled slightly laterally. Advanced to the previously measure depth.
4. **Leave applicator in place for 30–45 minutes.** The medication will be absorbed through the middle turbinate and lateral nasal mucosa to block the SPG.
5. **Remove the applicator.**

Tips

- Ensure the patient's neck remains extended throughout the entire procedure to allow for the local anesthetic to either diffuse across the mucosa to the SPG or spread along the sphenopalatine foramen into the PPF.

Safety Considerations

- Nasal epistaxis is a high-risk complication in patients who are thrombocytopenic or anticoagulated. Have suction or gauze available.

Infrazygomatic Fluoroscopic Approach

1. **Prepare equipment and supplies, position the patient supine, and clean the skin around the area of the block with antiseptic solution.**
2. **Obtain lateral fluoroscopy image of cranium.** Adjust head positioning until the PPF is clearly visualized with superimposed mandibular rami.
3. **Create skin wheal with 1% lidocaine at needle entry point inferior for the zygomatic arch and anterior to the mandible.**
4. **Insert spinal needle coaxially under lateral fluoroscopic guidance and direct superiorly and medially toward the PPF (Figure 2.6.9a).** Obtain intermittent anteroposterior (AP) fluoroscopic images to check needle depth. The needle tip should terminate immediately lateral to the ipsilateral nasal wall in the AP projection (Figure 2.6.9b).
5. **Inject 0.2 mL of contrast once needle tip is in the appropriate position under continuous fluoroscopic visualization to confirm correct localization in the PPF without intravascular contrast spread (Figure 2.6.9c).**
6. **Inject local anesthetic of choice with or without adjuvant steroid.**
7. **Flush and withdraw needle.** Apply bandage.

Postprocedure Management Considerations

Trigeminal Nerve Blocks

There are no special postoperative management considerations associated with this procedure. Complications from trigeminal nerve blocks can include intravascular injection or hematoma due to the close proximity of vascular structures. As the mandibular V3 nerve contains motor innervation, a well-performed nerve block may result in weakness of the muscles of mastication and facial asymmetry.

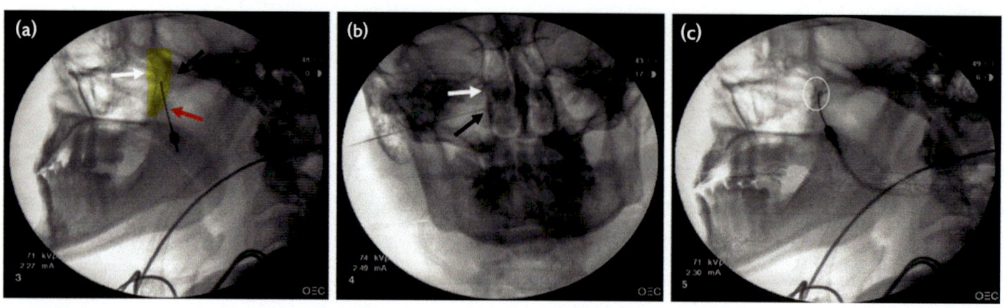

Figure 2.6.9 Fluoroscopic guided sphenopalatine ganglion block. **a,** Lateral fluoroscopic view with white arrow indicating the pterygopalatine fossa that is highlighted in yellow. Black arrow represents the pterygopalatine plate located posterior to the fossa. Red arrow represents the needle with tip being advanced superiorly and medially into the pterygopalatine fossa. **b,** Anteroposterior fluoroscopic view with white arrow representing the lateral nasal wall and black arrow denoting needle tip lateral to ipsilateral nasal wall. **c,** Lateral view of contrast spread with white circle showing dye spread with in the pterygopalatine fossa. (Images adapted from American Society of Regional Anesthesiology)

Sphenopalatine Ganglion Block

There are no special postoperative management considerations associated with this procedure. Adverse effects from the SPG block are minimal, but can include bitter taste, transient ipsilateral nostril burning sensation, and epistaxis.[3] Oropharyngeal numbness can occur, so patients should be instructed to avoid eating or drinking until the numbness passes. Hypotension and nausea are rare but potential adverse effects.[3]

References

1. Gupta R, Fisher K, Pyati S. Chronic Headache: A Review of Interventional Treatment Strategies in Headache Management. Curr Pain Headache Rep. 2019;23:68.
2. Gupta N, Dattatri R, Bharati SJ, et al. Ultrasound-Guided Real-Time Pterygopalatine Block for Analgesia in an Oral Cancer Patient. Indian J Palliat Care. 2018;24(1):112–114.
3. Robbins MS, Robertson CE, Kaplan E, et al. The Sphenopalatine Ganglion: Anatomy, Pathophysiology, and Therapeutic Targeting in Headache. Headache. 2016;56(2):240–258.
4. Levin M. Nerve Blocks in the Treatment of Headache. Neurotherapeutics. 2010;7(2):197–203.
5. Curatolo M. Regional Anesthesia in Pain Management. Curr Opin Anesthesiol. 2016;29:614–619.
6. Candido KD, Day M. Nerve Blocks of the Head and Neck. In: Benzon H, Rathmell JP, Wu CL, Turk DC, Argoff CE, Hurley RW (eds). Practical Management of Pain, 5th ed. Philadelphia: Mosby (Elsevier); 2014: 697–715.
7. Skulpoonkitti B, Day M. Sphenopalatine Ganglion Blocks. In: Manchikanti L, Kaye A, Falco F, Hirsch J (eds). Essentials of Interventional Techniques in Managing Chronic Pain. Cham: Springer (Switzerland); 2018: 519–30.

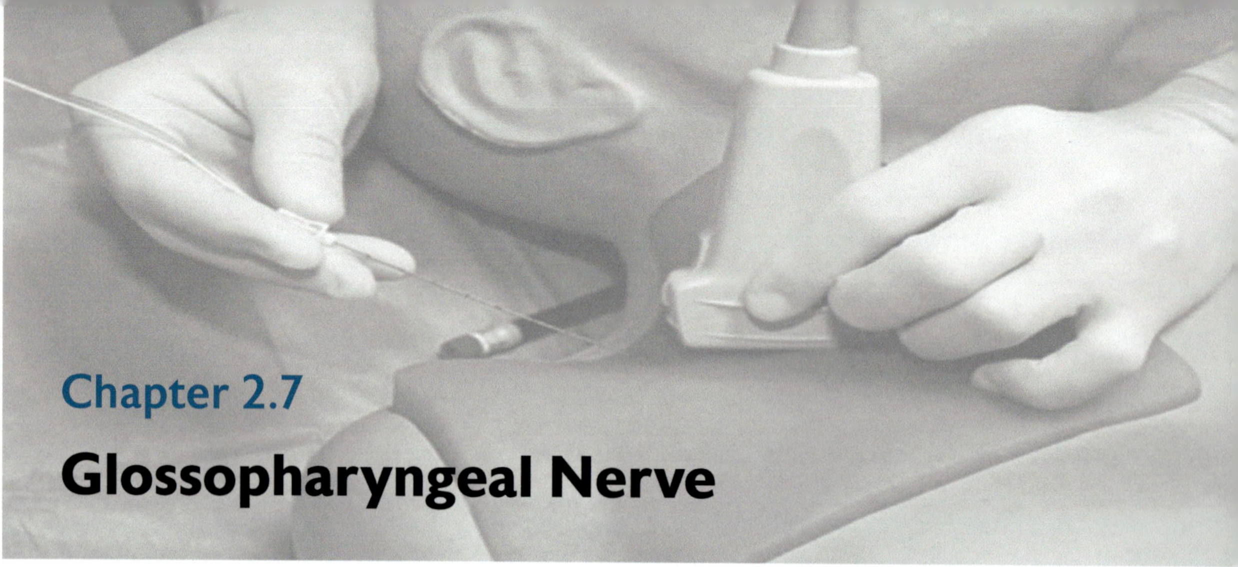

Chapter 2.7

Glossopharyngeal Nerve

Erdong Chen and Xiang Qian

Contents

Introduction and Critical Anatomy

Glossopharyngeal neuralgia (GPN) is a rare but debilitating condition that can lead to paroxysms of severe pain along the distribution of cranial nerve (CN) IX. It affects the throat, tongue, tonsillar fossa, pharynx, larynx, mandibular angle, and ear.[1] The glossopharyngeal nerve exits the skull base through the pars nervosa of the jugular foramen and courses adjacent to the styloid process (SP) of the temporal bone (Figure 2.7.1). It then courses along the side of the neck to pass under the hyoglossus muscle to its terminal distribution. It provides sensory innervation to the palatine tonsil, glands of the mouth, and base of the tongue.[2] Cranial nerve IX also provides motor innervation to the stylopharyngeus and parasympathetic innervation to the parotid gland via the otic ganglion. The incidence of GPN has been estimated to be 0.2–1.3 per 100,000 persons per year.[1,3,4] Pain associated with GPN is typically described as sharp, stabbing, or shooting pain that is incited by specific stimuli such as vocalization, mastication, swallowing, laughing, coughing, or yawning.[5] Cranial nerve IX also has afferent branches that communicate proximally with central vagal tracts at the spinal trigeminal nucleus and the nucleus solitarius. Hyperactivity of these interconnections explain rare cases of GPN causing hypotension, neurogenic syncope, bradycardia, and even cardiac arrest.[5–7] The symptoms of GPN lead to significant morbidity, including fear of alimentation and vocal communication that have led to psychiatric disorders and suicide.[8]

The cause of primary GPN can be multifactorial but is often poorly understood due to its low incidence. It can be due to vascular compression of the nerve and success has been achieved with

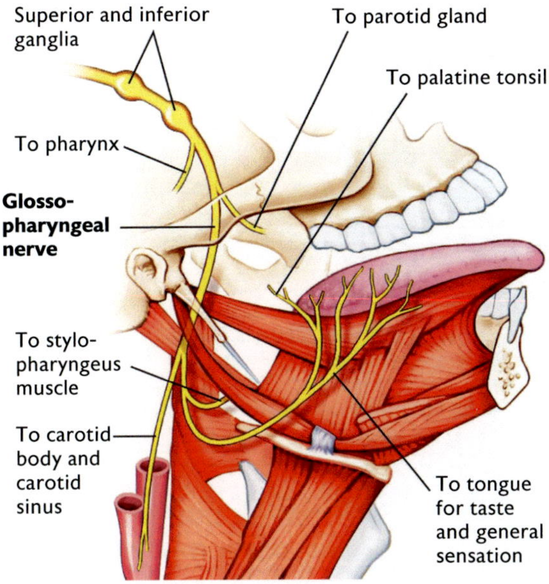

Figure 2.7.1 Glossopharyngeal nerve anatomy and innervation.

microvascular decompression in these cases. Glossopharyngeal neuralgia can also be secondary to head and neck cancer and case reports of various carcinomas compressing CN IX causing pain, bradycardia, and syncope.[2,6]

Indications

Current management strategies for GPN are similar to those for trigeminal neuralgia. Treatment can be tailored to the etiology of the neuralgia, but typically medical management is trialed first and followed by interventions. Pharmacotherapy with anticonvulsants (carbamazepine, oxcarbazepine, phenytoin, topiramate), gabapentinoids (gabapentin, pregabalin), and tricyclic antidepressants is typically effective in providing some degree of symptomatic relief, but these therapies are also limited by drug side effects and potential failure with medical therapy alone.

When medical management fails, a glossopharyngeal nerve block can be trailed to provide transient cessation of nerve impulse conduction. This involves injection of local anesthetic with or without the addition of steroids and is associated with a low incidence of adverse events. For patients with GPN secondary to vascular compression, microvascular decompression has been shown to provide long-lasting relief of pain paroxysms. However, decompression involves an open craniotomy and is associated with risk of intracranial hemorrhage and postoperative dysphagia.[9] Percutaneous rhizotomy of CN IX and the vagal afferents can also be performed with fluoroscopic guidance, but this procedure can be complicated by injury to the nearby vagus nerve, spinal accessory nerve, and internal carotid artery.[4] These risks are compounded by anatomic changes in oncologic pain. Gamma knife radiosurgery has also been performed for GPN with good tolerability and side effect profiles.[10] However, it has a higher failure ratio at follow-up and often requires repeat treatments.[11]

Glossopharyngeal nerve blocks are commonly performed with local anesthetic via four separate approaches: (1) topically, (2) intraoral injection, (3) parapharyngeal space injection, and (4) percutaneous peristyloid process injection.

Pulsed radiofrequency (PRF) modulation or radiofrequency ablation (RFA) rhizotomy has been reported to treat both primary and secondary GPN with sustained therapeutic benefit.[12,13] PRF delivers short pulses of high-frequency current to a peripheral nerve or ganglionic target and has demonstrated efficacy in treating neuropathic pain.[14–16] A 2020 study of 30 idiopathic GPN patients who received PRF under CT guidance showed pain relief survival of 93.3% at 1 year and 79.6% at 4 years.[12,13] Pulsed radiofrequency has also been shown to be effective and safe in treating chronic secondary GPN from oropharyngeal cancer[17] and tonsillectomy.[18]

The glossopharyngeal nerve passes through the pars nervosa of the jugular foramen, from which it exits the skull base and courses adjacent to the styloid process (SP). Peristyloid CN IX

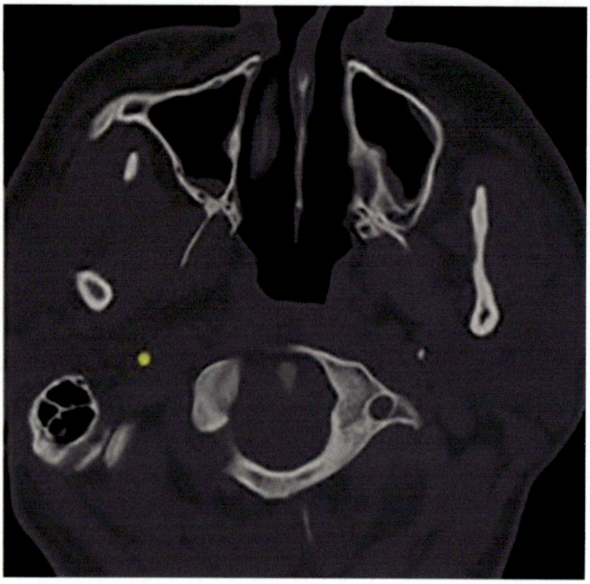

Figure 2.7.2 Styloid process normal anatomy. The styloid process (yellow) originates from the mastoid and travels anteromedially ending in the stylohyoid ligament and serves as the bony landmark for a glossopharyngeal nerve block. (Figure adapted from Telischak et al., Pain Medicine. January 2018, Pages 130–141)

blocks have been traditionally done under fluoroscopic guidance with a bony landmark-based technique with a target at the distal one third of the styloid process (SP). Ultrasound-based approaches have also been developed with advantages of being able to actively visualize needle trajectory, bone, soft tissue planes, vascular structures, and spread of injectate. However, the complexity of skull base anatomy makes ultrasound guidance challenging, especially when cancer has altered normal anatomy.

Recent technological advances have been described to improve navigation and positioning of therapeutic instruments, including fluoroscopy, computerized tomography (CT) guidance, 3D navigation techniques, and electrophysiological evoked potentials. More recently, a novel technique of flat-panel C-arm CT guidance has been described for intervention on the glossopharyngeal nerve that targets the nerve 5–10 mm posterior to the styloid process[19] (Figure 2.7.2).

Equipment and Patient Preparation

1. **Monitors and Sterility**
   a. No special monitors are needed for this procedure in an otherwise healthy patient.
   b. For patients with cardiac concerns, consider monitored anesthesia care in case of bradycardia and hypotension, which may result from activation of the trigeminal cardiac reflex.
   c. Emergency resuscitation equipment, supplemental oxygen, AMBU bag, suction, ACLS drugs and intralipid should be available immediately.
   d. Peripheral IV should be placed.
2. **Equipment**
   a. Imaging:
      i. Fluoroscopy/CT guided intervention: Fluoroscopy with C-arm CT capability and 3D navigation software such as Syngo Iguide
      ii. Ultrasound-guided block: Low-frequency (2–5 MHz) curvilinear array ultrasound probe

   b. Needle type:
      i. Fluoroscopy/CT guided intervention: 5 mm tip 21-gauge radiofrequency needle
      ii. Ultrasound guided block: 22-gauge 3.5-inch spinal needle
   c. Local anesthetic (1–2 mL): Lidocaine 1%–2%; ropivacaine 0.2%–0.5%; bupivacaine 0.25%–0.5%
   d. Adjuvant (0.5–1 mL): Nonparticulate steroid
3. **Position**
   a. Fluoroscopy/CT-guided intervention: supine with neck mildly extended and head gently secured with a soft strap.
   b. Ultrasound-guided block: supine or lateral position with a thin pillow under the head

Step-by-Step Technique

Glossopharyngeal Nerve Radiofrequency—Fluoroscopy/CT-Guided Approach

1. **Prepare equipment and supplies, position the patient in the supine position with the neck mildly extended, and clean the procedural area with antiseptic solution.**
2. **Determine location of initial needle insertion.** Place a radiopaque BB marker on the skin (Figure 2.7.3A). Measure target depth from the skin on processed CT images and mark needle to this depth (Figure 2.7.3B). The initial needle skin entry point is approximately 1 cm below the ipsilateral earlobe.
3. **Raise subcutaneous skin wheal with 1–2 mL 1% lidocaine at needle entry point.**
4. **Position the fluoroscopic C-arm so that a coaxial approach can be taken to advance the needle to the desired target.** A final needle position at or overshooting the styloid process posteriorly by 1–5 mm is ideal.
5. **Perform postpositioning CT to confirm the needle location prior to treatment (Figure 2.7.3c–d).**
6. **Replace the stylet with a RFA probe and perform electrostimulation to confirm the target.** A voltage of less than 0.2–0.3 volts confirms adequate proximity to the nerve for successful treatment.
7. **Inject 0.5 to 1 mL 1% lidocaine to the target to achieve a dense sensory block.**
8. **Perform radiofrequency ablation for 60 seconds at 60–80°C twice, with the needle tip turned 180° between cycles.** Needle turning is performed to take advantage of the needle curvature to increase the treatment area by creating overlapping lesions, increasing the likelihood of a successful treatment.
9. **After negative aspiration, inject 2 mL mixture of 1 mL bupivacaine 0.25% and 1 mL Decadron 10 mg to reduce the risk of postprocedural neuritis. Flush needle with 1% lidocaine and withdraw the needle**. Apply a bandage.

Glossopharyngeal Nerve Block—Ultrasound Approach

1. **Prepare equipment and supplies, position the patient in the supine position, and clean the procedural area with antiseptic solution.** Alternative positioning is lateral.
2. **Place the ultrasound probe in an oblique transverse orientation below the ear.** Locate the mastoid and the mandibular angle and draw a line between the two landmarks. Using deep pressure, the SP can be palpated just posterior to the angle of the jaw along this line.
3. **Draw a second line starting 1.5 cm above the posterior edge of the mandibular angle extending to the mastoid.** Scanning in this plane will visualize the SP[20] (Figure 2.7.4a–b).

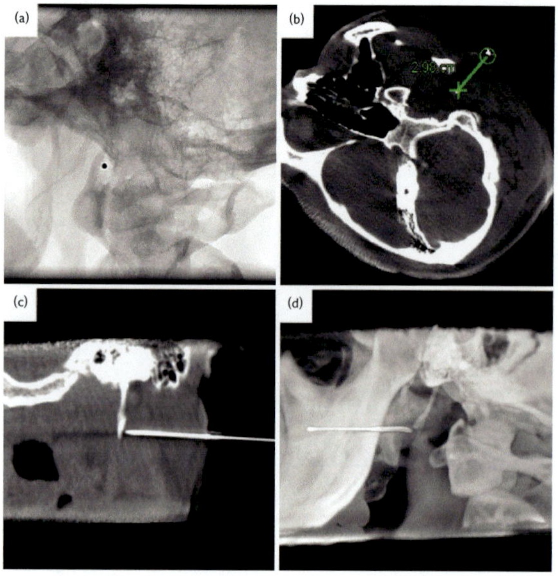

Figure 2.7.3 Fluoroscopy and CT-guided approach to the styloid process. A BB marker is placed on the skin (A), and a flat panel C-arm computerized tomography (CT) is performed. The C-arm CT is then used to select a needle path using needle-guidance software, and a lesion depth is calculated (B). The needle is then positioned in a bull's eye approach targeting the selected depth, with a postpositioning CT performed to confirm the needle location prior to treatment, as depicted on this multiplanar reformatted CT image abutting the styloid process (C). A 3D reconstructed image displays the needle in position adjacent to the styloid process (D). (Figure adapted from Telischak et al., Pain Medicine. January 2018, Pages 130–141)

4. **Use color flow doppler to identify the external carotid artery.** The internal carotid artery and internal jugular vein can be seen below or behind the SP[21] (Figure 2.7.5a–b).
5. **Raise subcutaneous skin wheal with 1–2 mL 1% lidocaine at needle entry point.**
6. **Under in-plane direct ultrasound visualization, introduce the procedural needle to the SP and direct the needle tip to the posterior portion of the SP (Figure 2.7.5b)**

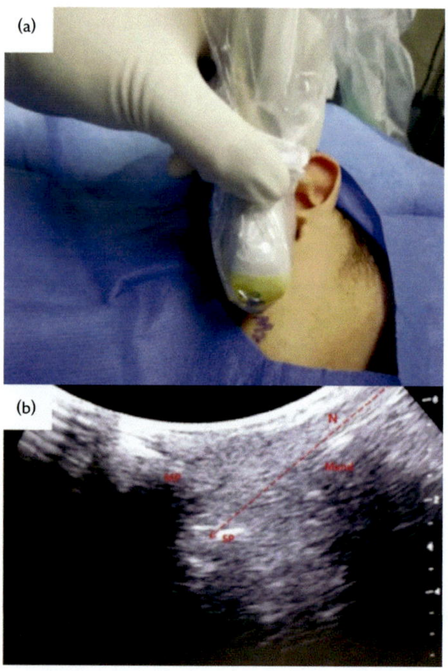

Figure 2.7.4 Identification of the styloid process and projected needle tract. (A) Ultrasound probe orientation. (B) Sagittal ultrasound image with view of the mastoid process (MP), the mandible (Mand), the styloid process (SP), and the ideal needle tract to the SP (N)[20]. (Figure adapted from Liu et al., J Pain Res. 2019;12:2503–2510)

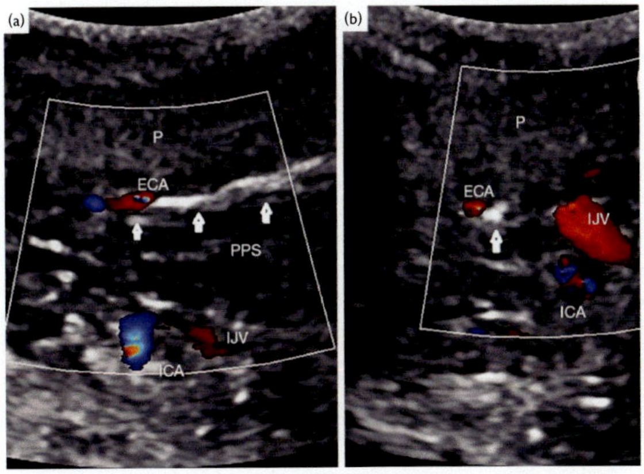

Figure 2.7.5 Ultrasound with color wave doppler vessels near the styloid process. Styloid process delineated by arrows. (A) Oblique coronal view of the mandibular ramus on ultrasound; (B) cross-sectional view of the styloid process via the transverse section of the mandibular ramus. arrows, styloid process; P, parotid gland; PPS, parapharyngeal space; ICA, internal carotid artery; ECA, external carotid artery; IJV, internal jugular vein; AIR, air in nasopharynx cavity. (Figure adapted from Zang et al., Ann Transl Med. 2020;8(24):1666.)

7. **After negative aspiration, inject 2 mL mixture of 1 mL bupivacaine 0.25% and 1 mL Decadron 10 mg**. Flush and remove the needle. Apply a bandage.

Safety Considerations

The classical jugular foramen approach to CN IX blocks can be complicated by violation of dura and injury to the nearby vagus nerve, spinal accessory nerve, and internal carotid artery. Therefore, the fluoroscopy-guided and CT-guided techniques described above target the SP via a lateral cervical approach. At the SP level, cranial nerves IX, X, and XI have separated from each other, with nerve IX being closest to the distal part of SP.

References

1. Rozen TD. Trigeminal neuralgia and glossopharyngeal neuralgia. *Neurolog Clin*. 2004;22(1):185–206.
2. Khan M, Nishi SE, Hassan SN, Islam MA, Gan SH. Trigeminal neuralgia, glossopharyngeal neuralgia, and myofascial pain dysfunction syndrome: an update. *Pain Res Manag*. 2017;2017:7438326. doi:10.1155/2017/7438326
3. Katusic S, Williams DB, Beard CM, Bergstralh E, Kurland LT. Incidence and clinical features of glossopharyngeal neuralgia, Rochester, Minnesota, 1945–1984. *Neuroepidemiology*. 1991;10(5–6):266–275.
4. Ma Y, Li Y-F, Wang Q-C, Wang B, Huang H-T. Neurosurgical treatment of glossopharyngeal neuralgia: analysis of 103 cases. *JNS*. 2016;124(4):1088. doi:10.3171/2015.3.Jns141806
5. Blumenfeld A, Nikolskaya G. Glossopharyngeal neuralgia. *Cur Pain and Head Rpts*. 2013;17(7):343.
6. Reddy GD, Viswanathan A. Trigeminal and glossopharyngeal neuralgia. *Neurol Clin*. 2014;32(2):539–52. doi:10.1016/j.ncl.2013.11.008
7. Metheetrairut C, Brown DH. Glossopharyngeal neuralgia and syncope secondary to neck malignancy. *J Otolaryngol*. 1993;22(1):18–20.
8. Albahkaly S, Alshehabi M, Al-Shmasi HS, Altaleb OA. Reappraisal of glossopharyngeal neuralgia. *Interdisciplinary Neurosurgery*. 2018;11:34–36. https://doi.org/10.1016/j.inat.2017.11.002
9. Zhao H, Zhang X, Zhu J, Tang YD, Li ST. Microvascular decompression for glossopharyngeal neuralgia: long-term follow-up. *World Neurosurg*. 2017;102:151–156. doi:10.1016/j.wneu.2017.02.106
10. Martínez-Álvarez R, Martínez-Moreno N, Kusak ME, Rey-Portolés G. Glossopharyngeal neuralgia and radiosurgery. *J Neurosurg*. 2014;121(Suppl):222–225. doi:10.3171/2014.8.Gks141273
11. Balossier A, Tuleasca C, Muracciole X, Donnet A, Levivier M, Régis J. The outcomes of a second and third Gamma Knife radiosurgery for recurrent essential glossopharyngeal neuralgia. *Acta Neurochir (Wien)*. 2020;162(2):271–277. doi:10.1007/s00701-019-04124-8

12. Jia Y, Shrestha N, Wang X, Wang T, Luo F. The long-term outcome of CT-guided pulsed radiofrequency in the treatment of idiopathic glossopharyngeal neuralgia: a retrospective multi-center case series. *J Pain Res*. 2020;13:2093–2102. doi:10.2147/jpr.S259994
13. van Tilburg CWJ. Percutaneous pulsed radiofrequency treatment in a patient with chronic bilateral painful glossopharyngeal neuropathy. *Am J Case Rep*. 2020 Feb 11;21:e920579. doi:10.12659/AJCR.920579. PMID: 32041932; PMCID: PMC7038638.
14. Ojango C, Raguso M, Fiori R, Masala S. Pulse-dose radiofrequency treatment in pain management-initial experience. *Skel Rad*. 2018;47(5):609–618. doi:10.1007/s00256-017-2854-8
15. Vanneste T, Van Lantschoot A, Van Boxem K, Van Zundert J. Pulsed radiofrequency in chronic pain. *Crnt Opin in Anaesth*. 2017;30(5):577–582. doi:10.1097/aco.0000000000000502
16. Chang MC. Efficacy of pulsed radiofrequency stimulation in patients with peripheral neuropathic pain: a narrative review. *Pain Physician*. 2018;21(3):E225–e234.
17. Bharti N, Chattopadhyay S, Singla N, Bala I, Batra YK, Bakshi J. Pulsed radiofrequency ablation for the treatment of glossopharyngeal neuralgia secondary to oropharyngeal carcinoma. *Pain Physician*. 2018;21(3):295–302.
18. Shah RV, Racz GB. Pulsed mode radiofrequency lesioning to treat chronic post-tonsillectomy pain (secondary glossopharyngeal neuralgia). *Pain Pract*. 2003;3(3):232–237. doi:10.1046/j.1533-2500.2003.03028.x
19. Telischak NA, Heit JJ, Campos LW, Choudhri OA, Do HM, Qian X. Fluoroscopic C-arm and CT-guided selective radiofrequency ablation for trigeminal and glossopharyngeal facial pain syndromes. *Pain Medicine*. 2017;19(1):130–141. doi:10.1093/pm/pnx088
20. Liu Q, Zhong Q, Tang G, He G. Ultrasound-guided glossopharyngeal nerve block via the styloid process for glossopharyngeal neuralgia: a retrospective study. *J Pain Res*. 2019;12:2503–2510. doi:10.2147/jpr.S214596
21. Zang Y, Chen S, Zang G, et al. The anatomic basis for ultrasound in the diagnosis and treatment of styloid process-related diseases. *Ann Transl Med*. 2020;8(24):1666. doi:10.21037/atm-20-7781

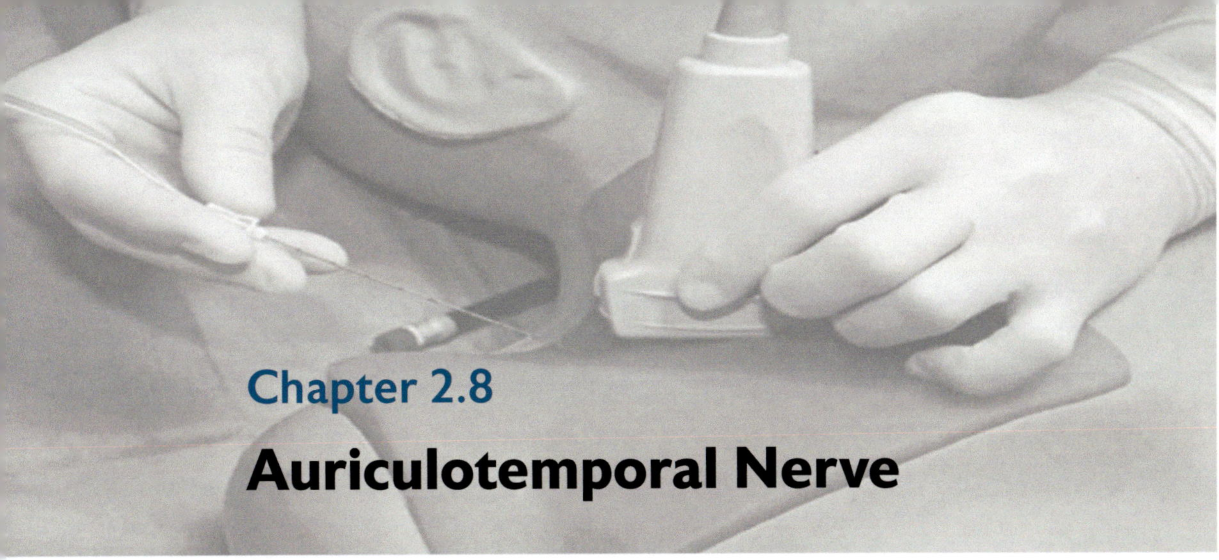

Chapter 2.8
Auriculotemporal Nerve

Richard J. Batka, Anthony Tran, and Neal Rakesh

Contents

Introduction

The auriculotemporal nerve (ATN) can be a source of pain in the regions of the external auditory meatus, base of the auricle, temporomandibular joint (TMJ), and skin of the posterior temporal region.[1–2] It can also result from TMJ dysfunction, parotid masses/tumors, surgery, and direct trauma.[3–5] Its susceptibility to compression by peri-auricular fascial bands and the superficial temporal artery (STA) can cause facial pain and serve as a trigger for chronic headaches.[6] Frey Syndrome (gustatory sweating and flushing) may arise after direct trauma, surgical manipulation, dorsal sympathectomy, or carotid endarterectomy due to aberrant reinnervation of the parotid gland. ATN blockade is a valuable tool for diagnosis of facial pain and recurrent headache. When combined with a corticosteroid, ATN blockade can be a treatment for neuritis. Landmark and fluoroscopy-guided approaches are well described; however, only ultrasound guidance offers live confirmation of needle placement and injectate delivery. This reduces the potential complication of intravascular infiltration and hematoma.

Indications

Cancer-related pain, postsurgical tumor resection neuralgia, chemotherapy/radiation-induced neuralgia, pain in the auricular and temporal regions of the face, recurrent migraine headaches, Frey Syndrome, Ramsay Hunt Syndrome, temporomandibular joint pain, auriculotemporal neuralgia.

Contraindications

The primary cancer-specific contraindication is the patient's current immune status, especially in the case of current or recent chemotherapy, given the risk of infection inherent with any invasive procedure. General contraindications include allergy to local anesthetics or corticosteroids, treatment with anticoagulation agents, and ongoing local or systemic infection. As always, a patient's refusal of or inability to consent for the procedure is an absolute contraindication.

Critical Anatomy

The auriculotemporal nerve (ATN) is formed from the posterior division of the mandibular branch of the trigeminal nerve (the fifth cranial nerve). It supplies cutaneous sensation of the posterior temple, TMJ, tragus, and auricle (Figure 2.8.1). It also carries parasympathetic fibers and secretomotor fibers to the parotid gland. Anatomical studies disclose considerable variation of the ATN with respect to the number of branches forming its root, course in relation to the middle meningeal artery in the infratemporal fossa, communication with other nerves, and location of its six named branches.[3–8] Almost invariably, the ATN enters the soft tissue of the face posterior to the TMJ through the parotid gland and ascends vertically over the zygomatic arch posterior and superficial to the superficial temporal artery.[6,9] The tragus is a reliable anatomic landmark for locating the ATN as it travels superficially to the zygomatic arch.

Equipment and Patient Preparation

1. **Monitors and Sterility**
   a. No specific monitors are needed for this procedure, but emergency resuscitation equipment should be available immediately. This includes ACLS drugs, supplemental oxygen, airway adjuncts, and suction.

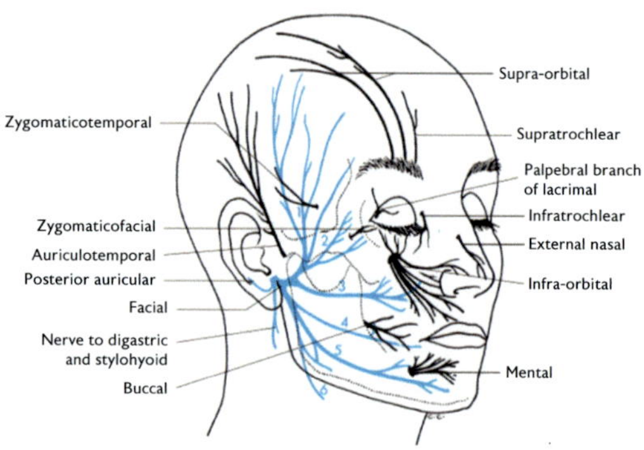

Figure 2.8.1 The nerves of the face. The motor facial nerve is shown in blue and the sensory trigeminal nerve is shown in black. (Reprinted with permission from Cunningham's Manual of Practical Anatomy: Head, Neck and Brain, 16th Edition)

   b. Strict antiseptic technique should be observed including sterile probe cover, ultrasound gel, and sterile gloves. Chlorhexidine or other skin prep agent should be used to clean the skin prior to commencing the procedure.

2. **Equipment**
   a. Probe: High-frequency linear array transducer (8–15 MHz)
   b. Needle type: 25- or 30-gauge, 1- to 1.5-inch needle
   c. Local anesthetic (0.5 mL): Lidocaine 1%–2%; ropivacaine 0.2%–0.5%; bupivacaine 0.25%–0.5%
   d. Adjuvant (0.5 mL): Particulate or nonparticulate steroid
3. **Position**
   a. Supine

Step-by-Step Technique

1. **Prepare equipment and supplies, position the patient in the prone position, and clean the procedural area with antiseptic solution.**
2. **Place the ultrasound probe anterior to the tragus such that it is superior and parallel to the zygomatic arch.**
3. **Identify the superficial temporal vasculature** (short-axis) using power doppler, color doppler, or B-flow (Figure 2.8.2).
4. **Translate the transducer anterior** such that there is adequate space to introduce the needle while maintaining visualization of the superficial temporal vasculature.
5. **Introduce the needle into the space anterior to the tragus (in-plane approach) and advance it toward the region just posterior to the superficial temporal vasculature (**Figure 2.8.2**).**
6. **Keeping the needle tip in view, deliver the injectate slowly and observe its spread in the target tissue.**
7. **Withdraw the needle and remove the ultrasound probe.** Clean the site with sterile gauze, apply a sterile adhesive dressing over the puncture site, then remove the window drape.

Tips

- Ensure the zygomatic arch is a bony backdrop to prevent inadvertent puncture of the needle into the oral cavity.
- Prior radiation and surgery may distort anatomy. The superficial temporal artery may be a landmark for the nerve if the nerve is not clearly visualized.
- Branches of the facial nerve are near the ATN, and injection can cause partial blockade of the facial nerve, resulting in facial muscle weakness.

Safety Considerations

- Use doppler to search for and identify the middle meningeal and temporal arteries near the target area to avoid during procedures

Postprocedure Management

Given the high vascularity of face and scalp tissue, the patient should be monitored for anesthetic or steroid toxicity. Additionally, the patient should be monitored for any signs of bleeding given the high vascularity and be treated accordingly.

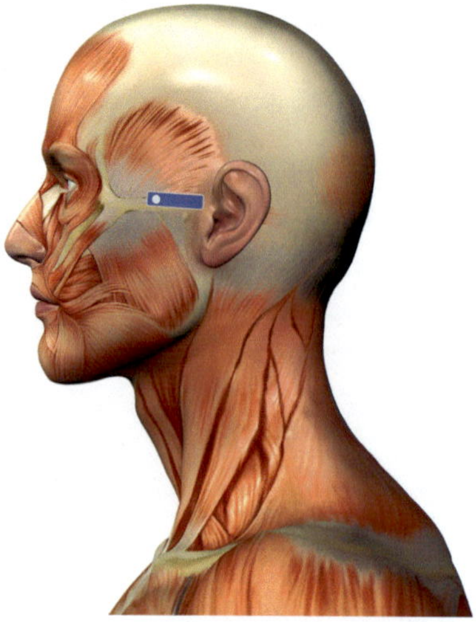

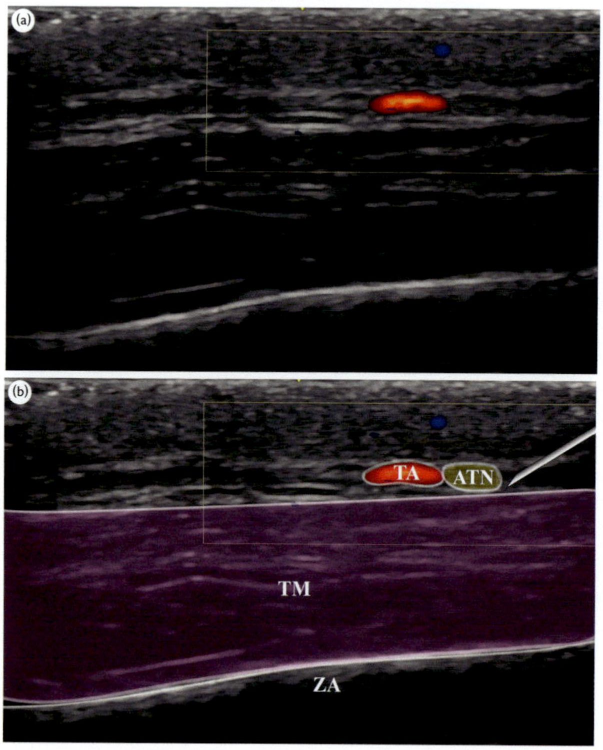

Figure 2.8.2 a, Ultrasound image of the lateral face in an axial plane over the zygomatic arch. **b,** Labeled ultrasound image of in-plane needle placement of the auriculotemporal nerve (ATN) in short-axis. *TA* temporal artery, *ATN* auriculotemporal nerve, *TM* temporalis muscle, *ZA* zygomatic arch bone.

Further Reading

- Blumenfeld A, Ashkenazi A, Napchan U, et al. Expert consensus recommendations for the performance of peripheral nerve blocks for headaches: a narrative review. *Headache J Head Face Pain*. 2013;53(3):437–446. doi:10.1111/head.12053

- Levin M. Nerve blocks in the treatment of headache. *Neurotherapeutics*. 2010;7(2):197–203. doi:10.1016/j.nurt.2010.03.001
- Trescot AM. Ultrasound for evaluation and treatment of headaches. *Anesthesia, Pain and Intensive Care*. Published online 2001.

References

1. Swendseid BP, Philips RHW, Rao NK, et al. The underappreciated role of auriculotemporal nerve involvement in local failure following parotidectomy for cancer. *Head Neck*. 2020;42(11):3253–3262. doi:10.1002/hed.26372
2. Thompson JD, Avey GD, Wieland AM, et al. Auriculotemporal nerve involvement in parotid bed malignancy. *Ann Otology Rhinology Laryngology*. 2019;128(7):647–653. doi:10.1177/0003489419837574
3. Baumel JJ, Vanderheiden JP, McElenney JE. The auriculotemporal nerve of man. *Am J Anat*. 1971;130(4):431–440. doi:10.1002/aja.1001300405
4. Fernandes PRB, Vasconsellos HA de, Okeson JP, Bastos RL, Maia MLT. The anatomical relationship between the position of the auriculotemporal nerve and mandibular condyle. *Cranio*. 2016;21(3):165–171. doi:10.1080/08869634.2003.11746246
5. Gülekon N, Anil A, Poyraz A, Peker T, Turgut HB, Karaköse M. Variations in the anatomy of the auriculotemporal nerve. *Clin Anat*. 2005;18(1):15–22. doi:10.1002/ca.20068
6. Janis JE, Hatef DA, Ducic I, et al. Anatomy of the auriculotemporal nerve: variations in its relationship to the superficial temporal artery and implications for the treatment of migraine headaches. *Plast Reconstr Surg*. 2010;125(5):1422–1428. doi:10.1097/prs.0b013e3181d4fb05
7. Schmidt BL, Pogrel MA, Necoechea M, Kearns G. The distribution of the auriculotemporal nerve around the temporomandibular joint. *Oral Surg Med Oral Path Oral Radiol Endodon*. 1998;86(2):165–168. doi:10.1016/s1079-2104(98)90119-6
8. Komarnitki I, Tomczyk J, Ciszek B, Zalewska M. Proposed classification of auriculotemporal nerve, based on the root system. *PLos One*. 2015;10(4):e0123120. doi:10.1371/journal.pone.0123120
9. Iwanaga J, Watanabe K, Saga T, Fisahn C, Oskouian RJ, Tubbs RS. Anatomical study of the superficial temporal branches of the auriculotemporal nerve: application to surgery and other invasive treatments to the temporal region. *J Plastic Reconstr Aesthetic Surg*. 2017;70(3):370–374. doi:10.1016/j.bjps.2016.10.025

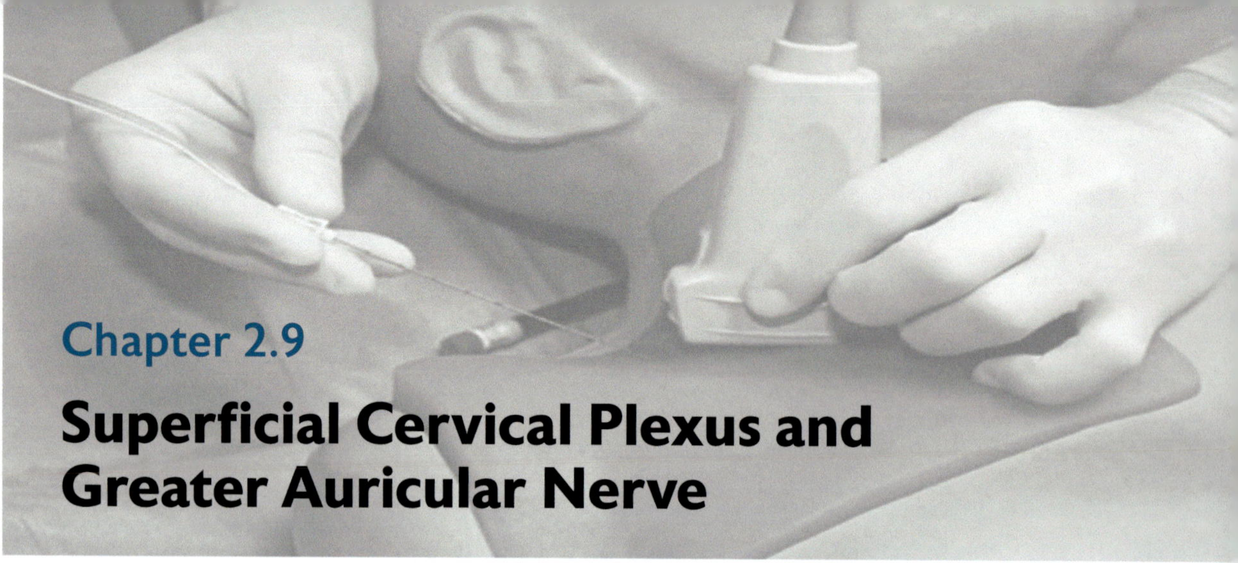

Chapter 2.9

Superficial Cervical Plexus and Greater Auricular Nerve

Anthony Tran

Contents

Introduction

A superficial cervical plexus block (CPB) provides analgesia for the anterolateral neck[1] and has been used for superficial neck surgery, lymph node dissection, external ear surgery, and carotid endarterectomy.[2] Furthermore, CPBs can provide analgesia for chronic pain syndromes related to structural alterations from cancer treatment (e.g., surgery, radiation) or cancer progression (e.g., intraneural tumor spread).[3–5] The cervical plexus is formed primarily by the anterior (ventral) rami of C1–C4 and divides into a deep motor branch and superficial sensory branch.[6] The superficial branch of the cervical plexus gives rise to the lesser occipital nerve, great auricular nerve, transverse cervical nerve, and supraclavicular nerve.[7] The cervical plexus block will be described along with a selective block of a direct branch (greater auricular nerve).

Critical Anatomy

A cervical plexus block is performed by blocking the contributing nerve roots as they emerge from the posterior border of the sternocleidomastoid muscle. The layers that are traversed to gain access to the target area (starting from most superficial) include the skin, subcutaneous tissue, and the superficial and deep layers of the deep cervical fascia. The depth of the needle and thereby delivery of anesthetics demarcates the various types of cervical plexus blocks: superficial, intermediate, and deep.[8] A superficial block is achieved by deposition of anesthetic directly below the subcutaneous layer. An intermediate block is achieved by deposition of anesthetic directly below the superficial layer of the deep cervical fascia. A deep block is achieved by deposition of anesthetic directly below the deep layer of the deep cervical fascia. Only the superficial and intermediate approaches are described in this chapter, as deep cervical plexus blocks have fallen out of favor due to respiratory-related complications from phrenic nerve involvement.[9] A selective block of the greater auricular nerve (GAN) can also be performed. This direct branch of the cervical plexus provides sensory innervation to the skin of the auricle, lower face and upper trunk.[10] The GAN can be blocked as it courses upward along the posterior aspect of the superficial sternocleidomastoid muscle prior to its bifurcation into anterior and posterior divisions.[11]

The anterolateral neck contains important neurovascular structures that will be reviewed to minimize inadvertent access. At the center of the procedural field and serving as the point of reference is the sternocleidomastoid muscle (SCM), which originates at the manubrium of the sternum and clavicle and travels obliquely along the side of the neck to insert at the mastoid process of the temporal bone.[12] Deep to the SCM lies the carotid sheath consisting of fibrous connective tissue encasing the common carotid artery, internal jugular vein, and vagus nerve.[13] Posterior to the carotid sheath lies the brachial plexus (cervical nerve roots C5–T1) which emerges between the anterior and middle scalene muscles.[14] These structures can be identified under ultrasound (Figure 2.9.1) and should be avoided.

Indications as Related to Cancer Pain

- Postoperative neuropathic pain
- Radiation-induced neuropathic pain
- Perineural tumor spread causing neuropathic pain
- Treatment-related headache in the distribution of the nerve[4,5]

Classic Indications

- Carotid Endarterectomy
- Superficial neck surgery
- External ear surgery
- Lymph node dissection[2]

Contraindications

- Patient refusal
- Overlying skin infection
- Local anesthetic allergy
- Contralateral phrenic nerve palsy

Equipment and Patient Preparation

1. **Monitors and Sterility**
   a. No specific monitors are needed for this procedure, but emergency resuscitation equipment should be available immediately. This includes ACLS drugs, supplemental oxygen, airway adjuncts, and suction.

b. Strict antiseptic technique should be observed including sterile probe cover, ultrasound gel, and sterile gloves. Chlorhexidine or other skin prep agent should be used to clean the skin prior to commencing the procedure.

2. **Equipment**
   a. Probe: High-frequency linear array transducer (8–12 MHz)
   b. Needle type: 2-5 or 30-gauge, 1- to 2-inch needle
   c. Local anesthetic (3–6 mL): Lidocaine 1%–2%; ropivacaine 0.2%–0.5%; bupivacaine 0.25%–0.5%
   d. Adjuvant (1 mL): Particulate or nonparticulate steroid
3. **Position**
   a. Supine (preferred) or lateral decubitus

Step-by-Step Technique

Cervical Plexus Approach

1. **Prepare equipment and supplies, position the patient supine with the head rotated away from the procedural side, and clean the skin around the area of the block with antiseptic solution.**
2. **Place the ultrasound probe in a transverse orientation along the midpoint of the SCM.**
3. **Translate the ultrasound probe laterally to the tapered border of the SCM.** With the lateral border of the SCM on screen, the cervical plexus may be seen resting between the hyperechoic fascial layer and above the hyperechoic prevertebral fascial layer (Figure 2.9.1).
4. **Insert the procedural needle using an in-plane approach from a posterior-to-anterior direction.** The target for the superficial CPB is inferior to the SCM. The target for the intermediate CPB is inferior to the superficial layer of the deep cervical fascia.
5. **Aspirate to rule out intravascular injection and deposit the injectate.** Remove the needle and apply a dressing.

Greater Auricular Nerve Approach

1. **Prepare equipment and supplies, position the patient supine with the head rotated away from the procedural side, and clean the skin around the area of the block with antiseptic solution.**
2. **Place the ultrasound probe in a transverse orientation along the upper third of the SCM.**
3. **Translate the ultrasound probe superiorly along the posterior edge of the SCM until visualizing the GAN.** The GAN will appear as a circular hypoechoic structure superficial to the SCM (Figure 2.9.2).
4. **Insert the procedural needle using an in-plane approach from a posterior-to-anterior direction to be adjacent to the GAN.**
5. **Aspirate to rule out intravascular injection and deposit the injectate.** Remove the needle and apply a dressing.

Tips

- Use doppler to search for and identify cervical radicular and satellite arteries near the target area to avoid.
- Identify cervical nerve roots and the brachial plexus prior to injection. Applying smaller volumes of injectate will prevent spread and leakage toward the brachial plexus, which would lead to a motor block.

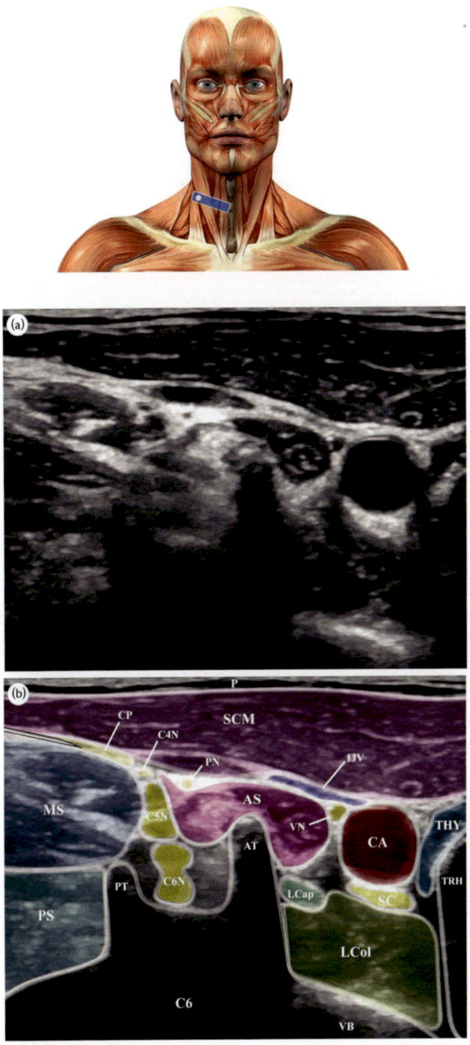

Figure 2.9.1 **a,** Ultrasound image of the anterolateral neck in an axial oblique plane at the C6 level. **b,** Labeled ultrasound image of in-plane needle placement of the cervical plexus (CP) between hyperechoic superficial layer of deep cervical fascia and above the deep layer of deep cervical fascia. *P* platysma, *SCM* sternocleidomastoid, *PN* phrenic nerve, *IJV* internal jugular vein, *MS* middle scalene, *CP* cervical plexus, *C4N* C4 nerve root, *C5N* C5 nerve root, *AS* anterior scalene, *VN* vagus nerve, *CA* carotid artery, *THY* thyroid, *TRH* trachea, *PS* posterior scalene, *C6 VB* vertebral body & *AT* anterior tubercle & *PT* posterior tubercle, *C6N* C6 nerve root, *LCap* longus capitus, *SC* location of sympathetic chain, *LCol* longus colli.

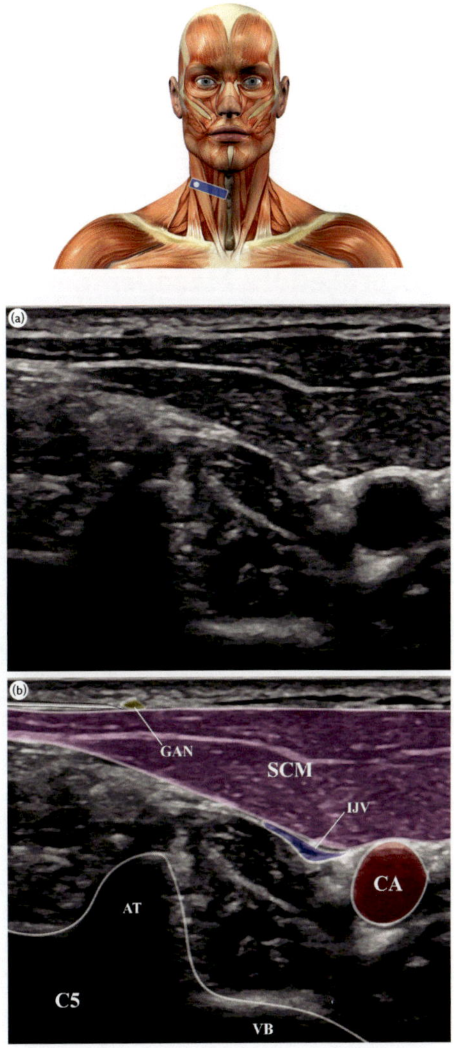

Figure 2.9.2 a, Ultrasound image of the anterolateral neck in an axial oblique plane at the C5 level. **b,** Labeled ultrasound image of in-plane needle placement of the greater auricular nerve (GAN) in short-axis. *SCM* sternocleidomastoid, *IJV* internal jugular vein, *CA* carotid artery, *C5 VB* vertebral body & *AT* anterior tubercle.

- The greater auricular nerve can be traced superiorly to observe for bifurcation into anterior and posterior divisions.
- Radiation and surgery may affect anatomy with scarring of dermal and muscular layers.

Safety Considerations

- Identify critical anatomy prior to beginning to ensure avoiding puncture of the carotid artery/internal jugular and spinal nerves.

Postprocedure Management

The cervical plexus and greater auricular nerve injections involve directing a needle in a highly vascularized and richly innervated region. Therefore, postprocedural concerns include infection, hematoma, local anesthetic systemic toxicity, and unintentional nerve involvement. Phrenic nerve involvement has been documented to occur approximately in 55% to 61% of cases with a deep cervical plexus block (not detailed in this chapter)[15,16] along with recurrent laryngeal nerve involvement.[17] Horner syndrome has been documented in superficial cervical plexus block[18] as a rare and self-limiting condition.

References

1. Ho B, De Paoli M. Use of ultrasound-guided superficial cervical plexus block for pain management in the emergency department. J Emerg Med. 2018;55(1):87–95.
2. Day M, Justiz R. Chapter 73—Head and neck block. In: Essentials of Pain Medicine (Third Edition). Editors: Benzon H, Raja S, Liu S, Fishman S, Cohen S, Hurley R, Narouze S, Malik K, Candido K. W.B. Saunders Ltd. 2011. 539–551.
3. Ginsberg L, Eicher S. Great auricular nerve: anatomy and imaging in a case of perineural tumor spread. Am J Neuroradiol. 2000;21(3):568–571.
4. Younghoon J, Saeyoung K. Treatment of great auricular neuralgia with real-time ultrasound-guided great auricular nerve block. Medicine. 2017;96(12):6325.
5. Orduña Valls J, Soto E, Ferrandis Martínez M, Nebreda C, Tornero Tornero C. Cervical plexus as anatomical target for the treatment of postoperative cervical neuropathic pain. J Pain Res. 2019;12:1217–1221.
6. Cesmebasi A. Chapter 31—Anatomy of the cervical plexus and its branches. In: Nerves and Nerve Injuries. Editors: Tubbs R, Rizk E, Shoja M, Loukas M, Barbaro N, Spinner R. Academic Press. 2015. 441–449.
7. Jankovic D., Peng P. Deep (and superficial) cervical plexus. In: Regional Nerve Blocks in Anesthesia and Pain Therapy. Springer. 2015. 211–222.
8. Kim J, Ko J, Bang S, Kim H, Lee S. Cervical plexus block. Korean J Anesthesiol. 2018;71(4):274–288.
9. Pandit J, Satya-Krishna R, Gration P. Superficial or deep cervical plexus block for carotid endarterectomy: a systematic review of complications. BJA. 2007; 99(2):159–169.
10. Peuker E, Filler T. The nerve supply of the human auricle. Clin Anat. 2002;15:35–37.
11. Thallaj A, Marhofer P, Moriggl B. Great auricular nerve blockade using high resolution ultrasound: a volunteer study. Anaesthesia. 2010;65(8):836–840.
12. Robinson J, Anderson E. Chapter 1—Skin structure and surgical anatomy. In: Surgery of the Skin. Editors: Robinson J, Sengelmann R, Hanke C, Siegel D. Mosby. 2014. 3–23.
13. Garner D, Kortz M, Baker S. Anatomy, head and neck, carotid sheath. In: StatPearls [Internet]. StatPearls Publishing; 2021.
14. Johnson E, Vekris M, Demesticha T, Soucacos P. Neuroanatomy of the brachial plexus: normal and variant anatomy of its formation. Surg Radiol Anat. 2010;32(3):291–297.

15. Emery G, Handley G, Davies MJ, Mooney PH. Incidence of phrenic nerve block and hypercapnia in patients undergoing carotid endarterectomy under cervical plexus block. Anaesth Intensive Care. 1998;26(4):377–381.
16. Castresana M, Masters R, Castresana E, Stefansson S, Shaker I, Newman W. Incidence and clinical significance of hemidiaphragmatic paresis in patients undergoing carotid endarterectomy during cervical plexus block anesthesia. J Neurosurg Anesthesiol. 1994;6(1):21–23.
17. Weiss A, Isselhorst C, Gahlen J, Freudenberg S, Roth H, Hammerschmitt N, Mattinger C, Kerger H. Acute respiratory failure after deep cervical plexus block for carotid endarterectomy as a result of bilateral recurrent laryngeal nerve paralysis. Acta Anaesthesiol Scand. 2005;49(5):715–719.
18. Flores S, Riguzzi C, Herring AA, Nagdev A. Horner's syndrome after superficial cervical plexus block. *West J Emerg Med*. 2015;16(3):428–431.

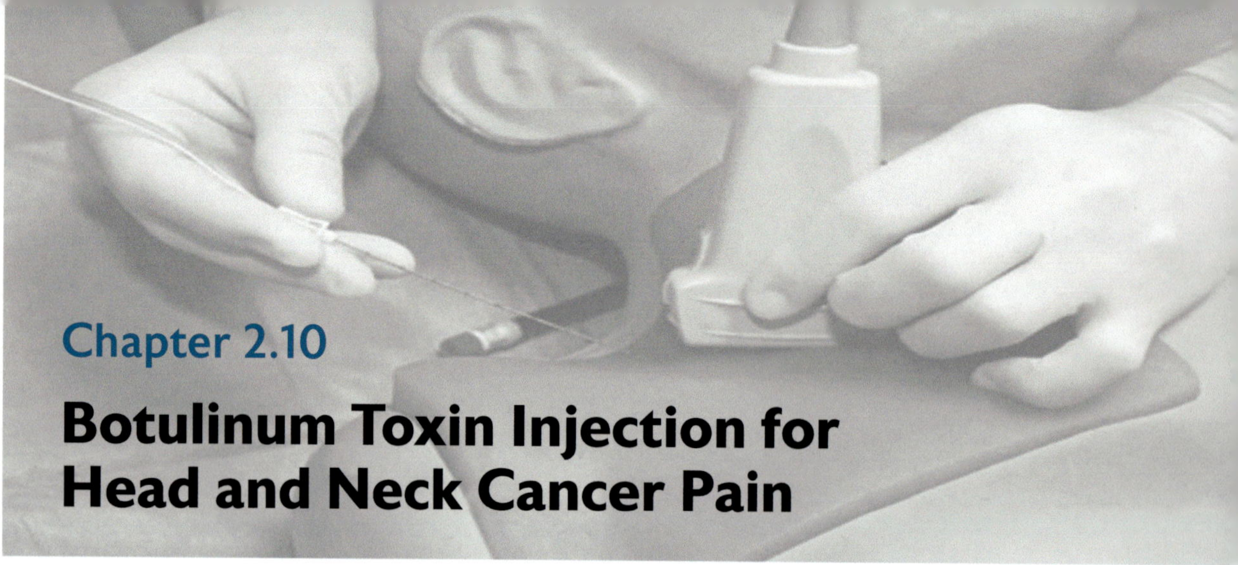

Chapter 2.10

Botulinum Toxin Injection for Head and Neck Cancer Pain

Franchesca König and A.C. Camargo

Contents

Introduction

Up to 80% of patients with head and neck cancer develop pain from the tumor itself or as a consequence of cancer treatment.[1] Both somatic and neuropathic pain after surgery or radiation can be difficult to treat, but botulinum neurotoxin (BoNT) injections have proven to be beneficial and well-tolerated interventions. Botulinum neurotoxin injections have been studied in several head and neck cancer treatment-related conditions including neuropathic and myofascial pain after neck dissections, myofascial pain after radiation therapy, and trismus (limited jaw range of motion) after radiation therapy.[2]

Botulinum neurotoxins are protein neurotoxins produced by the anaerobic bacteria *Clostridium botulinum*. There are seven distinct serotypes, alphabetically named A to G. There are two known mechanisms for analgesia: (1) Blockade of the synaptic release of acetylcholine, the principal neurotransmitter at the neuromuscular junction and (2) The inhibition of pain neurotransmitters at both the peripheral and central sensory levels (i.e., substance P and calcitonin gene–related peptide).[3] In the treatment of pain, injections may be intramuscular, intradermal, or subcutaneous. Desired effects may be first noted within 24–72 hours, peaking at approximately 2–3 weeks, and lasting up to 8–12 weeks and in some cases even longer.[4] Higher doses have been associated with a longer duration of effect.[5] Commercially available BoNT formulations in the United States include: onabotulinumtoxinA (Botox®), abobotulinumtoxinA (Dysport®), incobotulinumtoxinA (Xeomin®), and rimabotulinumtoxinB (Myobloc®/Neurobloc®).[6] Some formulations are not interchangeable, although onabotulinumtoxinA (Botox®) and incobotulinumtoxinA (Xeomin®) can be converted in 1:1 proportion. The conversion ratio of onabotulinumtoxinA (Botox®) and abobotulinumtoxinA (Dysport®) is 1:3.[7]

Indications

Botulinum neurotoxins are FDA-approved for painful conditions such as cervical dystonia, blepharospasm, spasticity, and for the prevention of chronic migraine; however, not all formulations have the same approved indications. For instance, Botox® is approved for the prevention of chronic migraine, whereas Dysport® is not. Additionally, not all formulations are approved for use in children.

Off-label indications include:

- Trismus
- Other temporomandibular joint disorders (i.e., Bruxism)
- Neuropathic conditions (i.e., incisional neuropathy, trigeminal neuralgia, postherpetic neuralgia, notalgia paresthetica)
- Other headaches (i.e., nummular headache)

Contraindications

Botulinum neurotoxins are contraindicated in patients with allergy or hypersensitivity to the toxin itself or components of the formulation, in local infection, and in pregnant and lactating females. Caution should be used in patients with motor neuron disease, neuromuscular junction disorders (e.g., myasthenia gravis and Lambert-Eaton syndrome), or amyotrophic lateral sclerosis. Relative contraindications include the use of several medications including aminoglycosides (i.e., gentamicin, polymyxin; may enhance the neuromuscular-blocking effect of BoNT), anticholinergic agents (may enhance anticholinergic effect), and anticoagulants (may result in bruising/bleeding).[4]

As with all injections, potential complications and adverse effects should be discussed with the patient prior to administration of the injection. Adverse effects are dependent on the site of injection and usually self-limited with time. These may include localized pain and bruising at the site of injection, infection, unintended temporary weakness/paralysis of nearby musculature, headache, and dry mouth (i.e., in the treatment of trismus with toxin diffusion to the parotid gland through the posterior part of the masseter). Potentially serious side effects may also occur secondary to systemic spread of the toxin, leading to severe systemic anaphylactic reactions and botulism-like symptoms (i.e., generalized muscular weakness leading to dysarthria, dysphagia, dysphonia, and respiratory distress). In the treatment of cervical dystonia, paralysis of unintended musculature can lead to dysphonia and dysphagia.[8]

Critical Anatomy

When treating muscular pain related to head and neck surgery or radiation treatments, identifying the responsible musculature is essential for proper treatment. Most commonly, treatment is guided by clinical examination, including palpation of individual muscles and observing specific patterns.[9] Ultrasound, electromyography, and electrical stimulation may be used to appropriately identify symptomatic muscles.[10] Occasionally, local anesthetic blockade of specific muscular targets may identify a painful target for the toxin treatment.

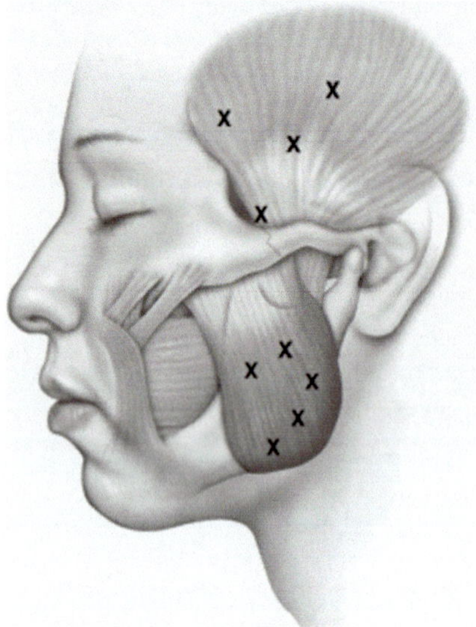

Figure 2.10.1 Diagram of needle placement for injection of botulinum toxin to the temporalis and masseter musculature. (Thambar S, Kulkarni S, Armstrong S, Nikolarakos D. Botulinum toxin in the management of temporomandibular disorders: a systematic review. Br J Oral Maxillofac Surg. 2020;58(5):508–519.)

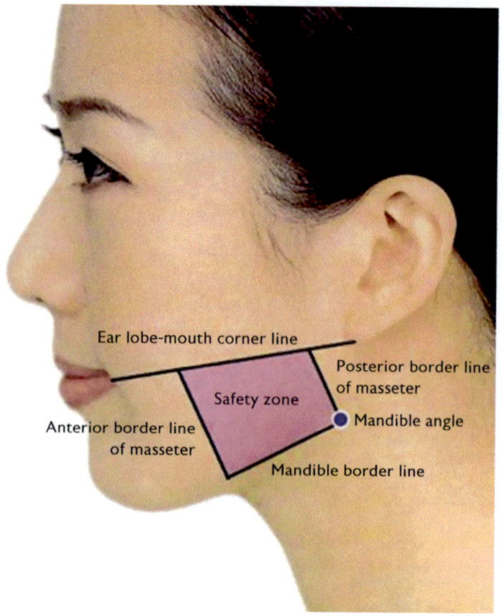

Figure 2.10.2 Masseter injection "safety zone" (Lee EI, et al. Botulinum toxin type A for treatment of masseter hypertrophy: volumetric analysis of masseter muscle reduction over time. Arch Aesthetic Plast Surg. 2016;22(2):79–86.)

Botulinum neurotoxin injections are helpful for trismus related to radiation effects and cervical dystonia after surgery and/or radiation. When treating trismus, the masseter and temporalis muscles are most commonly targeted (Figure 2.10.1).[11] The recommended safety zone for injection to the masseter is a rectangular shape with the upper border running from the oral commissure to the tragus of the ear, the lower border running along the mandibular angle, and the anterior and posterior borders running along the anterior and posterior margins of the masseter muscle (Figure 2.10.2).[12] Ultrasound may be used to visualize the masseter musculature and to ensure avoidance of the parotid gland (Figure 2.10.3).[13] Using electromyography, the lateral pterygoid may also be injected, either intra- or extra-orally (Figure 2.10.4).[14]

Electromyography and ultrasound may also be implemented for BoNT injections to the neck musculature for cervical dystonia or other neck muscular pain syndromes after head and neck surgery and radiation. The sternocleidomastoid and trapezius musculature are commonly targeted in these cases.[15] Again, knowledge of the anatomical landmarks is key. For clinically guided injections, activation of the sternocleidomastoid muscle is helpful to ensure avoidance of the external carotid artery. Other targeted muscles for cervical dystonia include splenius capitis, splenius cervicis, semispinalis capitis, longissimus, levator scapulae, and the scalene complex. Ultrasound with doppler may be used to identify vascular structures (Figure 2.10.5).[13] Ultrasound guidance can additionally be useful when injecting the trapezius musculature to reduce the possibility of pneumothorax (Figure 2.10.6).[16]

Lastly, distributing the total dose intended for each individual muscle between 1 to 4 injection areas is recommended. Multipoint injections may increase treatment effectiveness in regard to reducing pain, increasing range of motion, and lengthening the duration of the effect.[17]

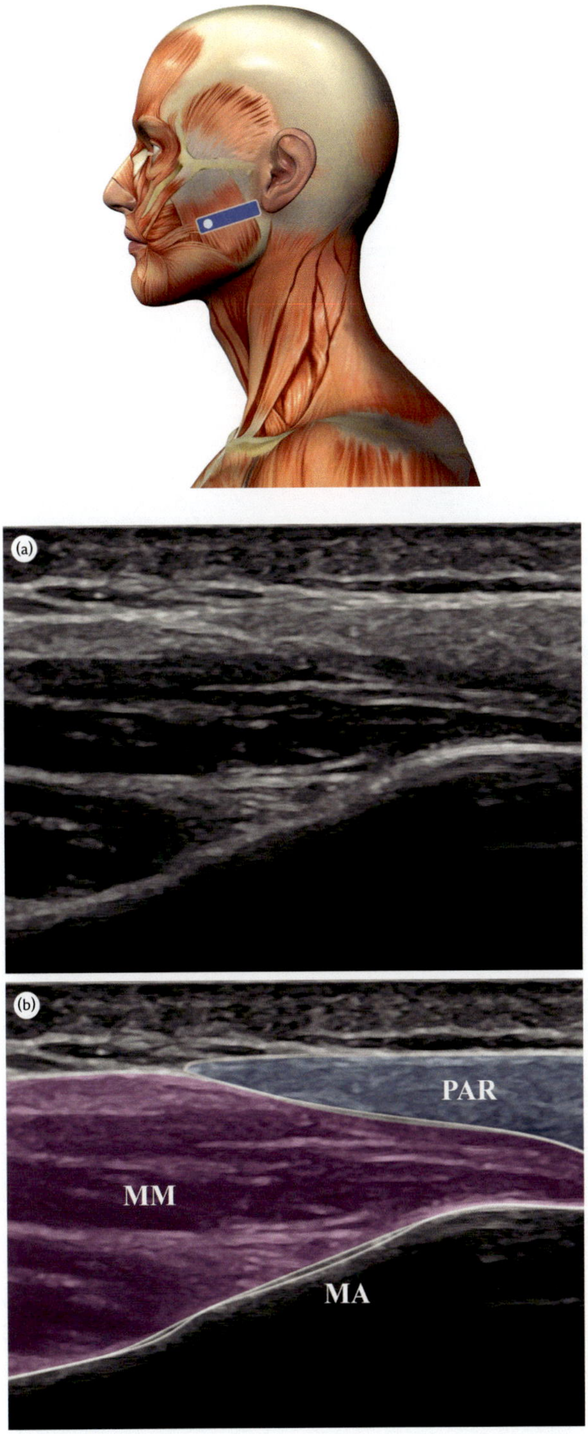

Figure 2.10.3 a, Unlabeled and **b,** labeled ultrasound image of the lateral face in axial oblique plane of the masseter muscle in short-axis. *MM* masseter muscle, *MA* maxilla, *PAR* parotid gland.

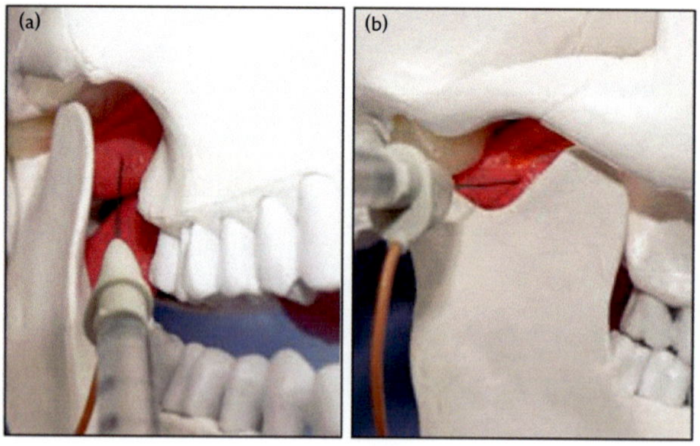

Figure 2.10.4 The intra-oral (A) and extra-oral (B) approaches for lateral pterygoid muscle injection. (Yoshida K. Botulinum neurotoxin injection for the treatment of recurrent temporomandibular joint dislocation with and without neurogenic muscular hyperactivity. Toxins (Basel). 2018;10(5):174.)

Equipment and Patient Preparation

1. Monitors and Sterility
   a. No specific monitors are needed for this procedure, but emergency resuscitation equipment should be available immediately. This includes ACLS drugs, supplemental oxygen, airway adjuncts, and suction.
   b. Strict antiseptic technique should be observed including sterile probe cover, ultrasound gel, and sterile gloves. Chlorhexidine or other skin prep agent should be used to clean the skin prior to commencing the procedure.
2. Equipment
   a. Guidance:[10]
      i. Anatomical (no additional equipment is required)
      ii. Ultrasound machine (with high-frequency linear array transducer [8–12 MHz])
      iii. Electromyography machine (with monopolar needle electrode)
      iv. Electrical stimulation machine (with monopolar needle)
   b. Needles type:
      i. Neck musculature: 25- to 30-gauge, 1.5-inch needle
      ii. Facial musculature: 30-gauge, 0.5- to 1.0-inch needle
   c. Botulinum toxin diluted in saline:
      i. 2 mL normal saline (0.9% sodium chloride injection) per 100-unit vial of onabotulinumtoxinA (Botox®) or incobotulinumtoxinA (Xeomin®)—resulting in concentrations of 5 units per 0.1 mL (total 50 units per 1 mL)
      ii. 1.5 mL normal saline (0.9% sodium chloride injection) per 300-unit vial of abobotulinumtoxinA (Dysport®)—resulting in concentrations of 20 units per 0.1 mL (total 200 units per 1 mL)
3. Position
   a. Supine or sitting, depending on target musculature and patient preference

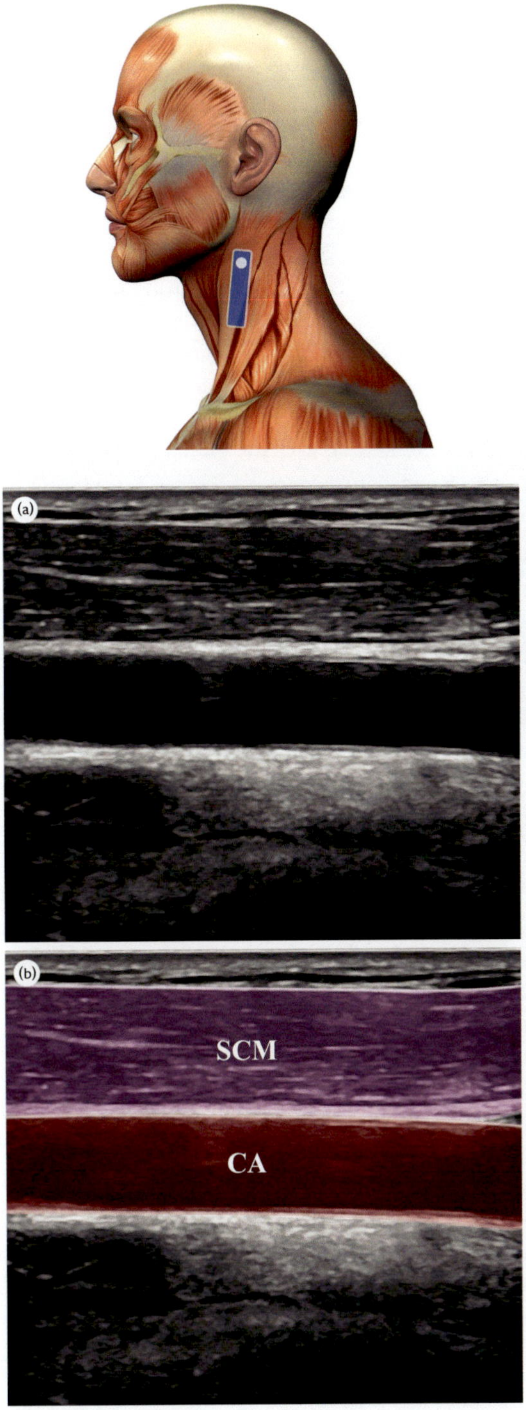

Figure 2.10.5 **a,** Unlabeled and **b,** labeled ultrasound image of the
lateral neck in a coronal plane. *SCM* sternocleidomastoid, *CA* common carotid artery.

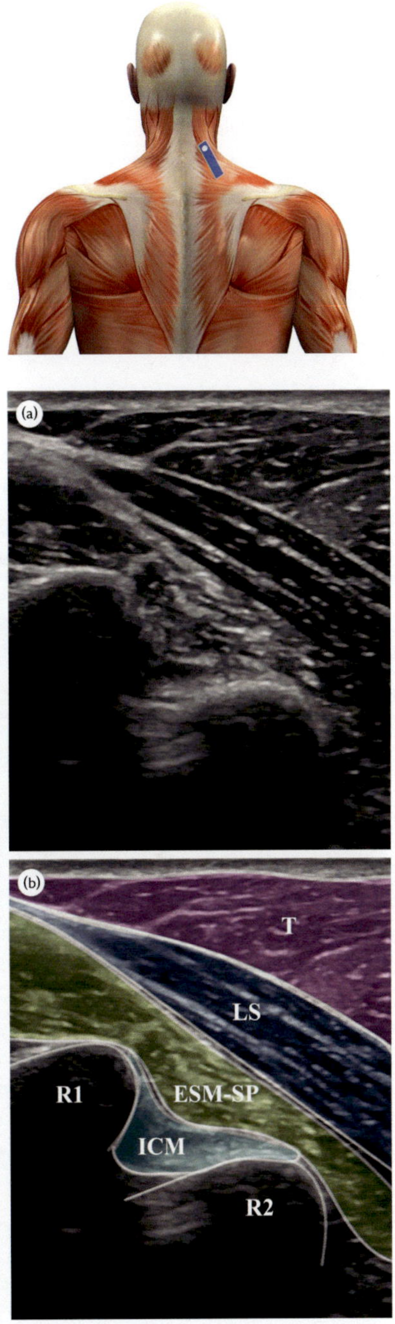

Figure 2.10.6 **a,** Unlabeled and **b,** labeled ultrasound image of the posterior neck in a sagittal oblique plane at the level of the 1st and 2nd ribs. *T* trapezius, *LS* levator scapulae, *ESM-SP* erector spinae serratus posterior muscle complex, *R1* 1st rib, *ICM* intercostal muscles, *R2* 2nd rib.

Procedure Technique

1. **Reconstitute the botulinum toxin, position the patient, prep the area with an antiseptic solution, and localize the target musculature**.
   a. For anatomical guidance of masseter musculature, identify the masseter safety zone, ask the patient to activate the masseter by "clenching the jaw," and palpate to feel for activation.
   b. The temporalis is similarly activated and palpated using the same techniques as with the masseter muscle.
   c. For anatomical guidance of the sternocleidomastoid muscle, ask the patient to rotate the head to the contralateral side and palpate musculature. Palpate for the carotid artery to ensure avoidance.
   d. For trapezius activation, ask patient to retract their scapula.
   e. For other muscles of cervical dystonia, ultrasound or electromyography is recommended to determine the appropriate muscles.
2. **Insert the needle perpendicularly** into the desired muscle**, aspirate, and inject the desired amount.** Normal dosage per muscle (specifically for onabotulinumtoxinA [Botox®]) is as follows:[18]
   a. Masseter—50 to 60 units (divided by 4 sites)
   b. Temporalis—20 units (divided by 4 sites)
   c. Sternocleidomastoid—15 to 100 units (divided by 3–4 sites)
   d. Trapezius—20 to 100 units (divided by 3 sites)
   e. Splenius Capitis—15 to 100 units
   f. Splenius Cervicis—20 to 60 units
   g. Scalene Complex—15 to 50 units
   h. Semispinalis Capitis—30 to 100 units
   i. Longissimus—30 to 100 units
   j. Levator Scapulae—20 to 100 units

Safety Considerations

- Ensure knowledge of important anatomic structures for each target, such as the carotid artery in the anterior neck, and the vertebral artery, nerve roots and cervical foramen in the lateral neck.
- Be aware that pneumothoraces may occur following injection of the trapezius musculature. Signs and symptoms of a pneumothorax may include dyspnea on exertion, tachypnea, chest pain, and decreased breath sounds on auscultation of the affected area.

Postprocedure Management

Normal postprocedure monitoring is advised after BoNT injections. Transient orthostatic hypotension may occur in some cases, for which lying in supine position for several minutes is usually sufficient for patient recovery. The patient should be advised that localized pain and bruising may occur at the site of injection and unintended temporary weakness/paralysis of nearby musculature may occur. Xerostomia may occur if the parotid gland is affected during injection of the masseter. Respiratory distress after injection of trapezius musculature should prompt evaluation for pneumothorax. More serious side effects, such as dysphagia, may occur with injections to anterior neck musculature. Dysphagia is typically self-limiting and resolves in about 2 weeks but may require speech-language pathology referral, diet changes, or even nasogastric tube insertion based on symptom severity. Neck weakness may occur with higher dosages, resulting in dropped head syndrome and instability. The responsible muscle should be identified, and dosage and injection technique revised in future injections. In very rare cases, patients may develop botulism with onset in the first days to week after injection. Symptoms include dysphagia, fatigue, headache, bilateral blepharoptosis, blurred vision, and even respiratory failure.[19] Most cases are mild, although some may require hospital admission for botulinum antitoxin serum, nasogastric tube, and respiratory support. After injection in-person follow up within 6–8 weeks is recommended to determine effectiveness and planning for potential repeat injection.

References

1. Bossi P, Giusti R, Tarsitano A, Airoldi M, De Sanctis V, Caspiani O, Alterio D, Tartaro T, Alfieri S, Siano M. The point of pain in head and neck cancer. Crit Rev Oncol Hematol. 2019;138:51–59. doi: 10.1016/j.critrevonc.2019.04.001. Epub 2019 Apr 5. PMID: 31092385.
2. Stubblefield MD, Levine A, Custodio CM, Fitzpatrick T. The role of botulinum toxin type A in the radiation fibrosis syndrome: a preliminary report. Arch Phys Med Rehabil. 2008;89(3):417–421. doi: 10.1016/j.apmr.2007.11.022. PMID: 18295617.
3. Mittal SO, Jabbari B. Botulinum neurotoxins and cancer: a review of the literature. Toxins (Basel). 2020;12(1):32. doi:10.3390/toxins12010032. PMID: 31948115; PMCID: PMC7020400.
4. Nigam PK, Nigam A. Botulinum toxin. Indian J Dermatol. 2010;55(1):8–14. doi: 10.4103/0019-5154.60343. PMID: 20418969; PMCID: PMC2856357.
5. Marsh WA, Monroe DM, Brin MF, Gallagher CJ. Systematic review and meta-analysis of the duration of clinical effect of onabotulinumtoxinA in cervical dystonia. BMC Neurol. 2014;14:91. doi: 10.1186/1471-2377-14-91. PMID: 24767576; PMCID: PMC4013807.
6. Dressler D. Botulinum toxin drugs: brief history and outlook. J Neural Transm (Vienna). 2016;123(3):277–279.
7. Scaglione F. Conversion ratio between Botox®, Dysport®, and Xeomin® in clinical practice. Toxins (Basel). 2016;8(3):65.
8. Witmanowski H, Błochowiak K. The whole truth about botulinum toxin: a review. Postepy Dermatol Alergol. 2020;37(6):853–861. doi:10.5114/ada.2019.82795
9. Jost WH, Tatu L. Selection of muscles for botulinum toxin injections in cervical dystonia. Mov Disord Clin Pract. 2015;2(3):224–226.
10. Walker HW, Lee MY, Bahroo LB, Hedera P, Charles D. Botulinum toxin injection techniques for the management of adult spasticity. PM R. 2015;7(4):417–427. doi: 10.1016/j.pmrj.2014.09.021. Epub 2014 Oct 8. PMID: 25305369.
11. Thambar S, Kulkarni S, Armstrong S, Nikolarakos D. Botulinum toxin in the management of temporomandibular disorders: a systematic review. Br J Oral Maxillofac Surg. 2020;58(5):508–519.
12. Lee EI, et al. Botulinum toxin type A for treatment of masseter hypertrophy: volumetric analysis of masseter muscle reduction over time. Arch Aesthetic Plast Surg. 2016;22(2):79–86. doi.org/10.14730/aaps.2016.22.2.79
13. Jecker P. Ultrasound anatomy of the head and the neck. In: Welkoborsky H., Jecker P. (eds.), Ultrasonography of the Head and Neck. Springer, Cham (Switzerland); 2019: 30–40. https://doi.org/10.1007/978-3-030-12641-4_3
14. Yoshida K. Botulinum neurotoxin injection for the treatment of recurrent temporomandibular joint dislocation with and without neurogenic muscular hyperactivity. Toxins (Basel). 2018;10(5):174. doi: 10.3390/toxins10050174. PMID: 29693593; PMCID: PMC5983230.
15. Stathakios J, Carron MA. Anatomy, head and neck, posterior cervical region. [Updated 2020 Jul 31]. In: StatPearls [Internet]. Treasure Island (FL): StatPearls Publishing; 2021.
16. Chu H. et al. Change of safe needling depth at acupoint GB21 according to posture and breathing. Evidence-Based Complementary and Alternative Medicine; 2018: 2308102.

17. Tyślerowicz M, Kiedrzyńska W, Adamkiewicz B, Jost WH, Sławek J. Cervical dystonia: improving the effectiveness of botulinum toxin therapy. Neurol Neurochir Pol. 2020;54(3):232–242. doi: 10.5603/PJNNS.a2020.0021. Epub 2020 Apr 14. PMID: 32285434.
18. Allergan. BOTOX® Prescribing Information, February 2021.
19. Bai L, Peng X, Liu Y, Sun Y, Wang X, Wang X, et al. Clinical analysis of 86 botulism cases caused by cosmetic injection of botulinum toxin (BoNT). Medicine (Baltimore). 2018;97(34):e10659.

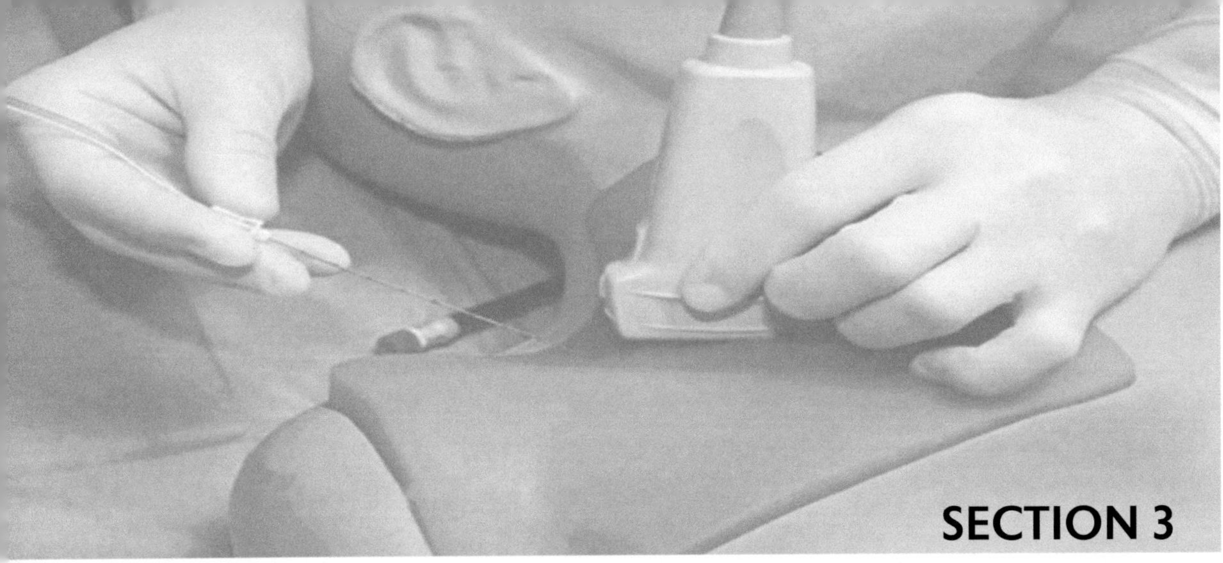

SECTION 3

BREAST AND CHEST WALL SECTION

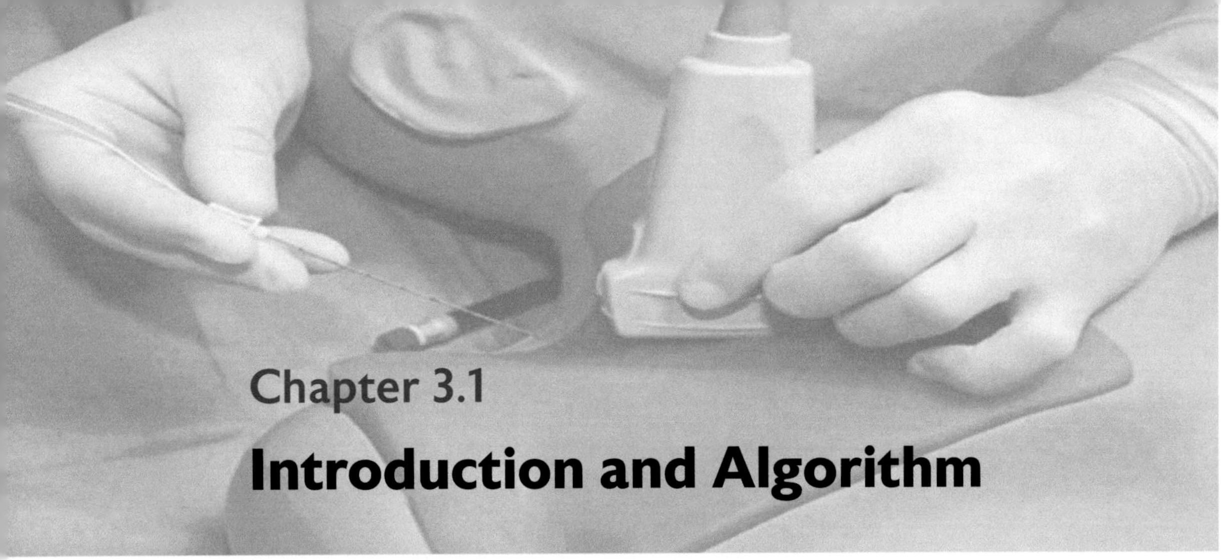

Chapter 3.1

Introduction and Algorithm

Amitabh Gulati

Contents

Introduction

Breast and lung cancers constitute a large proportion of total cancer deaths in the United States. The 5-year survival rate for breast cancer is 89.1% compared to lung cancer, which is 19.6%.[1] However, both cancers present with pain syndromes that are related to direct tumor involvement or due to treatment- (surgery, chemotherapy, or radiation) associated complications.

Breast Cancer Pain

The cutaneous innervation of the breast arises from the anterior and lateral branches of intercostal nerves T1–T6.[2] The lateral cutaneous branch arises at the midaxillary line (MAL) and splits into anterior and posterior branches. These branches innervate the skin of the lateral thoracic wall from the scapular line to midclavicular line. The anterior cutaneous branch of the intercostal nerve arises at the parasternal line and supplies the anterior portion of the thoracic wall.[3] A specific band-like dermatomal distribution of the skin is innervated by each intercostal nerve, which is critical in helping delineate the anatomic distribution of pain and determine the appropriate interventional treatment approach. The intercostobrachial nerve, a lateral branch of the second intercostal nerve, does not divide into anterior and posterior portions. Instead, it and the medial brachial cutaneous nerve provide sensation to the superior medial aspect of the arm and axilla.[4] Cutaneous innervation

Table 3.1.1 Breast Cancer Pain Syndromes Classified by Anatomical Location

Chest	Shoulder	Arm
Myofascial pain	Adhesive capsulitis	Lymphedema
Costochondritis	Subacromial bursitis	Neuropathy
Tumor-related pain	Scapulothoracic bursitis	Intercostobrachial neuralgia
Postmastectomy pain	Contractures	Complex regional pain syndrome
Radiation-induced fibrosis	Brachial plexopathy	Axillary web syndrome
Contractures	Rotator cuff tendinopathy	
HRT myalgias		
Persistent post-op pain		
Cervical radiculopathy		
Phantom breast pain		
Radiation dermatitis		
Fibromyalgia		

of the superior aspect of the chest and shoulders is also supplied by the supraclavicular nerves that originate from C3 and C4.

The medial pectoral, lateral pectoral, and long thoracic nerves are associated with anterior chest wall and breast pain.[2,3] The medial pectoral nerve branches from the medial cord of the brachial plexus and is derived from ventral rami of C8–T1 to innervate both the pectoralis minor muscle and part of the pectoralis major muscle. The lateral pectoral nerve branches from the lateral cord of the brachial plexus and is derived from the ventral rami of C5–C7 to innervate the pectoralis major muscle. The long thoracic nerve is also derived from the ventral rami of C5–C7 and traverses the anterolateral aspect of the first rib into the axilla to innervate the serratus anterior muscle.

Common breast cancer–associated pain syndromes can be classified in various ways including temporal (acute, subacute, chronic), organ system (neurologic, musculoskeletal, lymphatic, and cutaneous), or anatomic location (chest, shoulder, and arm).[5] Presented below is an anatomic location classification (Table 3.1.1).

Thoracic Cancer Pain

Cancer-related pain may originate from tumors invading the lungs, heart, esophagus, central neuraxis, brachial plexus, peripheral nerves, bony structures, and lymph nodes.[6] Cancer pain syndromes due to underlying thoracic neoplasms can be highly variable, but the most involved anatomic regions include the chest wall and spine. Metastatic disease is frequently encountered in the thoracic cavity and is most associated with lung, colon, prostate, and breast cancer.[7]

Branches of the intercostal nerves innervate the thoracic wall and parietal pleura. The intercostal nerves originate from the anterior primary rami of T1 to T12 and then emerge through the intervertebral foramen to enter the paravertebral space.[3] After traversing the paravertebral space, the thoracic spinal nerve roots divide into anterior and posterior branches. The intercostal nerves arise from the anterior branches and give off four main branches: gray rami communicans that interface with the sympathetic chain, a posterior cutaneous branch, a lateral cutaneous branch, and an anterior cutaneous branch.[8] The lateral cutaneous branch of each intercostal nerve is given off near the anterior axillary line and supplies most of the sensation to the chest wall. Each intercostal nerve terminates as an anterior cutaneous branch which supplies the anterior chest wall near midline. Muscular sub-branches supply the intercostal muscles, while pleural sensory and peritoneal sensory branches (from T7 to T11 primarily) innervate the parietal pleura and parietal peritoneum.

Table 3.1.2 Thoracic Cancer Pain Syndromes

Visceral Pain Syndromes	Lung cancer associated pleural pain Cardiac tumor-related chest pain
Nociceptive Pain Syndromes	Chest wall pain Pancoast tumor SVC obstruction Bony metastatic disease Paraneoplastic pain Skull base disease
Neuropathic Pain Syndromes	Intercostal neuralgia Brachial plexopathy Suprascapular entrapment Spinal cord compression
Treatment-Related Pain Syndromes	Radiation-associated pain Postsurgical pain Chemotherapy-associated pain

The intercostal nerves are overall responsible for supplying sensation from the skin, parietal pleura, intercostal spaces, and chest wall musculature including the intercostal and serratus posterior muscles.[9]

Thoracic neoplasm-associated pain syndromes can also be classified by various schema. These include etiology (direct tumor invasion or treatment related), pain characteristics (visceral, nociceptive, or neuropathic), and anatomic (chest wall with intrinsic pathology, chest wall with arm symptoms, and chest wall with spine disease) (Table 3.1.2).

Treatment Algorithm

Recent literature published provides an algorithmic approach to interventional treatment for thoracic and breast cancer patients.[10–13] Chest pain algorithms initially divide patients based on the anatomic cause of pain: lung and pleural pathology, Pancoast tumor, and spine disease. Each etiology can be further subdivided into distinct anatomic regions of the chest, which dictates which interventional strategies can be trialed. Similarly, breast pain can be approached based on the initial distribution of pain (Figure 3.1.1). Progressing from peripheral nerve and fascial plane blocks, neurolytic blocks and neuromodulation therapies can be employed depending on the therapeutic response.

Interventional Treatment Contraindications

Refusal for the procedure, infection at the needle entry site, severe coagulopathy, bleeding diathesis, and empyema should be considered absolute contraindications to chest wall pain interventions. Relative contraindications include thrombocytopenia, anticoagulation, immunocompromised status, distorted anatomy, prior nerve injury, local anesthetic allergy, implanted pacemaker, and inability to consent to the procedure (Table 3.1.3). Extra caution must be taken in patients with kyphoscoliosis, as chest wall deformity may predispose them to thecal or pleural puncture. Other patients who require extra caution are those in whom pneumothorax may be life-threatening: patients with a single lung on the procedural side, on mechanical positive pressure ventilation, or with neuromuscular disease. Additionally, patients who underwent thoracotomy may have obliteration of the paravertebral space by scar tissue and adhesions of the lung to the chest wall, predisposing patients to pleural or

Table 3.1.3 **Contraindications to Breast and Chest Wall Injections**

Contraindications	Related Types
Absolute	Refusal for the procedure Localized or systemic infection Severe coagulopathy Substantial bleeding diathesis Empyema
Relative	Thrombocytopenia Anticoagulation Immunocompromised patients Distorted anatomy Prior nerve injury or damage Allergy to anesthetics Implanted pacemaker Allodynia Inability to consent the procedure
Extra Caution	Kyphoscoliosis Single lung on the side of procedure Mechanically ventilated with positive pressure ventilation Postsurgical/Prior thoracotomy Neuromuscular disease in the area

pulmonary puncture. Notably, paravertebral blocks can be used in patients undergoing pleurectomy if the parietal pleura over the paravertebral space that is medial to the angle of the rib is intact.

Conclusions

The diverse pain syndromes that breast and lung cancer patients suffer with necessitate a comprehensive pain-management strategy that employs pharmacologic and interventional strategies. As outlined, an anatomic approach to interventional treatment allows for algorithmic but individualized treatment plans for patients.

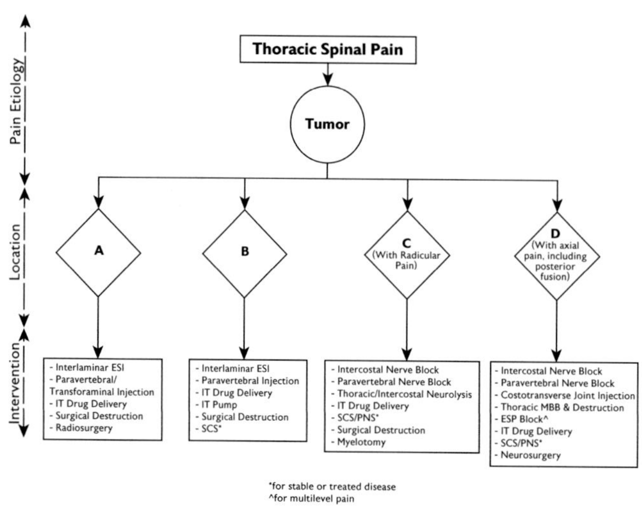

Figure 3.1.1 Interventional algorithm for breast and chest wall pain. a, Chest wall pain due to lung pathology. b, Chest wall pain due to a Pancoast tumor. c, Chest wall pain due to neuraxial metastases. d, Chest wall pain due to neuropathic pain.

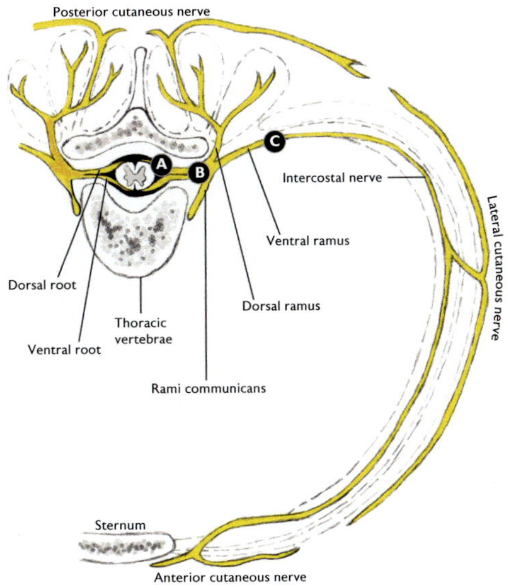

Figure 3.1.2 a, Interventional algorithm for thoracic spine pain based on location of the tumor represented by (A) - (C). b, Illustration representing tumor location of intraspinal (A), foraminal (B), and intercostal.

References

1. U.S. Cancer Statistics Working Group. U.S. Cancer Statistics Data Visualizations Tool, based on 2019 submission data (1999–2017): U.S. Department of Health and Human Services, Centers for Disease Control and Prevention and National Cancer Institute; www.cdc.gov/cancer/dataviz, released in June 2020.
2. Moore KL et al. Clinically Oriented Anatomy. Lippincott Williams & Wilkins; 2013.
3. Agur AMR et al. Grant's Atlas of Anatomy. Lippincott Williams & Wilkins; 2013.
4. Henry BM et al. Origin, branching, and communications of the intercostobrachial nerve: a meta-analysis with implications for mastectomy and axillary lymph node dissection in breast cancer. Cureus. 2017;9(3):e1101.
5. Valimahomed A, et al. Chapter 9: Breast cancer pain: a review of pathology and interventional techniques. Gulati A, et al. (eds.), Essentials of Interventional Cancer Pain Management. 1st ed. Springer Nature Switzerland; 2019: 63–84.
6. Mercadante S et al. Pain in patients with lung cancer: pathophysiology and treatment. Lung Cancer. 2010;68(1):10–15.
7. Teunissen SCCM et al. Symptom prevalence in patients with incurable cancer: a systematic review. J Pain Symptom Manage. 2007;34(1):94–104.
8. Waldman SD. Atlas of Interventional Pain Management. 3rd ed. Saunders/Elsevier; 2009.
9. Snell RS. Clinical Anatomy by Regions. Lippincott Williams & Wilkins; 2012.
10. Gulati A, et al. A retrospective review and treatment paradigm of interventional therapies for patients suffering from intractable thoracic chest wall pain in the oncologic population. Pain Med. 2015;16(4):802–810.
11. Rispoli L, et al. Interventional pain treatments in the management of oncologic patients with thoracic spinal tumor–related pain: a case series. Pain Pract. 2019;19(8):866–874.
12. Piracha MM, et al. A tale of two planes: deep versus superficial serratus plane block for postmastectomy pain syndrome. Reg Anesth Pain Med. 2017;42(2):259–262.
13. Zocca JA, et al. Ultrasound-guided serratus plane block for treatment of postmastectomy pain syndromes in breast cancer patients: a case series. Pain Pract. 2017;17(1):141–146.

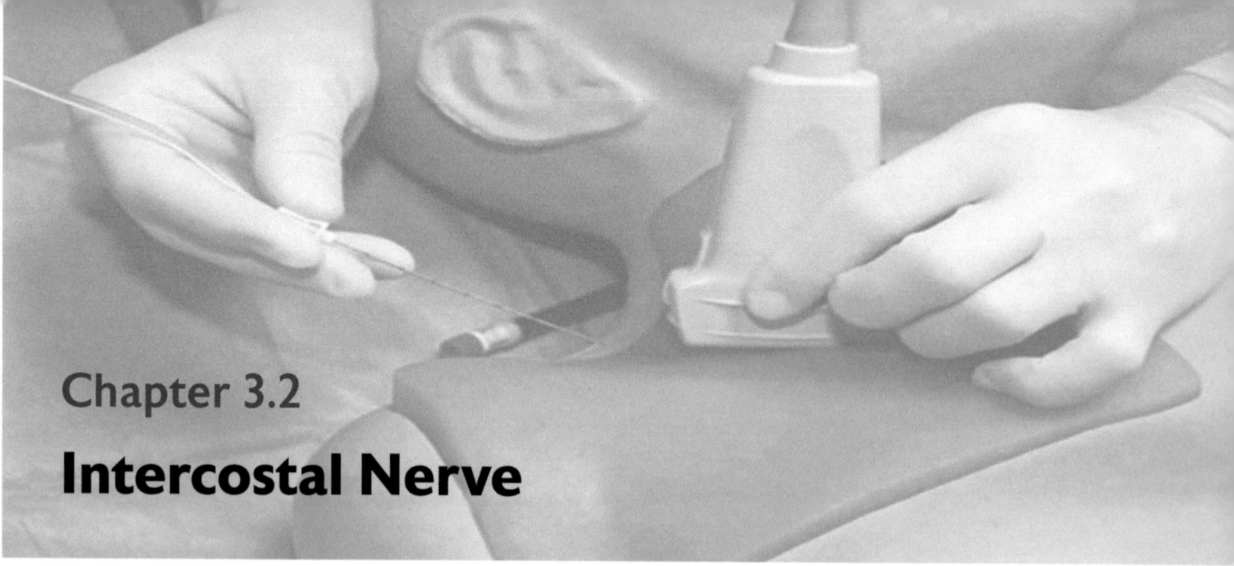

Chapter 3.2
Intercostal Nerve

Ehtesham Baig

Contents

Introduction

The intercostal nerves supply sensation to the skin and muscles of the chest and abdominal wall.[1] These nerves can serve as a target for blockade for a variety of acute and chronic oncologic pain conditions involving the thorax and upper abdomen. Advantages of intercostal nerve block include ease of procedure, decreased use of opioids and reduced associated side effects, and an improvement in respiratory function in the perioperative period.[2]

Indications

Intercostal nerve blocks can relieve pain originating from conditions including pathologic rib fractures, rib and pleural tumors, dislocation of costochondral joint, acute herpes zoster and postherpetic neuralgia, perioperative pain (thoracotomy, mastectomy, sternotomy, abdominal surgery), idiopathic and postoperative intercostal neuropathic pain (post-thoracotomy pain), and somatic pain from in-dwelling catheters (chest tubes, gastrectomy and nephrostomy tubes).[3-7]

Critical Anatomy

The thoracic spinal nerves (T1–T12) give rise to the intercostal nerves. Once the respective spinal nerves have passed through the intervertebral foramina, they divide into the ventral and dorsal rami (Figure 3.2.1). The dorsal rami course posteriorly and innervate the skin and muscles in the paravertebral region. The ventral rami of T1–T11 form the intercostal nerves entering the intercostal spaces; and the ventral ramus of T12 forms the subcostal nerve that is located inferior to the corresponding 12th rib. Of note, T1–12 are usually collectively referred to as the intercostal nerves. The intercostal nerves are mixed sensory-motor nerves composed of dorsal horn sensory fibers, ventral horn motor efferent fibers, and postganglionic sympathetic fibers.

Upon exiting from the spine, each intercostal nerve runs between the pleura and posterior intercostal membrane. The nerve eventually pierces the membrane to lie between the internal intercostal and innermost intercostal muscles. Within this space, the nerve runs with its associated artery and vein just inferior to the rib. As the intercostal nerve moves anteriorly, the lateral cutaneous branch splits off and piercesthrough the external intercostal muscle posteriorly to the midaxillary line. The lateral branch innervates the skin of the chest. Further anteriorly at the level of the midaxillary line, the intercostal nerve piercesthrough the internal and external intercostal muscles to terminate as the anterior cutaneous branch.[8]

Equipment and Patient Preparation

1. Monitors and Sterility

a. No specific monitors are needed for this procedure, but emergency resuscitation equipment should be available immediately. This includes ACLS drugs, supplemental oxygen, airway adjuncts, and suction.

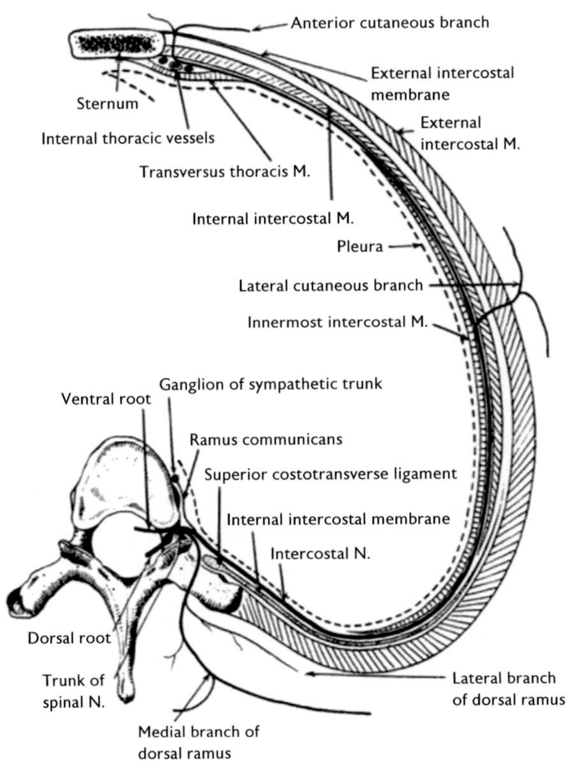

Figure 3.2.1 A diagram of the upper thoracic spinal nerve illustrating the ventral/dorsal rami and intercostal nerve. (Reprinted with permission from Cunningham's Manual of Practical Anatomy: Thorax and Abdomen, 16th Edition)

   b. Strict antiseptic technique should be observed including sterile probe cover, ultrasound gel, and sterile gloves. Chlorhexidine or other skin prep agent should be used to clean the skin prior to commencing the procedure.

2. **Equipment**
   a. Probe: High-frequency linear array transducer (8–12 MHz)
   b. Needle type: 22- or 25-gauge, 1.5- to 2-inch needle (ideally short bevel or blunt tip needle for safety)
   c. Local anesthetic (1–2 mL per site): Lidocaine 1%–2%; ropivacaine 0.2%–0.5%; bupivacaine 0.25%–0.5%
   d. Adjuvant (0.5 mL per site): Particulate or nonparticulate steroid

3. **Position**
   a. Prone (preferred) or sitting

Step-by-Step Technique

Intercostal Block—Sagittal Approach

1. **Prepare equipment and supplies, position the patient prone, and sterilize the procedural area with antiseptic solution.**
2. **Identify the correct rib level by counting caudally from the 1st rib or cephalad from the 12th rib.** Take note that patients may have anatomic variations in their number of ribs.
3. **Place the ultrasound probe in a parasagittal position to visualize the rib in short axis.** The optimal view will clearly see the rib, intercostal muscles, and pleura (Figure 3.2.2).
4. **Visualize the target for intercostal nerve block.** Moving the cephalad portion of the ultrasound probe laterally may improve visualization due to the angulation of the ribs. The target is below the inferior portion of the rib and deep to the internal intercostal muscle.
5. **Inject local anesthetic subcutaneously for analgesia at the procedural site.** With an in-plane approach, deposit the injectate at the location of the intercostal nerve.
6. **Repeat the procedure at various levels as required.**

Intercostal Block—Transverse Approach

1. **Prepare equipment and supplies, position the patient prone, and sterilize the procedural area with antiseptic solution.**
2. **Identify the correct rib level by counting caudally from the 1st rib or cephalad from the 12th rib.** Take note that patients may have anatomic variations in their number of ribs.
3. **Rotate the ultrasound probe to a transverse position to visualize the rib in long axis (Figure 3.2.3).** The rib will appear as a hyperechoic bone with an osseous shadow.
4. **Visualize the target for intercostal nerve block (Figure 3.2.4**). Move the ultrasound probe caudally to visualize the external, internal, and innermost internal intercostal muscles overlying the pleura. The target plane lies between the internal and innermost intercostal muscles.
5. **Inject local anesthetic subcutaneously for analgesia at the procedural site.** With an in-plane approach, deposit the injectate at the location of the intercostal nerve.
6. **Repeat the procedure at various levels as required.**

Tips

- A shallow approach toward the inferior border of the corresponding rib is preferred.
- Correct placement is confirmed when the injectate is seen to push the innermost intercostal muscle and pleura away from the injected solution.

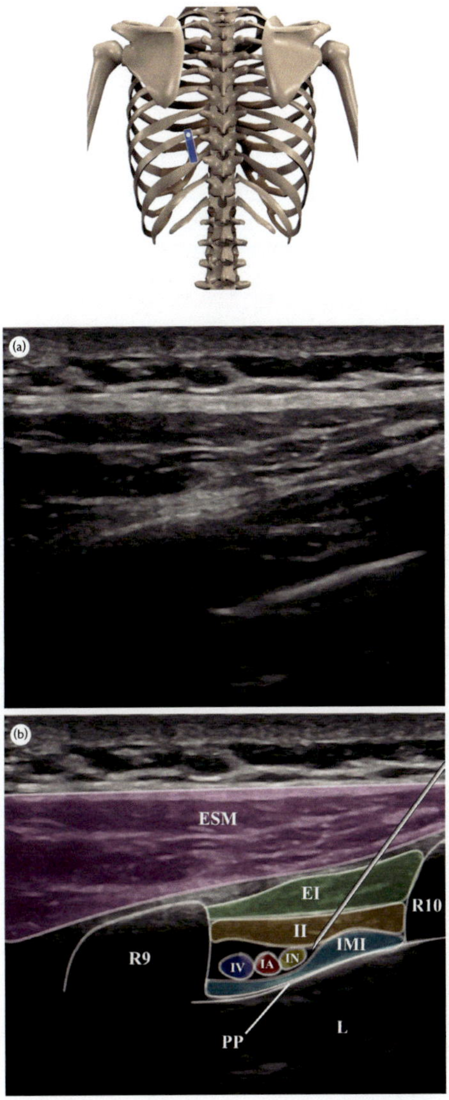

Figure 3.2.2 a, Ultrasound image of the posterior thoracic spine at T9–10 level in a sagittal plane. **b,** Labeled ultrasound image of in-plane needle placement for a T9 intercostal nerve block in short-axis. *ESM* erector spinae muscle, *R9* 9th rib, *EI* external intercostal muscle, *II* internal intercostal muscle, *IV* intercostal vein, *IA* intercostal artery, *IN* intercostal nerve, *IMI* innermost intercostal muscle, *R10* 10th rib, *PP* parietal pleura, *L* lung.

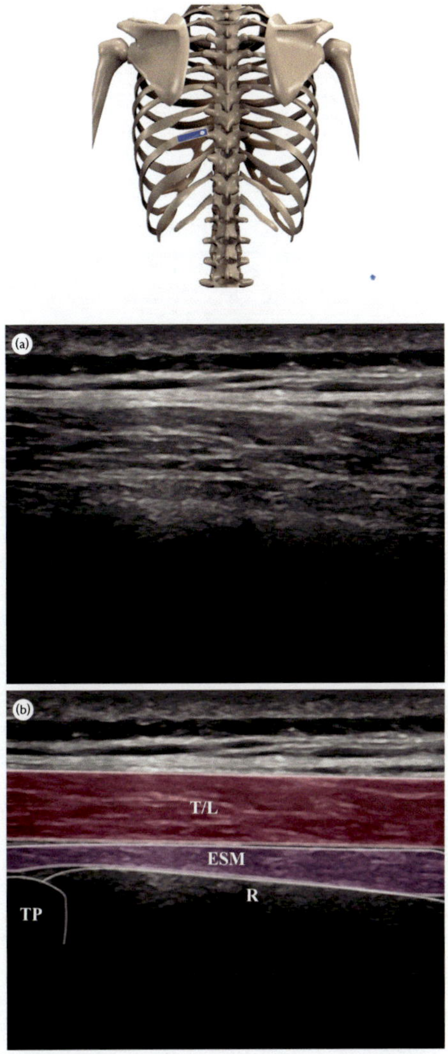

Figure 3.2.3 a, Unlabeled and **b,** Labeled ultrasound image of the posterior thoracic spine at T9 level showing the transverse process and rib articulation. *T/L* trapezius & latissimus muscles, *ESM* erector spinae muscles, *TP* transverse process, *R* rib.

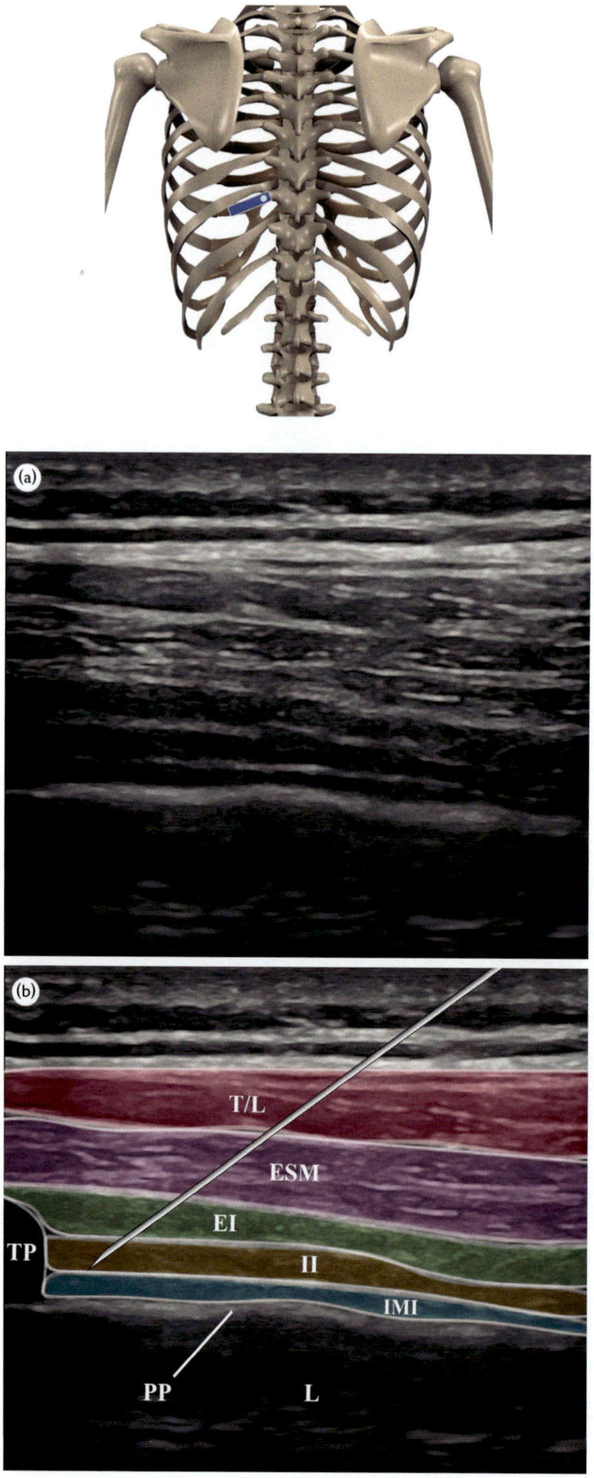

Figure 3.2.4 a, Ultrasound image of the posterior thoracic spine at T9 level in an axial oblique plane. **b,** Labeled ultrasound image of in-plane needle placement for a T9 intercostal nerve block in long-axis. *T/L* trapezius & latissimus muscles, *ESM* erector spinae muscle, *TP* transverse process, *EI* external intercostal muscle, *II* internal intercostal muscle, *IMI* innermost intercostal muscle, *PP* parietal pleura, *L* lung.

Safety Considerations

- A steep and ventral approach beyond the rib border may result in lung tissue penetration and pneumothorax.
- Avoid leaving the needle open to air to decrease the risk of pneumothorax.

Postprocedure Management

Although the risk of developing pneumothorax is low after intercostal block, any difficulty in breathing after the procedure should be evaluated by obtaining a bedside chest X-ray. Supplemental oxygen should be made available to the patient and if required, a chest tube can be inserted if pneumothorax is suspected.

Further Reading

- Bhatia A, Peng PWP. Chapter 25: Ultrasound-guided peripheral nerve blockade in chronic pain management. In: Narouze SN, ed., Atlas of Ultrasound-Guided Procedures in Interventional Pain Management. Springer Science and Business Media; 2011:243–254.
- Cousins MJ, Carr DB, Horlocker TT, Bridenbaugh PO. Intercostal, intrapleural, and peripheral blockade of the thorax and abdomen. In: Harmon DC, Shorten GD, eds., Cousins and Bridenbaugh's Neural Blockade in Clinical Anesthesia and Pain Medicine, 4th ed. Lippincott Williams and Wilkins; 2009:386–390.
- Gulati A. Chapter 57: Intercostal nerve block. In: Diwan S, Staats P, eds., Atlas of Pain Medicine Procedures. McGraw-Hill Education; 2014:400–410.
- Moore KL, Agur AMR. Essential Clinical Anatomy. Lippincott Williams & Wilkins; 2006.
- Mulroy MF, Bernards CM, McDonald SB, Salina FV. Intercostal and terminal nerve anesthesia of the trunk. In: Mulroy MF, ed., Regional Anesthesia, 4th ed. Lippincott Williams & Wilkins; 2009:137–146.

References

1. Byas-Smith MG, Gulati A. Ultrasound-guided intercostal nerve cryoablation. Anesth Analg. 2006;103:1033–1035.
2. Dowling R, Thielmeier K, Ghaly A, Barber D, Dine A. Improved pain control after cardiac surgery: results of a randomized, double-blind, clinical trial. J Thorac Cardiovasc Surg. 2003;126(5):1271–1279.
3. Moore DC, Bridenbaugh LD. Intercostal nerve block in 4333 patients: indications, technique and complications. Anesth Analg. 1962;41:1–10.
4. Karmakar MK, Ho AMH. Acute pain management of patients with multiple fractured ribs. J Trauma. 2003;54:612–615.
5. Kopacz DJ, Thompson GE. Intercostal blocks for thoracic and abdominal surgery. Tech Reg Anesth Pain Manag. 1998;2:25–29.
6. Shanti CM, Carlin AM, Tyburski JG. Incidence of pneumothorax from intercostal nerve block for analgesia in rib fractures. J Trauma. 2001;51:536–539.
7. Cohen SP, Sireci A, Wu CL, Larkin TM, Williams KA, Hurley RW. Pulsed radiofrequency of the dorsal root ganglia is superior to pharmacotherapy or pulsed radiofrequency of the intercostal nerves in the treatment of chronic postsurgical thoracic pain. Pain Physician. 2006;9:227–235.
8. Bhatia A, Gofeld M, Ganapathy S, Hanlon J, Johnson M. Comparison of anatomic landmarks and ultrasound guidance for intercostal nerve injections in cadavers. Reg Anesth Pain Med. 2013;38:503–507.

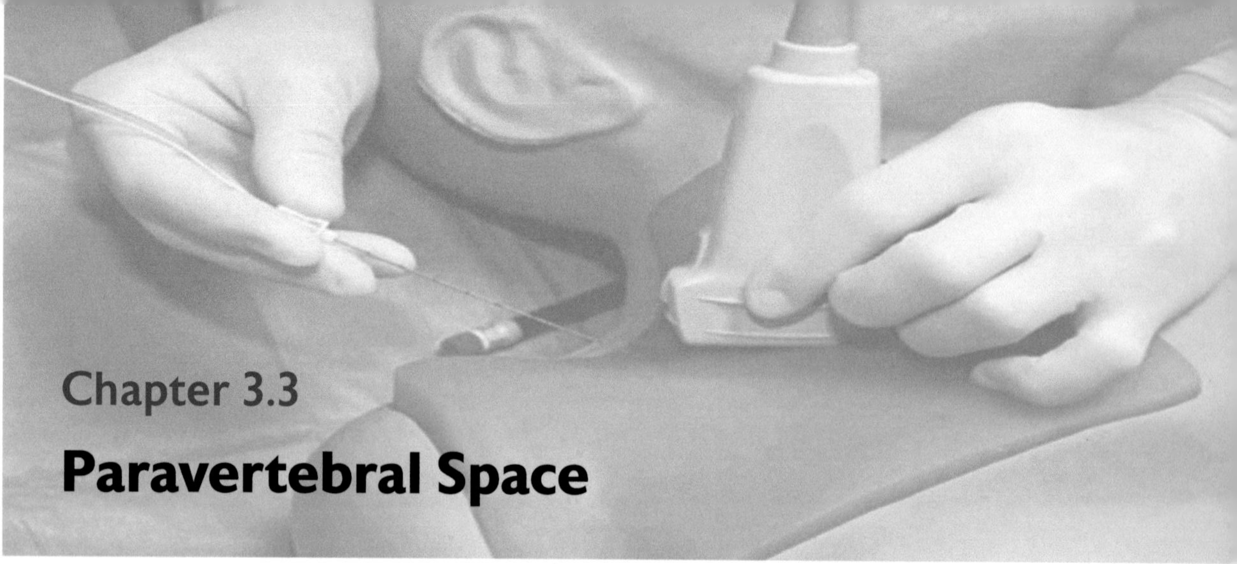

Chapter 3.3

Paravertebral Space

Daniel Chun-suk Oh

Contents

Introduction

Thoracic paravertebral blocks (TPVBs) target the spinal nerves as they emerge from the intervertebral foramina within the paravertebral space. A single injection can provide ipsilateral, segmental, somatic and sympathetic nerve blockade of 3 to 6 dermatomes, which has been useful for regional anesthesia.[1] Paravertebral block is particularly useful to treat acute and chronic unilateral chest wall and spine pain. Indications include, but are not limited to, perioperative pain control for breast and chest wall surgery, benign and malignant neuralgia, rib fractures, tumor pain of the spine and ribs, and postherpetic neuralgia.[1–4] Additional indications include treatment-associated pain syndromes such as postmastectomy or post-thoracotomy pain. Bilateral use of TPVB has also been described, particularly in the setting of bilateral breast and thoracic surgeries.[4–6] Paravertebral blocks confer similar pain relief compared to epidural blocks while resulting in fewer side effects.[7]

Critical Anatomy

The thoracic paravertebral space is a wedge-shaped space that lies on either side of the vertebral column and is wider on the left than the right.[8] The boundaries are (Figure 3.3.1):

- Medial: vertebrae, intervertebral foramina
- Lateral: parietal pleura

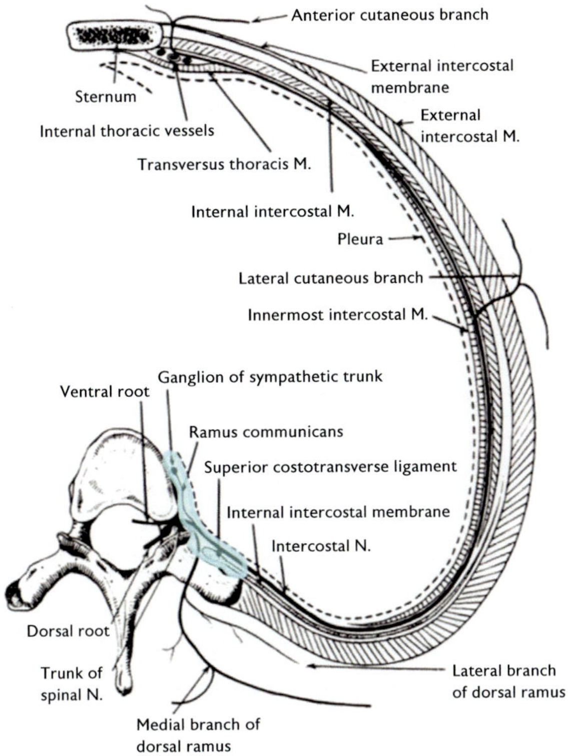

Figure 3.3.1 A diagram of the upper thoracic spinal nerve illustrating the paravertebral space in light blue. (Adapted with permission from Cunningham's Manual of Practical Anatomy: Thorax and Abdomen, 16th Edition)

- Anterior: parietal pleura
- Posterior: superior costotransverse ligament
- Superior: inferior portion of rib
- Inferior: lateral portion of the transverse process and superior portion of rib

The spinal root emerges from the intervertebral foramen and divides into the dorsal and ventral rami. The sympathetic chain is just anterior to the intercostal nerve and connects via the rami communicantes. Notably, the paravertebral space spans the vertebral column and across the heads and necks of the ribs. The endothoracic fascia which lies between the parietal pleura and the superior costotransverse ligament divides the space into the anterior and posterior compartments. The nerves are located in this posterior compartment.[2]

The paravertebral space is continuous with the intercostal space laterally, the epidural space medially, and the contralateral paravertebral space through the paravertebral and epidural space.

Clinical Applications

Paravertebral blocks result in unilateral, segmental, somatic, and sympathetic nerve blockade. They effectively treat acute and chronic unilateral pain from the spine and chest wall. Thoracic paravertebral blocks are indicated for perioperative regional blockade of the thorax and for treating thoracic pain from chronic pain syndromes. These include postmastectomy pain syndrome, post-thoracotomy pain syndrome, postherpetic neuralgia, benign and malignant neuralgias, rib fractures, tumor pain of the spine and ribs, and visceral pain from the lungs or liver capsule.

Equipment and Patient Preparation

1. **Monitors and Sterility**
   a. No specific monitors are needed for this procedure, but emergency resuscitation equipment should be available immediately. This includes ACLS drugs, supplemental oxygen, airway adjuncts, and suction.
   b. Strict antiseptic technique should be observed including sterile probe cover, ultrasound gel, and sterile gloves. Chlorhexidine or other skin prep agent should be used to clean the skin prior to commencing the procedure.
2. **Equipment**
   a. Probe: High-frequency linear array transducer (8–12 MHz)
   b. Needle type: 22- or 25-gauge, 1.5 to 2 to 2 - 3.5 inch needle
   c. Local anesthetic (2–4 mL per site): Lidocaine 1%–2%; ropivacaine 0.2%–0.5%; bupivacaine 0.25%–0.5%
   d. Adjuvant (0.5–1 mL per site): Particulate or nonparticulate steroid
3. **Position**
   a. Prone (preferred) or lateral decubitus

Procedure Technique

Paravertebral—Sagittal Approach

1. **Prepare equipment and supplies, position the patient prone, and sterilize the procedural area with antiseptic solution.**
2. **Identify the correct rib level.** Count caudally from the 1st rib or cephalad from the 12th rib. Take note that patients may have anatomic variations in their number of ribs.
3. **Place the ultrasound probe in a parasagittal orientation to visualize the desired transverse process.** Laterally, the ribs, intercostal muscles, and pleura will be observed (Figure 3.3.2). Translate medially to see the costotransverse joint (Figure 3.3.3). Further medial, the transverse process, which appears flatter and less rounded than the rib surface, will come into view (Figure 3.3.4). If the probe is too medial, the lamina will be observed (Figure 3.3.5).
4. **Inject local anesthetic subcutaneously for analgesia at the procedural site.**
5. **Insert the procedural needle with an in-plane approach from a caudad-to-cephalad direction (Figure 3.3.4).** Place the needle through the erector spinae muscles and below the transverse process. There may be loss-of-resistance as the needle punctures the superior costotransverse ligament. Consider using hydrodissection during needle advancement to verify needle tip position.
6. **Inject the medication into the paravertebral space while aspirating every 2–3 mL.** Remove the needle and apply a dressing.

Paravertebral—Axial Approach

1. **Prepare equipment and supplies, position the patient prone, and sterilize the procedural area with antiseptic solution.**
2. **Identify the correct rib level.** Count caudally from the 1st rib or cephalad from the 12th rib. Take note that patients may have anatomic variations in their number of ribs.
3. **Rotate the ultrasound probe to a transverse orientation while keeping the desired rib in view.** A boney acoustic shadow will be cast deep to the ribs, obstructing visualization of the pleura.
4. **Move the ultrasound probe medially until the rib articulates with the transverse process (Figure 3.3.6**). Of note, this is the costotransverse joint.

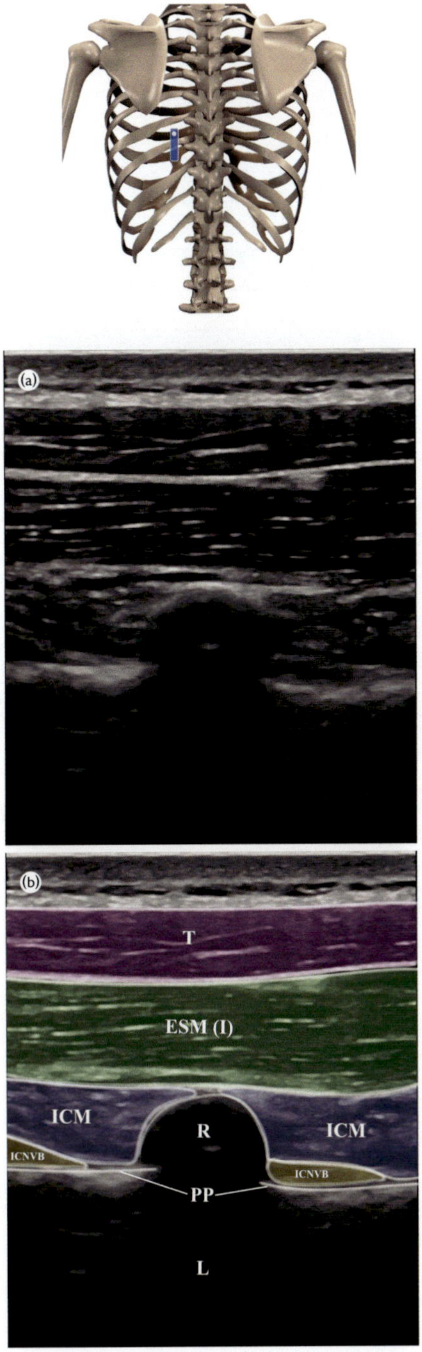

Figure 3.3.2 a, Unlabeled and **b,** labeled ultrasound image of the posterior thorax at the level of the T8 rib in a sagittal plane. *T* trapezius, *ESM (I)* erector spinae muscle—iliocostalis muscle, *ICM* intercostal muscles, *R* rib, *ICNVB* intercostal neurovascular bundle, *PP* parietal pleura, *L* lung.

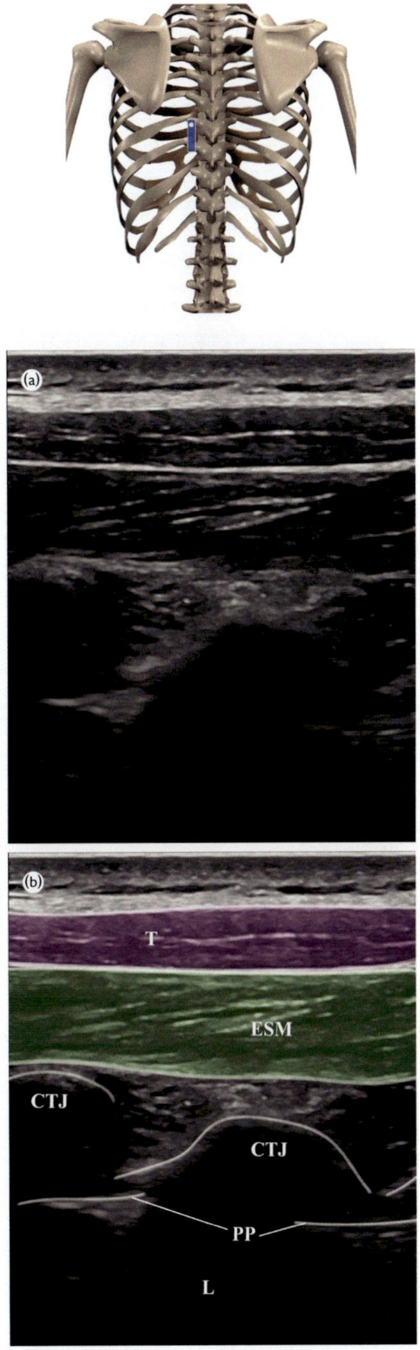

Figure 3.3.3 a, Unlabeled and **b,** labeled ultrasound image of the posterior thorax at the level of the T8–9 in a sagittal plane at the costotransverse joint. *T* trapezius, *ESM* erector spinae muscle, *CTJ* costotransverse joint, *PP* parietal pleura, *L* lung.

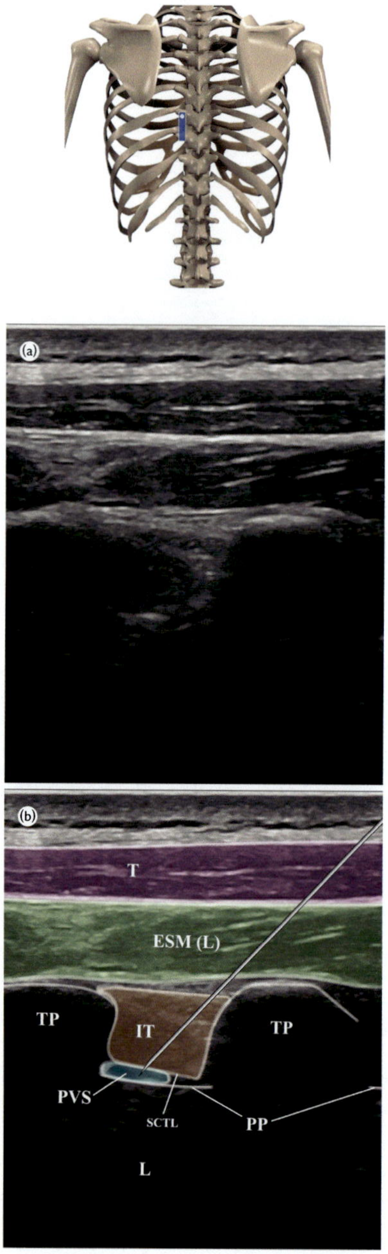

Figure 3.3.4 **a,** Ultrasound image of the posterior thorax at the level of the T8–9 in a sagittal plane. **b,** Labeled ultrasound image of in-plane needle placement for a paravertebral block at the transverse process. *T* trapezius, *ESM (L)* erector spinae muscle—longissimus muscle, *TP* transverse process, *IT* intertransverse muscles and ligaments, *SCTL* superior costotransverse ligament, *PVS* paravertebral space, *PP* parietal pleura, *L* lung.

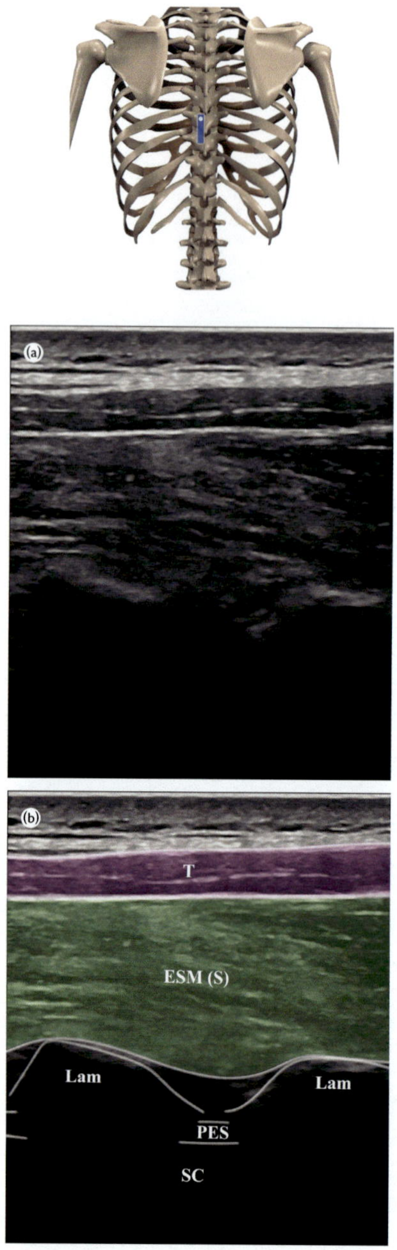

Figure 3.3.5 **a,** Unlabeled and **b,** labeled ultrasound image of the posterior thorax at the level of the T8–9 in a sagittal plane at the lamina. *T* trapezius, *ESM (S)* erector spinae muscle—spinalis muscle, *Lam* lamina, *PES* posterior epidural space, *SC* spinal cord.

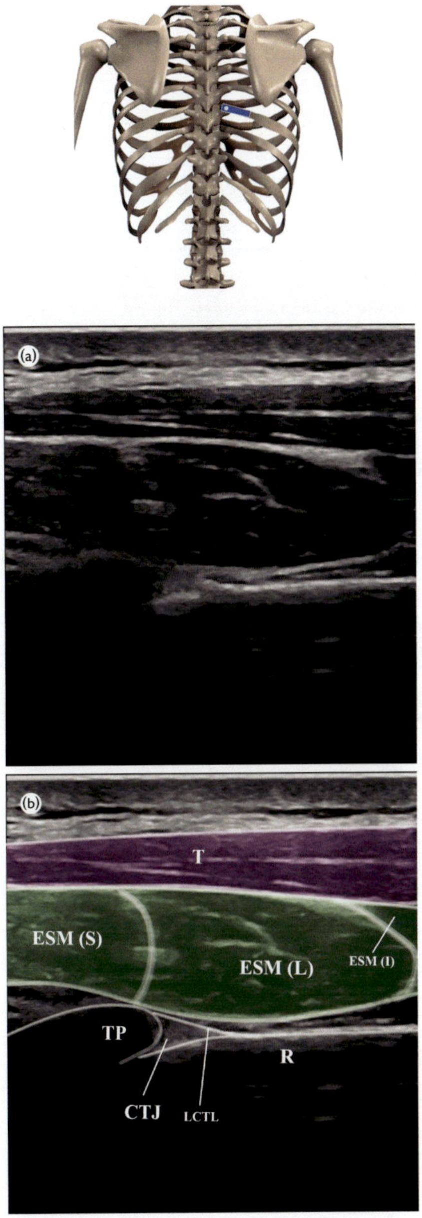

Figure 3.3.6 **a,** Unlabeled and **b,** labeled ultrasound image of the posterior thorax at the level of the T7 in an axial oblique plane showing the transverse process and rib articulation. *T* trapezius, *ESM (S)* erector spinae muscle—spinalis muscle, *ESM (L)* erector spinae muscle—longissimus muscle, *ESM (I)* erector spinae muscle—iliocostalis muscle, *TP* transverse process, *LCTL* lateral costotransverse ligament, *CTJ* costotransverse joint, *R* rib.

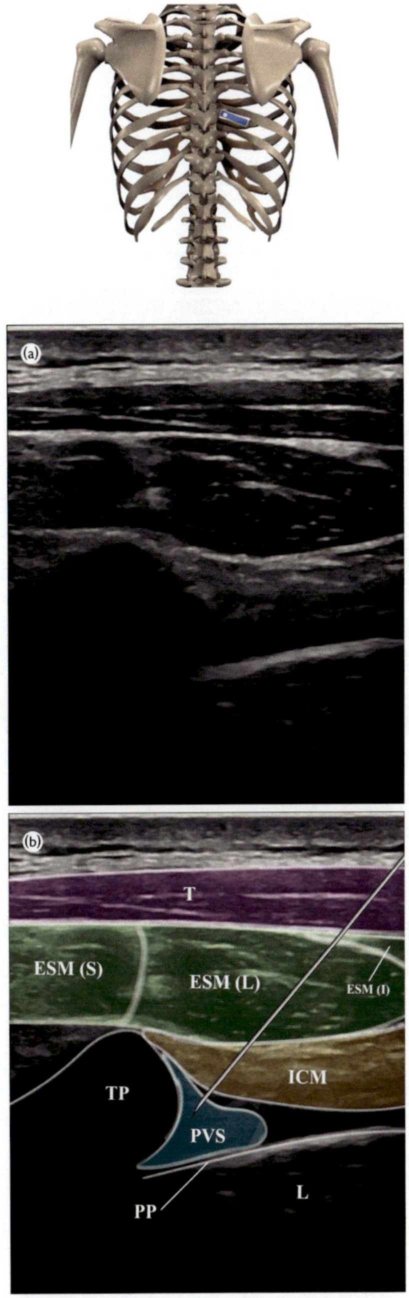

Figure 3.3.7 **a,** Ultrasound image of the posterior thorax at the level of the T7 in an axial oblique plane. **b,** Labeled ultrasound image of in-plane needle placement for a paravertebral block. *T* trapezius, *ESM (S)* erector spinae muscle—spinalis muscle, *ESM (L)* erector spinae muscle—longissimus muscle, *ESM (I)* erector spinae muscle—iliocostalis muscle, *TP* transverse process, *ICM* intercostal muscles, *PVS* paravertebral space, *PP* parietal pleura, *L* lung.

5. **Move the ultrasound probe caudally until the rib leaves the field of view.** The transverse process or lamina should still be visualized medially and the pleura should be seen laterally and inferiorly (Figure 3.3.7). The triangular paravertebral space is outlined by the boney acoustic shadow of the transverse process medially, the costotransverse ligament superiorly, and the pleura inferiorly.
6. **Inject local anesthetic subcutaneously for analgesia at the procedural site.**
7. **Insert the procedural needle with an in-plane approach from a lateral-to-medial direction (Figure 3.3.7).** Advance the needle through the erector spinae muscles and below the transverse process. There may be loss-of-resistance as the needle punctures the superior costotransverse ligament. Consider using hydrodissection during needle advancement to verify needle tip position.
8. **Inject the medication into the paravertebral space while aspirating every 2–3 mL.** The pleura should be displaced inferiorly by the injection of medication into the paravertebral space. Remove the needle and apply a dressing.

Tips

- A shallow approach toward the inferior border of the corresponding transverse process is preferred. For beginners, the needle can contact the inferolateral aspect of the transverse process. The needle is then withdrawn to be lateral to the transverse process, and redirected anteriorly to the paravertebral space.
- A lateral-to-medial approach is preferred for the axial approach to avoid lung puncture.
- Correct placement is confirmed when the injectate is seen to push the pleura away from the injected solution.

Safety Considerations

- A steep and ventral approach may result in lung tissue penetration and pneumothorax.
- Avoid leaving the needle open to air to decrease the risk of pneumothorax
- If the needle tip is advanced too medially the needle tip may injure the exiting thoracic nerve root or enter the thoracic foramen, resulting in possible epidural injection or dural puncture.

Post-Op Management Considerations

Primary concerns with TPVBs are vascular puncture, hypotension, epidural or intrathecal injection, pleural puncture, and pneumothorax.[9]Vascular puncture is more likely in bilateral blocks. Pulmonary hemorrhage has been reported in thoracic PVB in patients with previous thoracic surgery.[10]

Although the risk of developing pneumothorax is low after TPVB block, any difficulty in breathing after the procedure should be evaluated by obtaining a bedside chest X-ray. Supplemental oxygen should be made available to the patient and if required, a chest tube can be inserted if pneumothorax is suspected.

Further Reading

- Karmakar MK. Chapter 9: Ultrasound-Guided Thoracic Paravertebral Block in: Narouze S. *Atlas of Ultrasound-Guided Procedures in Interventional Pain Management*, 2nd ed. New York, NY: Springer; 2018:103–116.
- Valimahomed A, Zocca J, Gulati A. Chapter 9: Breast Cancer Pain: A Review of Pathology and Interventional Techniques in: Gulati A, Puttanniah V, Bruel BM, Rosenberg WS, Hung JC. *Essentials of Interventional Cancer Pain Management*. New York, NY: Springer; 2019:63–84.
- Krediet AC, Moayeri N, van Geffen G-J, et al. Different approaches to ultrasound-guided thoracic paravertebral block: an illustrated review. Anesthesiology. 2015;123(2):459–74.
- NYSORA. Thoracic paravertebral block. http://www.nysora.com/techniques/neuraxial-and-perineuraxial-techniques/landmark-based/3077-thoracic-paravertebral-block.html. Published May 9, 2013.

References

1. Gilbert J, Hultman J. Thoracic paravertebral block: A method of pain control. Acta Anaesthesiol Scand. 1989; 33: 142–5.
2. Tenicela R, Pollan SB. Paravertebral-peridural block technique: A unilateral thoracic block. Clin J Pain. 1990; 6: 227–34.
3. Karmakar MK. Chapter 9: Ultrasound-Guided Thoracic Paravertebral Block in: Narouze S. *Atlas of Ultrasound-Guided Procedures in Interventional Pain Management*, 2nd ed. New York, NY: Springer; 2018:103–116.
4. Klein SM, Bergh A, Steele SM, Georgiade GS, Greengrass RA. Thoracic paravertebral block for breast surgery. Anesth Analg. 2000; 90: 1402–5.
5. Coveney E, Weltz CR, Greengrass R, Iglehart JD, Leight GS, Steele SM, Lyerly HK: Use of paravertebral block anesthesia in the surgical management of breast cancer: Experience in 156 cases. Ann Surg. 1998; 227: 496–501.
6. Richardson J, Vowden P, Sabanathan S. Bilateral paravertebral analgesia for major abdominal vascular surgery: A preliminary report. Anaesthesia. 1995; 50: 995–8.
7. Biswas S, Verma R, Bhatia VK, et al. Comparison between thoracic epidural block and thoracic paravertebral block for post thoracotomy pain relief. J Clin Diagn Res. 2016; 10(9): UC08-UC12.
8. MacIntosh R, Bryce-Smith R. *Local Analgesia and Abdominal Surgery*. Edinburgh, E&S Livingstone, 1962, 26–32.
9. Naja Z, Lönnqvist PA. Somatic paravertebral nerve blockade: Incidence of failed block and complications. Anaesthesia. 2001; 56(12): 1184–1188.
10. Thomas PW, Sanders DJ, Berrisford RG. Pulmonary haemorrhage after percutaneous paravertebral block. Br J Anaesth. 1999; 83(4): 668–669.

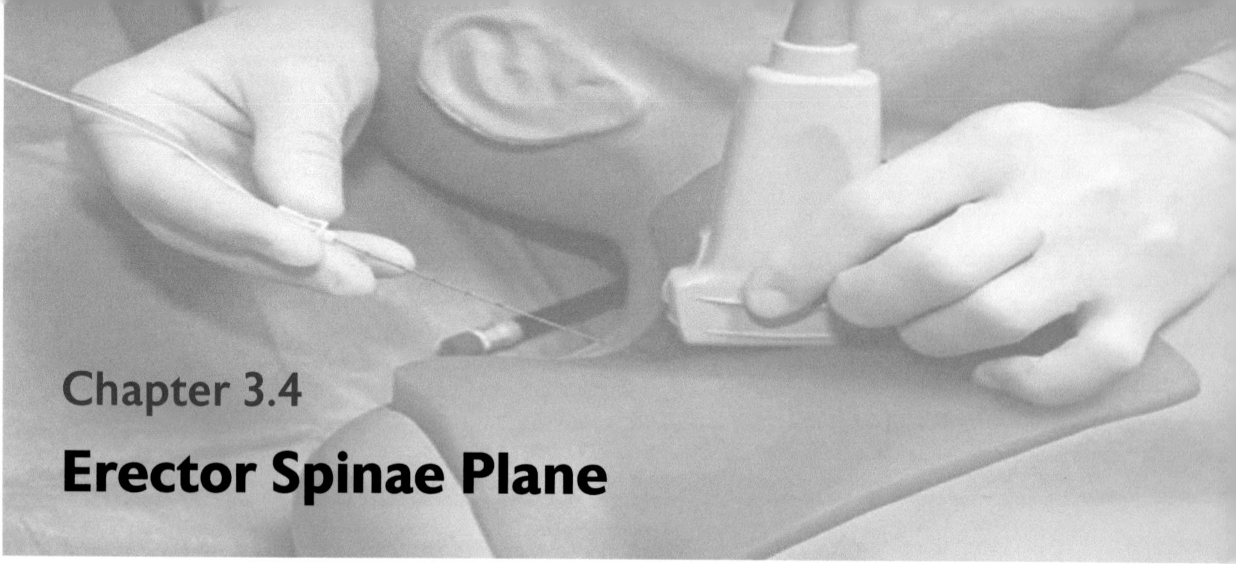

Chapter 3.4

Erector Spinae Plane

Akshat Gargya

Contents

Introduction

The thoracic erector spinae plane is a fascial plane field block and has been proven useful for acute and chronic thoracic pain syndromes. Although exact mechanism is unknown, the erector spinae plane (ESP) block is theorized to target spinal nerves similar to paravertebral block.[1–4] Additionally, the posterior thoracic elements are likely targeted in this plane.

Indications

The ESP block is a useful block to manage pain related to the chest wall. It is also used for postoperative pain management for breast, thoracic, and abdominal surgeries including video-assisted thoracotomy surgery (VATS), esophagectomy, radical mastectomy, and abdominoplasty.[5] This block can also be offered to cancer patients suffering pain from low cervical lymphadenopathy, bone metastases, and thoracic neuropathy.[6] Additionally, the block is helpful for patients with thoracic myofascial pain from surgeries, radiation therapy, tumors, or sudden weight loss.

Critical Anatomy

The spinalis, longissimus thoracis, and iliocostalis are vertically running muscles that are collectively referred to as the erector spinae muscles (Figure 3.4.1). Motor and sensory innervation to the erector spinalis muscles and the posterior wall is provided by the dorsal rami branches of the thoracolumbar nerves (Figure 3.4.2). In an ESP block, local anesthetic is deposited in the fascial plane inferior to the erector spinae muscles usually just lateral to the tip of the transverse process of the vertebra. Local anesthesia in this plane is proposed to have effect on the ventral and dorsal ramus of the spinal nerves. The ramus further divides to sensory branches and hence provide analgesia to anterolateral wall. Cadaveric studies have shown that diffusion of medication to the paravertebral space can provide both visceral and somatic analgesia.[1]

In our experience, targeting the fascial plane between the spinalis thoracis and the thoracic lamina (medial ESP block) has been effective in managing midline thoracic spinal pain. Presumably the thoracic medial branches are anesthetized during the injection. The injection is ideally performed at the lateral position where the bone of the medial transverse process and lamina connect in order to reduce the chance of epidural spread. The classic lateral ESP, along the lateral transverse process or rib, block will likely target posterior and lateral branches of the intercostal nerve and the thoracic lateral branch nerves. This approach will target posterolateral thoracic chest wall pain. Of note, at the level of T11 and T12, the planes begin to resemble the lumbar fascial planes.

Equipment and Patient Preparation

1. Monitors and Sterility

a. No specific monitors are needed for this procedure but emergency resuscitation equipment should be available immediately. This includes ACLS drugs, supplemental oxygen, airway adjuncts, and suction.

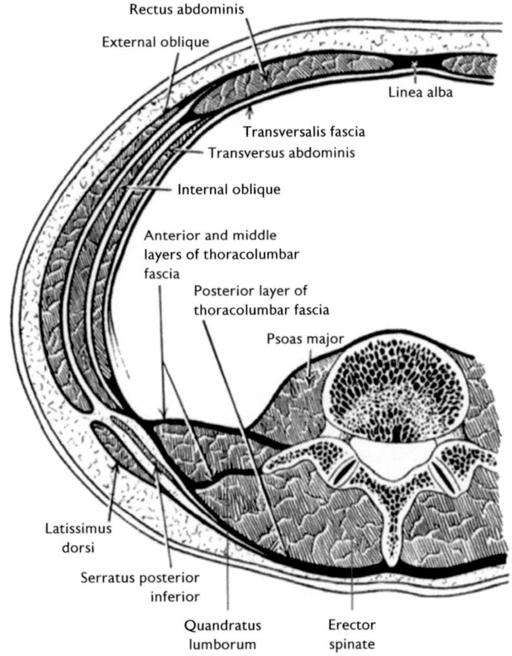

Figure 3.4.1 A horizontal section through the abdominal walls at the level of the second lumbar vertebra illustrating the locations of the erector spinae and quadratus lumborum muscles. (Reprinted with permission from Cunningham's Manual of Practical Anatomy: Thorax and Abdomen, 16th Edition)

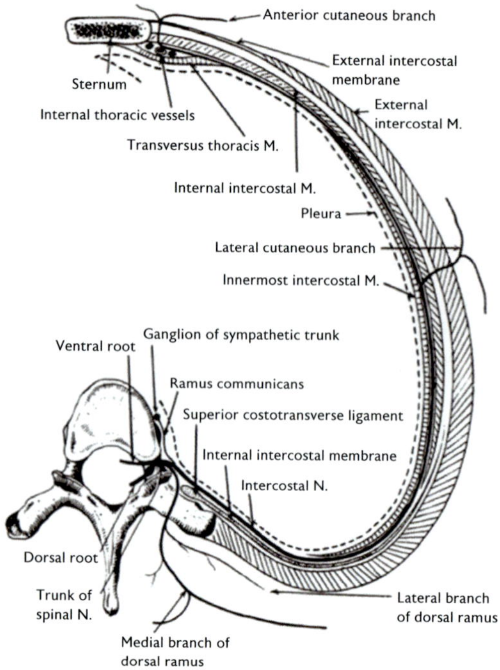

Figure 3.4.2 A diagram of the upper thoracic spinal nerve in an intercostal space. (Reprinted with permission from Cunningham's Manual of Practical Anatomy: Thorax and Abdomen, 16th Edition)

b. Strict antiseptic technique should be observed including sterile probe cover, ultrasound gel, and sterile gloves. Chlorhexidine or other skin prep agent should be used to clean the skin prior to commencing the procedure.

2. **Equipment**
   a. Probe: High-frequency linear array transducer (8–12 MHz)
   b. Needle type: 22- or 25-gauge, 1.5- to 3.5-inch needle
   c. Local anesthetic (9 mL per side): Lidocaine 1%–2%; ropivacaine 0.2%–0.5%; bupivacaine 0.25%–0.5%
   d. Adjuvant (1 mL per side): Particulate or nonparticulate steroid
3. **Position**
   a. Prone (preferred) or lateral decubitus

Procedure Technique

ESP Block—Sagittal Approach

1. **Prepare equipment and supplies, position the patient in the prone position, and clean the skin around the area of the block with antiseptic solution**
2. **Place the transducer in a sagittal orientation over the back.** Count the ribs down from the 1st rib or up from the 12th rib to identify the target level, understanding that some patients may have anatomical variations with 11 or 13 ribs. Move the ultrasound probe medially to identify the spinous process
3. **Translate laterally to identify the lamina (Figure 3.4.3)**. The probe can be further translated laterally to visualized the transverse process (Figure 3.4.4), costotransverse junction (Figure 3.4.5),

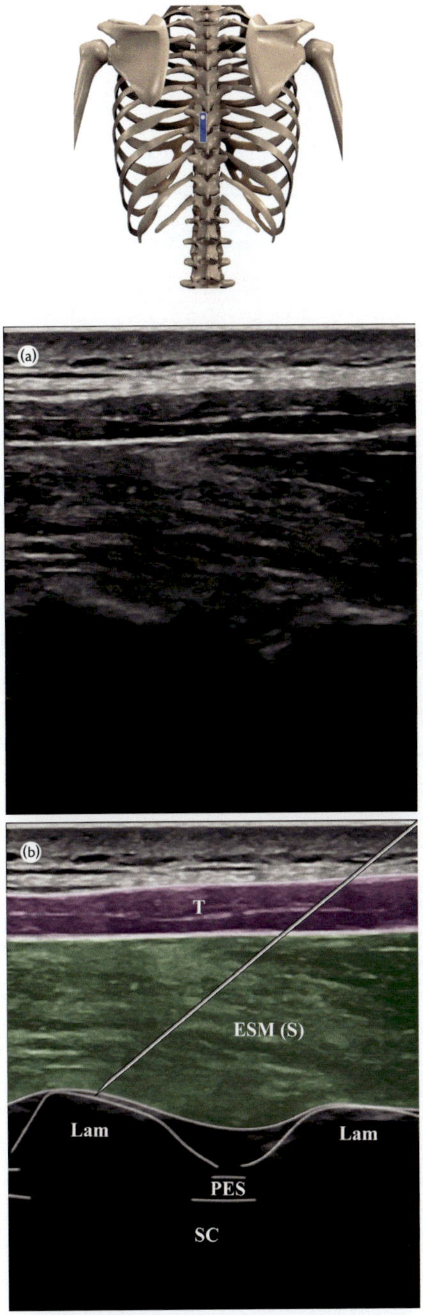

Figure 3.4.3 a, Ultrasound image of the posterior thorax at the level of the T8–9 in a sagittal plane. **b,** Labeled ultrasound image of in-plane needle placement for an erector spinae plane block at the lamina. *T* trapezius, *ESM (S)* erector spinae muscle—spinalis muscle, *Lam* lamina, *PES* posterior epidural space, *SC* spinal cord.

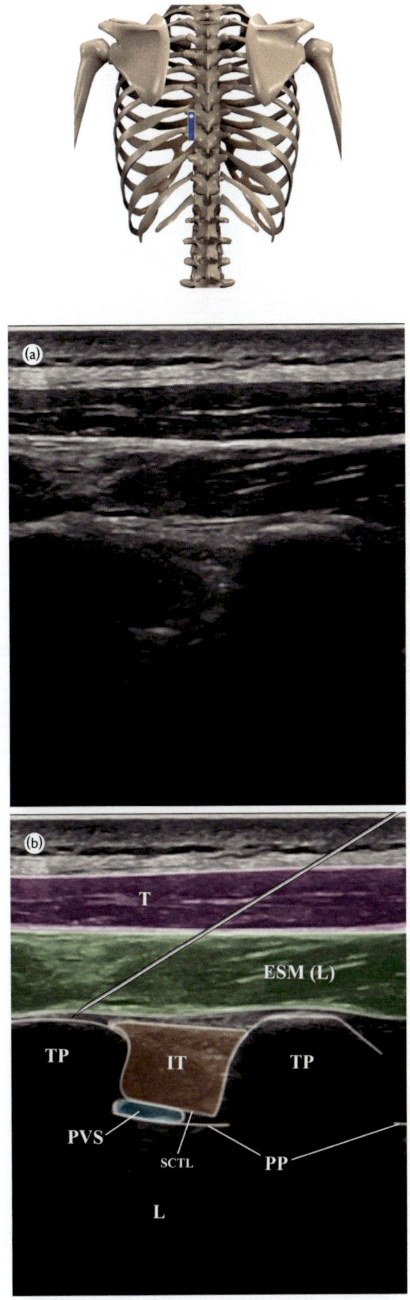

Figure 3.4.4 a, Ultrasound image of the posterior thorax at the level of the T8-9 in a sagittal plane. **b,** Labeled ultrasound image of in-plane needle placement for an erector spinae plane block at the transverse process. *T* trapezius, *ESM (L)* erector spinae muscle—longissimus muscle, *TP* transverse process, *IT* intertransverse muscles and ligaments, *SCTL* superior costotransverse ligament, *PVS* paravertebral space, *PP* parietal pleura, *L* lung.

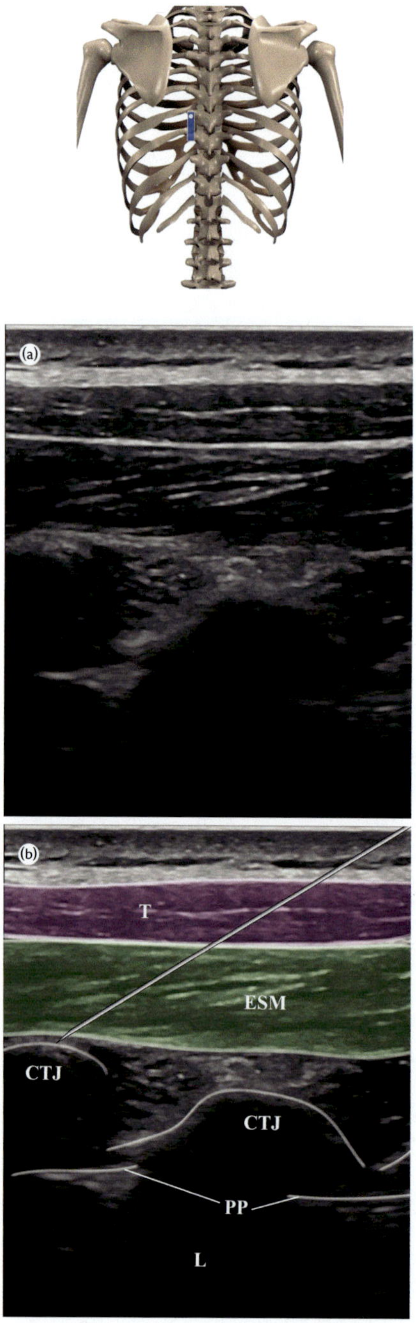

Figure 3.4.5 a, Ultrasound image of the posterior thorax at the level of the T8–9 in a sagittal plane. **b,** Labeled ultrasound image of in-plane needle placement for an erector spinae plane block at the costotransverse joint/junction. *T* trapezius, *ESM* erector spinae muscle, *CTJ* costotransverse joint, *PP* parietal pleura, *L* lung.

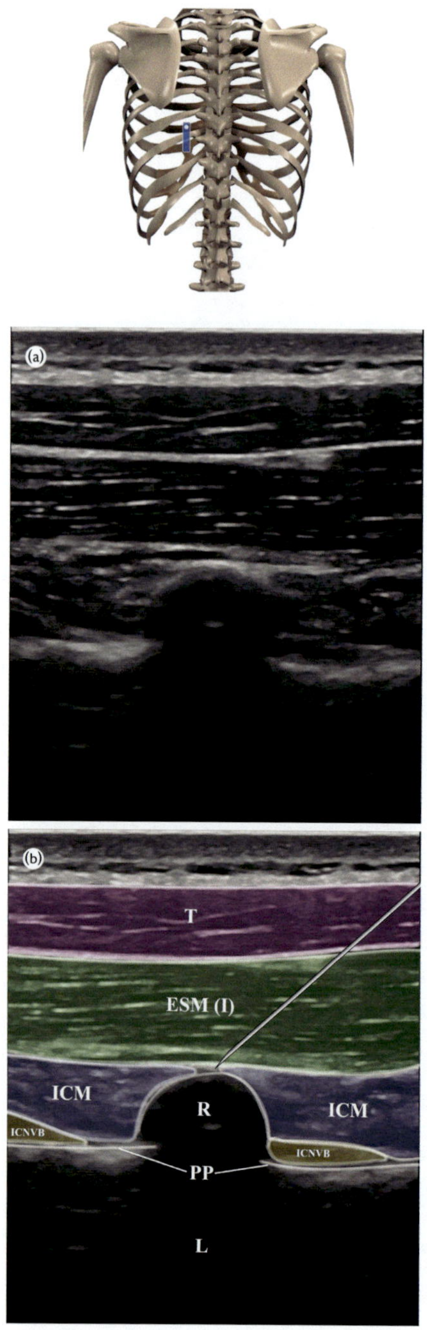

Figure 3.4.6 a, Ultrasound image of the posterior thorax at the level of the T8 in a sagittal plane. **b,** Labeled ultrasound image of in-plane needle placement for an erector spinae plane block at the rib. *T* trapezius, *ESM (I)* erector spinae muscle—iliocostalis muscle, *ICM* intercostal muscles, *R* rib, *ICNVB* intercostal neurovascular bundle, *PP* parietal pleura, *L* lung.

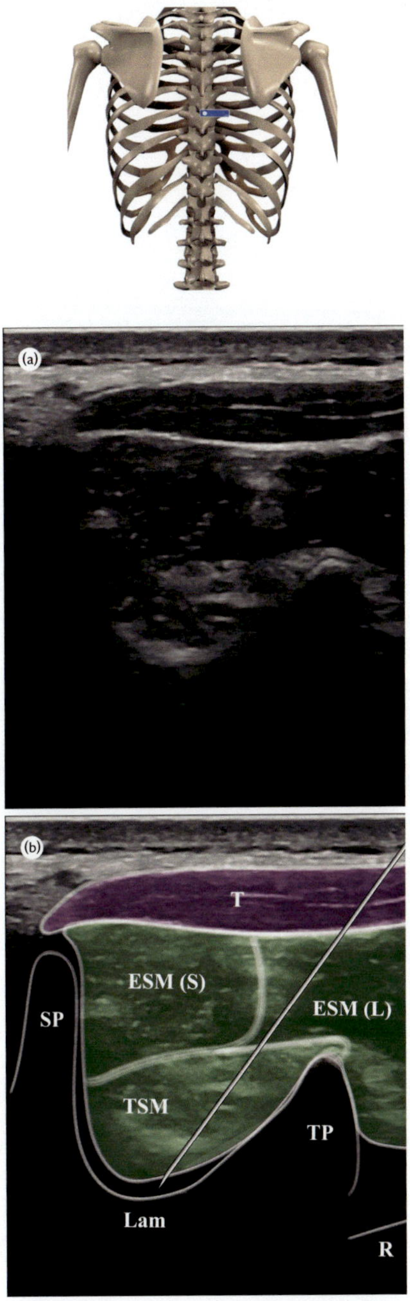

Figure 3.4.7 **a,** Ultrasound image of the posterior thorax at the level of the T7 in an axial plane. **b,** Labeled ultrasound image of in-plane needle placement for an erector spinae plane block at the lamina. *T* trapezius, *SP* spinous process, *ESM (S)* erector spinae muscle—spinalis muscle, *ESM (L)* erector spinae muscle—longissimus muscle, *TSM* transversospinalis muscles—semispinalis/multifidus/rotatores, *TP* transverse process, *Lam* lamina, *R* rib.

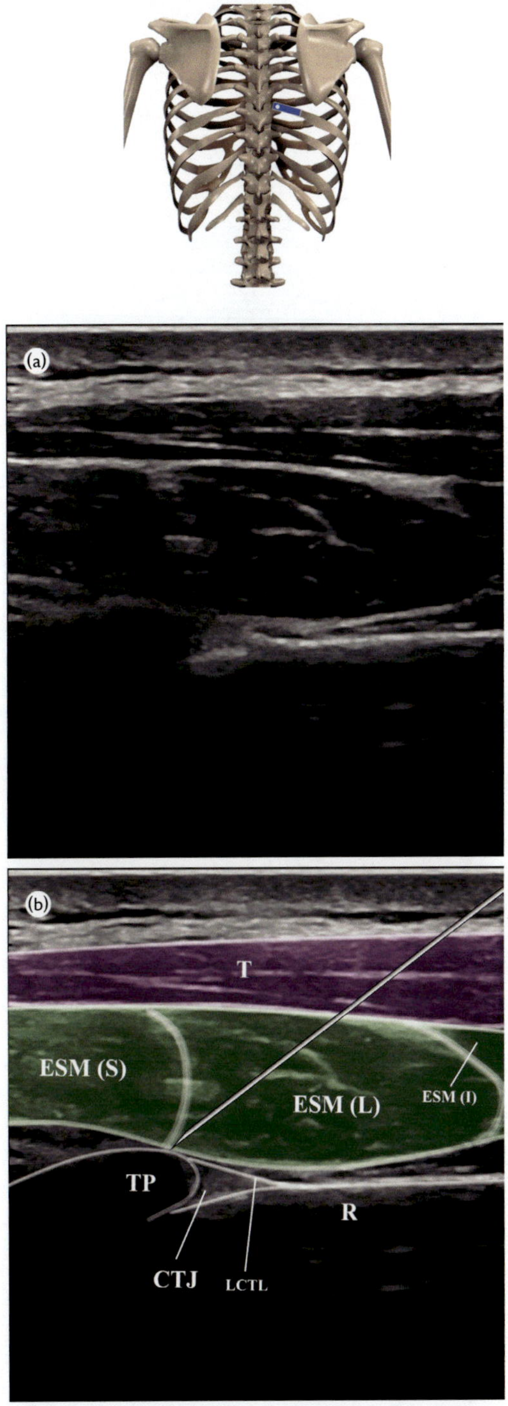

Figure 3.4.8 **a,** Ultrasound image of the posterior thorax at the level of the T7 in an axial oblique plane. **b,** Labeled ultrasound image of in-plane needle placement for an erector spinae plane block at the transverse process. *T* trapezius, *ESM (S)* erector spinae muscle—spinalis muscle, *ESM (L)* erector spinae muscle—longissimus muscle, *ESM (I)* erector spinae muscle—iliocostalis muscle, *TP* transverse process, *LCTL* lateral costotransverse ligament, *CTJ* costotransverse joint, *R* rib.

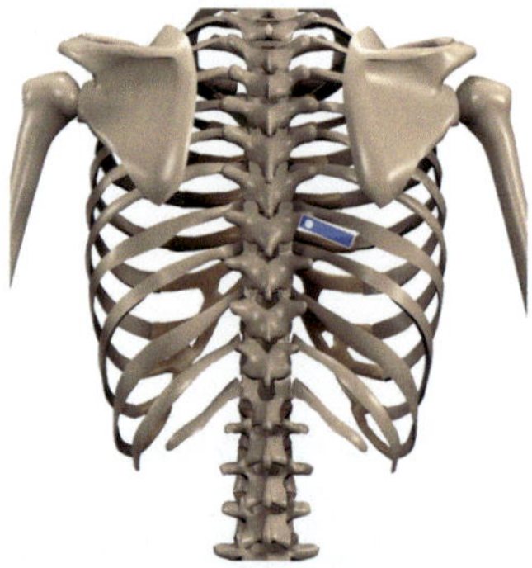

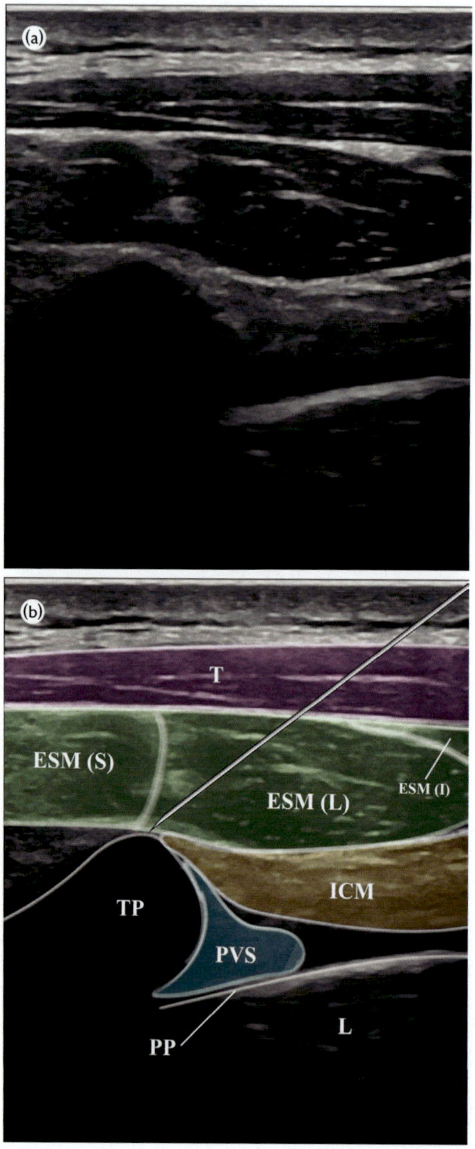

Figure 3.4.9 a, Ultrasound image of the posterior thorax at the level of the T7 in an axial oblique plane. **b,** Labeled ultrasound image of in-plane needle placement for an erector spinae plane block at the transverse process. *T* trapezius, *ESM (S)* erector spinae muscle—spinalis muscle, *ESM (L)* erector spinae muscle—longissimus muscle, *ESM (I)* erector spinae muscle—iliocostalis muscle, *TP* transverse process, *ICM* intercostal muscles, *PVS* paravertebral space, *PP* parietal pleura, *L* lung.

and ribs (Figure 3.4.6). Care must be taken to identify and differentiate it from the associated rib. The underlying pleura should also be visualized.

4. **Insert the needle in an in-plane approach to reach either the lamina, transverse process, costotransverse junction, or ribs.** Depending on the location of injection (medial or lateral ESP), the injectate may spread in different directions to capture different pain distributions. Hydrodissection can be used at this location to visualize the fluid lifting the erector spinae muscle off the bone.

ESP Block—Axial Plane

1. **Place the transducer in a sagittal orientation over posterior abdominal wall and count the ribs from caudad to cephalad to identify the target level**. Move the ultrasound probe medially and identify the spinous process.
2. **Rotate 90 degrees on the spinous process to have an axial image of the spinous process, lamina, and transverse process (Figure 3.4.7).** Translate the probe further laterally to identify the costotransverse joint and rib (Figure 3.4.8). Care must be taken to identify and differentiate it from the associated rib. The underlying pleura should also be visualized (Figure 3.4.9).
3. **Insert the needle in an in-plane approach from lateral to medial to reach the lamina, transverse process, or rib.** Depending on the location of injection, the injectate (medial or lateral) may spread in different directions to capture different pain distributions. Hydrodissection can be used at this location to visualize the fluid lifting the erector spinae muscle off the bone.

Tips and Safety Considerations

- Use doppler imaging to identify satellite vessels to avoid inadvertent puncture and intravascular injection.

Postprocedure Management

The patient should be monitored for possible total spinal anesthesia after an ESP block, and hence care must be taken to monitor mental status of the patient and vital signs. Although the risk of developing pneumothorax is low after ESP block, any difficulty in breathing after the procedure should be evaluated by obtaining a bedside chest X-ray. Supplemental oxygen should be made available to the patient and if required, a chest tube can be inserted if a pneumothorax is suspected.

References

1. Vidal E, Giménez H, Forero M, Fajardo M. Erector spinae plane block: a cadaver study to determine its mechanism of action. Revista Española de Anestesiología y Reanimación (English Edition). 2018;65(9):514–519.
2. Elsharkawy, H, El-Boghdadly, K, Kolli, S, Esa, WAS, DeGrande, S, Soliman, LM, Drake, RL. Injectate spread following anterior sub-costal and posterior approaches to the quadratus lumborum block: a comparative cadaveric study. Eur J Anaesthesiol. 2017;34:587–595.
3. Elsharkawy H, El-Boghdadly K, Barrington M. Quadratus lumborum block: anatomical concepts, mechanisms, and techniques. Anesthesiology. 2019;130(2):322–335. doi: 10.1097/ALN.0000000000002524
4. Kot P, Rodriguez P, Granell M, et al. The erector spinae plane block: a narrative review. Korean J Anesthesiol. 2019;72(3):209–220. doi:10.4097/kja.d.19.00012
5. Jain K, Jaiswal V, Puri A. Erector spinae plane block: relatively new block on horizon with a wide spectrum of application; a case series. Indian J Anaesth. 2018;62(10):809–813. doi:10.4103/ija.IJA_263_18
6. Forero M, Adhikary SD, Lopez H, Tsul C, Chin KJ. The erector spinae plane block: a novel analgesic technique in thoracic neuropathic pain. Reg Anaesth Pain Med. 2016;41:621–627.

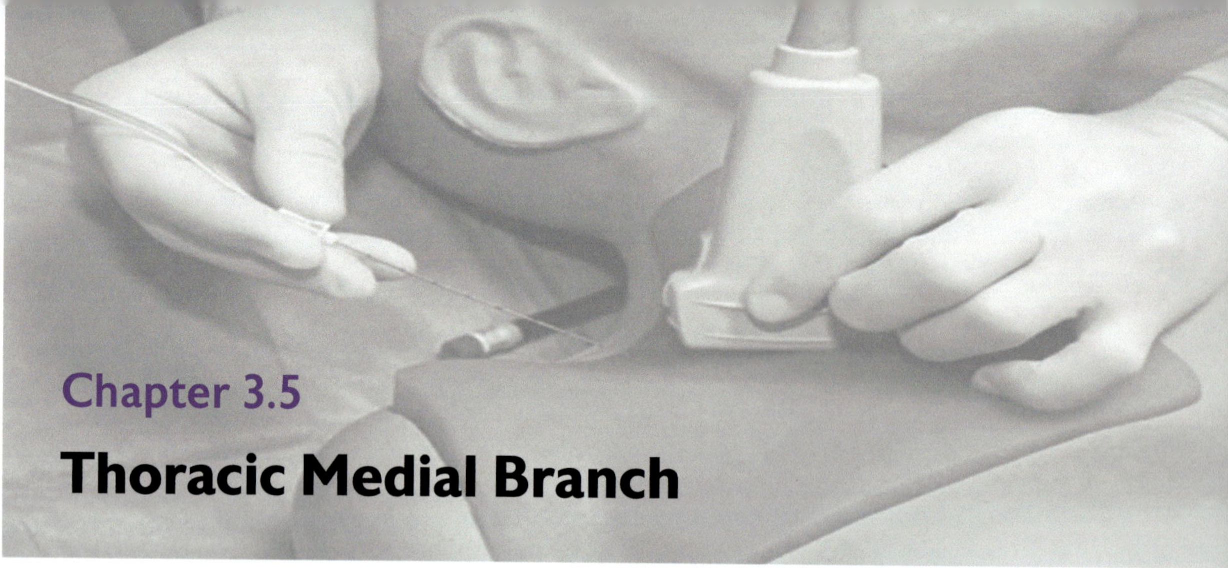

Chapter 3.5

Thoracic Medial Branch

Daniel Chun-suk Oh

Contents

Introduction

Using the thoracic medial branch block (TMBB) to target the innervation to thoracic facet joints is helpful for treating oncologic causes of posterior thoracic axial back pain. Common causes of axial pain in this region include metastatic disease to the posterior thoracic spinal elements; post-thoracic fusion; radiation injuries to bone, nerve, and muscle; muscle spasms; and dermatologic conditions such as postherpetic neuralgia and notalgia paresthetica. Chronic conditions can also affect facet joints and include osteoarthritis, inflammatory arthritis, synovial impingement, and meniscoid entrapment. Common physical exam signs of facetogenic pain are tenderness to palpation over the facet joints and pain with back extension and rotation.[1]

Diagnostic or therapeutic blocks can help the pain by targeting either facet joint, costotransverse joint or medial branch nerve.[2–4] Thoracic axial back pain can be targeted by direct intra-articular injections into the facet or costotransverse joints; however, medial branch blocks have multiple advantages over targeting joints. These include procedural ease and safety of reaching a transverse process and the possibility of radiofrequency ablation as a long-lasting pain intervention. Compared to the superior-medial location of lumbar dorsal ramus and medial branch nerves, the thoracic medial branch (TMB) nerves are near the superior lateral border of the thoracic transverse processes. Therefore, they can be targeted for intervention even after thoracic spinal fusions as the rods and pedicle screws are typically medial to the nerve location.[5,6] Additionally, targeting the TMB instead of the thoracic facet joint may be safer as there is a reduced risk of epidural or spinal injection.[7]

Critical Anatomy

As the nerve root exits the neuroforamen, it divides into ventral and dorsal rami (Figure 3.5.1). The dorsal ramus gives off three branches: the medial, intermediate, and lateral branches. Each thoracic facet joint is innervated by the medial branch at the corresponding level and from the level above. For example, the T–T6 facet joint is innervated by the ipsilateral T4 and T5 medial branches. As it branches off the dorsal ramus, the thoracic medial branches travel inferoposteriorly in variable locations based on the level. Typically, C8–T3 and T9–10 medial branches travel posteriorly on the superolateral aspect of the transverse process. From T4–T8, the medial branches may overlie the superolateral aspect of the transverse process, but sometimes are suspended within the intertransverse space as they travel posteriorly. The T11 branch runs across the lateral surface of the root of the short T12 transverse process. At T12, the medial branch runs a course similar to that of lumbar medial branches, which would be at the junction between the superior articular process (SAP) and the transverse process.[1] All thoracic medial branches will then course caudally and posteriorly to the multifidus and semispinalis muscles before further running inferiorly and medially over the dorsal aspect of the multifidus.[5,6] Risk of pneumothorax and vascular puncture is heightened with thoracic MBB compared to other levels given the vicinity to pleura.

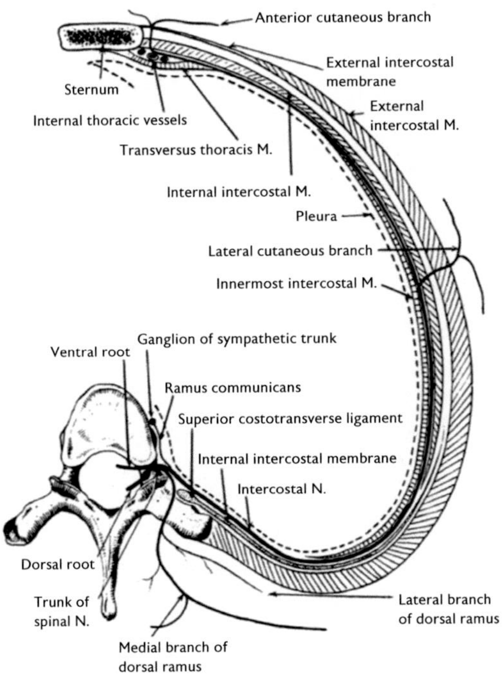

Figure 3.5.1 A diagram of the upper thoracic spinal nerve illustrating the ventral branch/intercostal nerve and dorsal ramus. (Reprinted with permission from Cunningham's Manual of Practical Anatomy: Thorax and Abdomen, 16th Edition)

Equipment and Patient Preparation

1. **Monitors and Sterility**
   a. No specific monitors are needed for this procedure, but emergency resuscitation equipment should be available immediately. This includes ACLS drugs, supplemental oxygen, airway adjuncts, and suction.
   b. Strict antiseptic technique should be observed including sterile probe cover, ultrasound gel, and sterile gloves. Chlorhexidine or other skin prep agent should be used to clean the skin prior to commencing the procedure.
2. **Equipment**
   a. Probe: High-frequency linear array transducer (8–12 MHz)
   b. Needle type: 22- or 25-gauge, 1.5- to 3.5-inch needle
   c. Local anesthetic (0.5–1 mL per nerve): Lidocaine 1%–2%; ropivacaine 0.2%–0.5%; bupivacaine 0.25%–0.5%
   d. Adjuvant (0.5–1 mL per nerve): Particulate or nonparticulate steroid
3. **Position**
   a. Prone

Procedure Technique

1. **Prepare equipment and supplies, position the patient prone, and sterilize the procedural area with antiseptic solution.**
2. **Identify the correct rib level by counting caudally from the 1st rib or cephalad from the 12th rib.** Take note that patients may have anatomic variations in their number of ribs.
3. **Place the ultrasound probe in a transverse orientation to visualize the desired rib and its articulation with the transverse process.** Desired needle location depends on the targeted spinal level. The C8–T3 and T9–10 medial branches course along the superior lateral borders of the transverse processes for T1–4 and T10–11. T4–8 medial branches may be difficult to target, as they are often localized within the intertransverse space. The T11 medial branch courses along the root of the SAP on T12. The T12 medial branch courses along the junction of the SAP and transverse process of L1 (Figure 3.5.2).
4. **Inject local anesthetic subcutaneously for analgesia at the procedural site.** Insert the needle with an in-plane approach to deposit injectate at the location of the MBB as described above.
5. **Repeat the procedure at various levels as required.**

Tips and Safety Considerations

- Avoid advancing the needle past the transverse process to prevent lung or thoracic nerve root injury.
- Use doppler imaging to identify satellite vessels to avoid inadvertent puncture and intravascular injection.

Post-Op Management Considerations

Although the risk of developing pneumothorax is low after TMBB, any difficulty in breathing after the procedure should be evaluated by obtaining a bedside chest X-ray. Supplemental oxygen should be made available to the patient and if required, a chest tube can be inserted if pneumothorax is suspected.

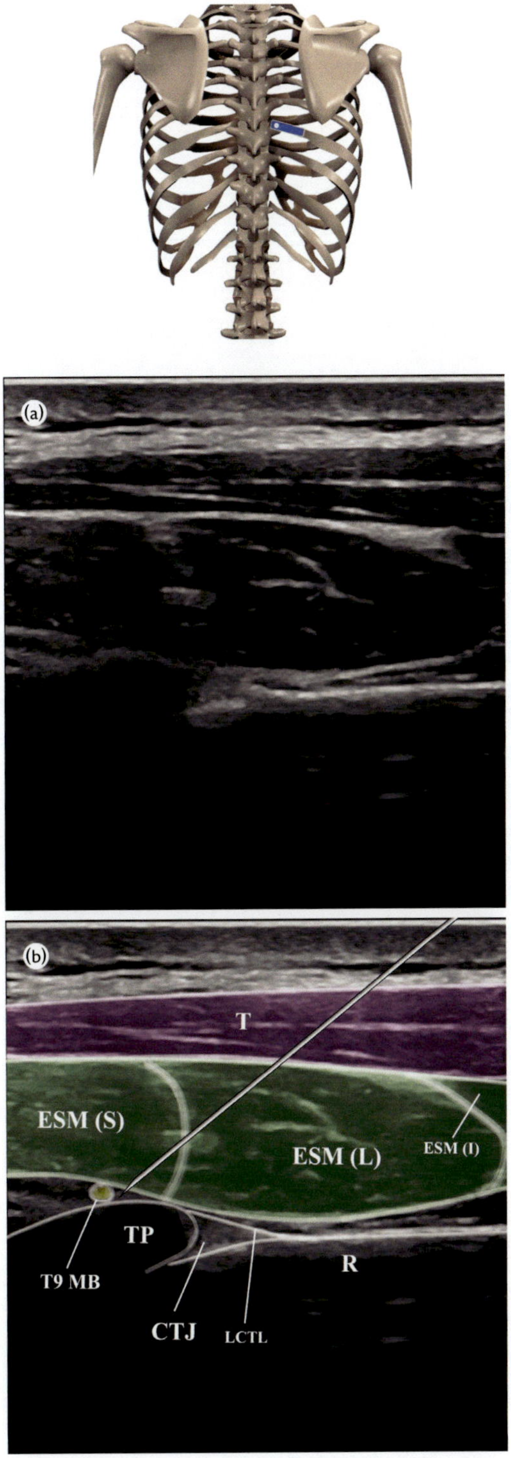

Figure 3.5.2 **a,** Ultrasound image of the posterior thorax at the level of the T7 in an axial oblique plane. **b,** Labeled ultrasound image of in-plane needle placement for an erector spinae plane block at the transverse process. *T* trapezius, *ESM (S)* erector spinae muscle—spinalis muscle, *ESM (L)* erector spinae muscle—longissimus muscle, *ESM (I)* erector spinae muscle—iliocostalis muscle, *T9 MB* T9 medial branch location, *TP* transverse process, *LCTL* lateral costotransverse ligament, *CTJ* costotransverse joint, *R* rib.

Further Reading

- Bogduk N. *Practice Guidelines for Spinal Diagnostic and Treatment Procedures.* International Spine Intervention Society; 2013.

References

1. Manchikanti L, Singh V, Pampati V, Beyer CD, Damron KS. Evaluation of the prevalence of facet joint pain in chronic thoracic pain. Pain Physician. 2002;5:354–359.
2. Masharawi Y, Rothscild B, Dar G, et al. Facet orientation in the thoracolumbar spine: three-dimensional anatomic and biochemical analysis. Spine. 2004;29:1755–1763.
3. Bogduk N. On the rational use of diagnostic blocks for spinal pain. Neurosurgery Quarterly. 2009;19:88–100.
4. Barnsley L, Lord S, Bogduk N. Comparative local anaesthetic blocks in the diagnosis of cervical zygapophysial joints pain. Pain. 1993:55:99–106.
5. Chua WH. Clinical Anatomy of the Thoracic Dorsal Rami. BMedSci Thesis. University of Newcastle, Newcastle, Australia; 1994.
6. Chua WH, Bogduk N. The surgical anatomy of thoracic facet denervation. Acta Neurochir. 1995;136:140–144.
7. Manchikanti L, Singh V, Falco F, Cash K, Pampati V. Effectiveness of thoracic medial branch blocks in managing chronic pain: a preliminary report of a randomized, double-blind controlled trial. Pain Physician. 2008;11(4):491–504.

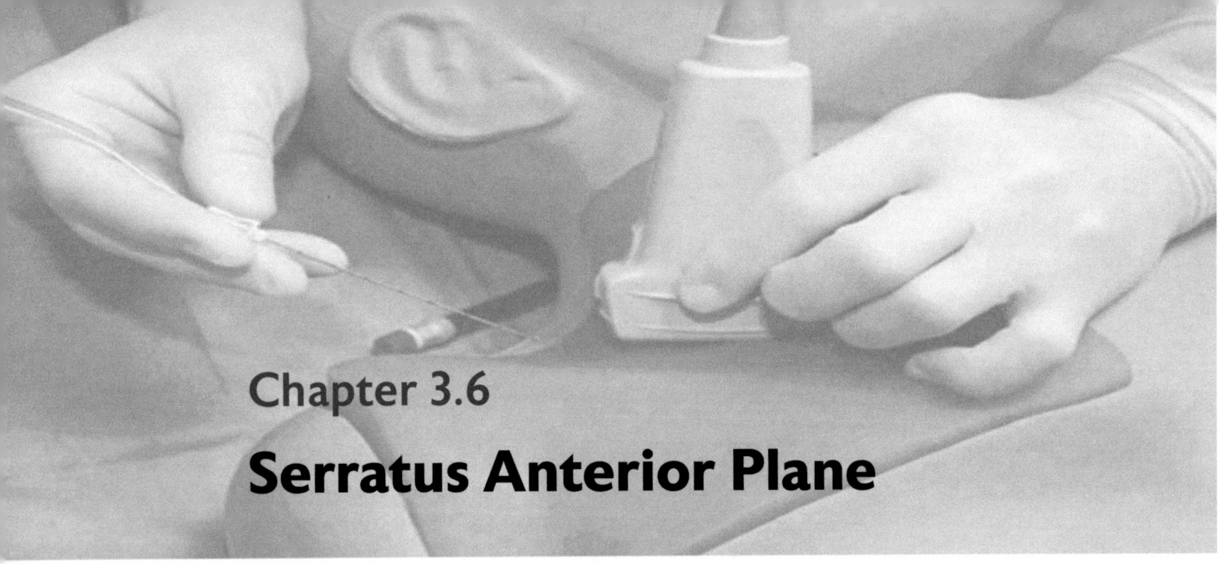

Chapter 3.6
Serratus Anterior Plane

Daniel Chun-suk Oh

Contents

Introduction

The serratus anterior plane (SAP) approach can be performed superficial and/or deep to the serratus anterior muscle to treat lateral chest wall pain. Additionally, the superficial block may provide analgesia to the axillary region and upper proximal arm to target the lateral cutaneous branches of the intercostal nerves as well as the intercostobrachial, long thoracic, and thoracodorsal nerves. Both planes are similar to the pectoralis plane (PECS) blocks in that they target the anterolateral chest wall, but the effect of the SAP block is greatest in the lateral and anterior chest wall. In contrast, a PECS block has the greatest effect on the upper anterior chest wall.

The deep SAP block is believed to cover intercostal nerves in the T2–T9 dermatomes, which may provide a wider blockade than the PECS blocks.[1] Thus, indications include pain from post-thoracotomy syndrome, rib fractures, postmastectomy syndrome, chest tubes, drainage tubes, tumors originating from the lateral chest wall, and post-tissue expanders.[1–3] In addition to the aforementioned indications, SAP may also be useful for neuropathic pain from radiation neuritis or tumor compression.

Critical Anatomy

Chest wall plane interventions target the innervation of the anterolateral chest wall by depositing medication between the various muscle plane layers of the pectoralis major/minor, serratus anterior, and transversus thoracis muscles (Figures 3.6.1–2). The anterior chest wall is innervated by the lateral and medial pectoral nerves, T2–T6 spinal nerves, long thoracic nerve, and thoracodorsal nerve (Figure 3.6.3). The lateral pectoral nerve originates from C5–C7 and runs between the pectoralis major and minor to supply the pectoralis major. The medial pectoral nerve originates from C8–T1 and runs deep to the pectoralis minor to supply the pectoralis major and minor. The T2–T6 spinal nerves run between the intercostal muscles and give off lateral and anterior branches. The lateral branch pierces the intercostal muscles and serratus anterior muscle in the midaxillary line to give off anterior and posterior cutaneous branches. The anterior branch pierces the intercostal muscles and serratus anterior muscle anteriorly to supply the medial breast. The long thoracic nerve originates from C5–C7 and runs on the outer surface of the serratus anterior to the axilla, where it supplies the serratus anterior. The thoracodorsal nerve originates from C6–C8 and runs deep in the posterior axillary wall to supply the latissimus dorsi.[1,4–6]

The superficial SAP (sSAP) injection is into the fascial plane between the latissimus dorsi and serratus anterior muscles at the level of the 4th or 5th rib in the midaxillary line. The sSAP primarily targets the thoracodorsal and long thoracic nerves, and may also cover the intercostobrachial nerve and lateral cutaneous branches of the intercostal nerves (T3–T9). The block provides axillary analgesia and is especially useful before axillary node dissection.[1,6]

The deep SAP (dSAP) injection targets the fascial plane between the serratus anterior muscle and the ribs. At the 2nd or 3rd rib, the intercostobrachial nerve is targeted. Deep breast pain may be better targeted at the 4th or 5th rib.[1,6]

Choosing the correct plane for intervention depends on anatomic changes due to surgery and patient symptomology. Reconstruction and surgical technique may alter the available planes for injection. In these cases, posterior thoracic injections may be preferred.

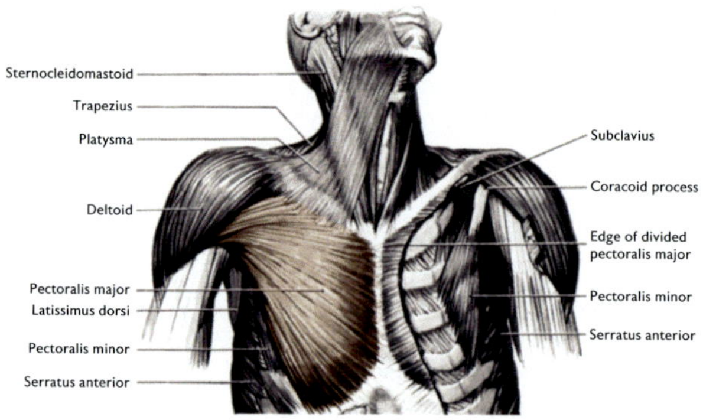

Figure 3.6.1 Muscles of the anterior wall of the thorax. On the anatomical left side, the pectoralis major is removed to show the pectoralis minor and serratus anterior. (Reprinted with permission from Cunningham's Manual of Practical Anatomy: Thorax and Abdomen, 16th Edition)

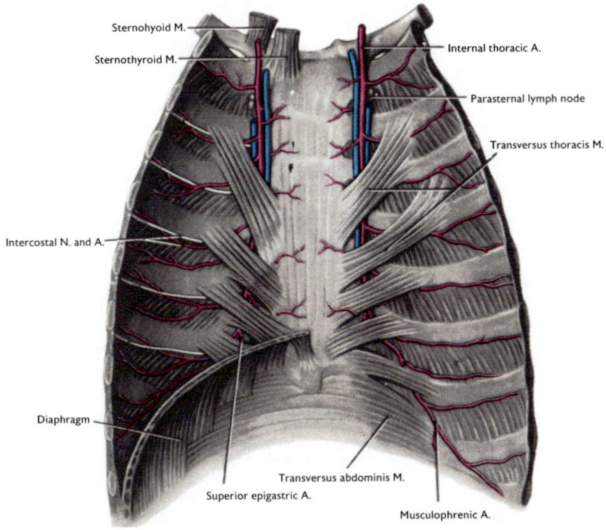

Figure 3.6.2 Posterior surface of the anterior thoracic wall, revealing the transversus thoracis muscle. (Reprinted with permission from Cunningham's Manual of Practical Anatomy: Thorax and Abdomen, 16th Edition)

Equipment and Patient Preparation

1. Monitors and Sterility

a. No specific monitors are needed for this procedure, but emergency resuscitation equipment should be available immediately. This includes ACLS drugs, supplemental oxygen, airway adjuncts, and suction.

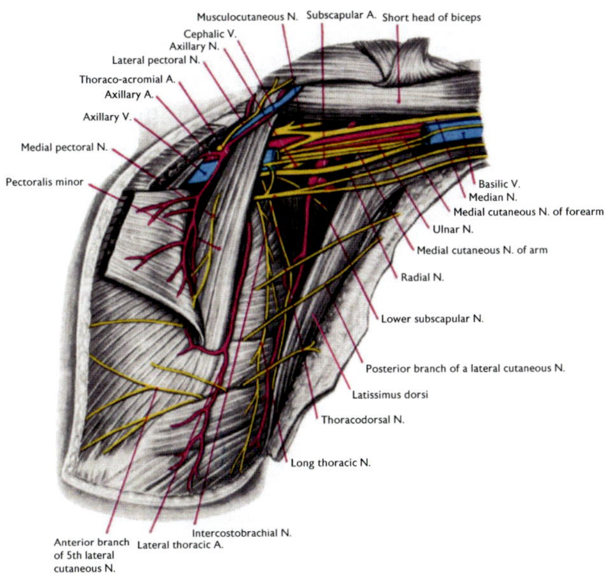

Figure 3.6.3 Contents of the axilla exposed by reflection of the pectoralis major, revealing anterior chest wall innervations. (Reprinted with permission from Cunningham's Manual of Practical Anatomy: Thorax and Abdomen, 16th Edition)

b. Strict antiseptic technique should be observed including sterile probe cover, ultrasound gel, and sterile gloves. Chlorhexidine or other skin prep agent should be used to clean the skin prior to commencing the procedure.

2. **Equipment**
   a. Probe: High-frequency linear array transducer (8–12 MHz)
   b. Needle type: 22- or 25-gauge, 1.5- to 3.5-inch needle
   c. Local anesthetic (6–9 mL per plane): Lidocaine 1%–2%; ropivacaine 0.2%–0.5%; bupivacaine 0.25%–0.5%
   d. Adjuvant (0.5–1 mL per plane): Particulate or nonparticulate steroid
3. **Position**
   a. Prone (preferred) or lateral decubitus

Procedure Technique

1. **Prepare equipment and supplies, position the patient in lateral decubitus, and sterilize the procedural area with antiseptic solution.**
2. **Identify the correct rib level by counting caudally from the 1st rib or cephalad from the 12th rib.** Take note that patients may have anatomic variations in their number of ribs.
3. **Place the ultrasound probe in a transverse orientation in the midaxillary line at the level of the 5th rib.** The hyperechoic pleural line and ribs should be easily identified. The serratus anterior muscle lies superficially above the ribs. The latissimus dorsi muscle lies superficially and superiorly above the serratus anterior muscle.
4. **The target for the sSAP is the fascial plane superficial to the serratus anterior and between the serratus anterior and latissimus dorsi (Figure 3.6.4—needle placement #2).** This blocks the long thoracic nerve and thoracodorsal nerve. Use a needle with an in-plane approach to deposit injectate in the sSAP.
5. **The target for the dSAP is the plane between the serratus anterior and external intercostal (Figure 3.6.4—needle placement #1).** Use a needle with an in-plane approach to deposit injectate in the dSAP.
6. **To block the intercostobrachial nerve (ICBN), target the superior border of the 2nd or 3rd rib in the fascial plane between the serratus anterior and intercostal muscles (Figure 3.6.5).** The injectate will track in this plane to the nerve at the level of the 2nd rib. Use a needle with an in-plane approach to deposit injectate.

Tips and Safety Considerations

- Use doppler imaging to identify satellite vessels to avoid inadvertent puncture and intravascular injection.

Post-Op Management Considerations

Although the risk of developing pneumothorax is low after SAP block, any difficulty in breathing after the procedure should be evaluated by obtaining a bedside chest X-ray. Supplemental oxygen should be made available to the patient and if required, a chest tube can be inserted if pneumothorax is suspected.

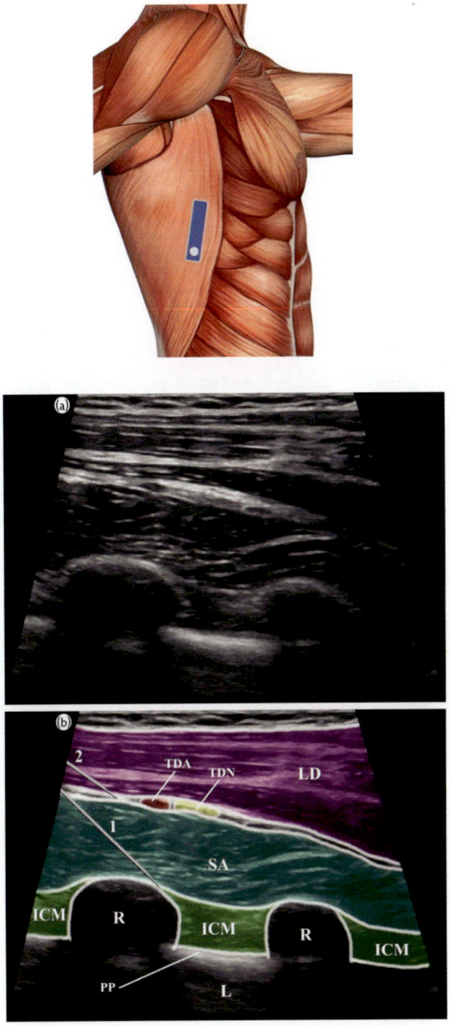

Figure 3.6.4 **a,** Ultrasound image of the lateral thorax at the level of the 4th–5th ribs in a coronal oblique plane. **b,** Labeled ultrasound image of in-plane needle placement for a deep serratus plane block (1) and superficial serratus plane and thoracodorsal nerve block (2) in short-axis. *LD* latissimus dorsi, *TDA* thoracodorsal artery, *TDN* thoracodorsal nerve, *SA* serratus anterior, *ICM* intercostal muscles, *R5* 5th rib, *R4* 4th rib, *PP* parietal pleura, *L* lung.

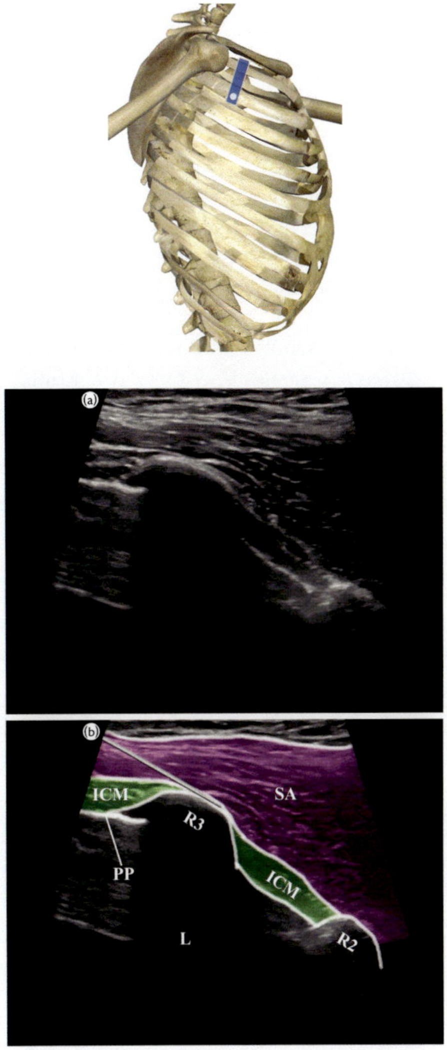

Figure 3.6.5 **a,** Ultrasound image of the lateral thorax at the level of the 2nd–3rd ribs in a coronal oblique plane. **b,** Labeled ultrasound image of in-plane needle placement for a deep serratus plane block targeting the intercostobrachial nerve (ICBN) in short-axis. *SA* serratus anterior, *ICM* intercostal muscles, *R3* 3rd rib, *R2* 2nd rib, *PP* parietal pleura, *L* lung.

Further Reading

- NYSORA. Pectoralis and Serratus Plane Blocks; 2023. https://www.nysora.com/regional-anesthesia-for-specific-surgical-procedures/thorax/pectoralis-serratus-plane-blocks/.

References

1. Blanco R, Parras T, McDonnell JG, Prats-Galino A. Serratus plane block: a novel ultrasound-guided thoracic wall nerve block. Anaesthesia. 2013;68:1107–1113.
2. Madabushi R, Tewari S, Gautam SK, Agarwal A, Agarwal A. Serratus anterior plane block: a new analgesic technique for post-thoracotomy pain. Pain Physician. 2015;18:E421–424.
3. Kunhabdulla NP, Agarwal A, Gaur A, Gautam SK, Gupta R, Agarwal A. Serratus anterior plane block for multiple rib fractures. Pain Physician. 2014;17:E651–653.
4. Biswas A, Castanov V, Li Z, Perlas A, Kruisselbrink R, Agur A, Chan V. Serratus plane block: a cadaveric study to evaluate optimal injectate spread. Reg Anesth Pain Med. 2018;43(8):854–858.
5. Piracha MM, Thorp SL, Puttanniah V, Gulati A. "A tale of two planes": deep versus superficial serratus plane block for postmastectomy pain syndrome. Reg Anesth Pain Med. 2017;42(2):259–262.
6. Mayes J, Davison E, Panahi P, Patten D, Eljelani F, Womack J, Varma M. An anatomical evaluation of the serratus anterior plane block. Anaesthesia. 2016;71(9):1064–1069.

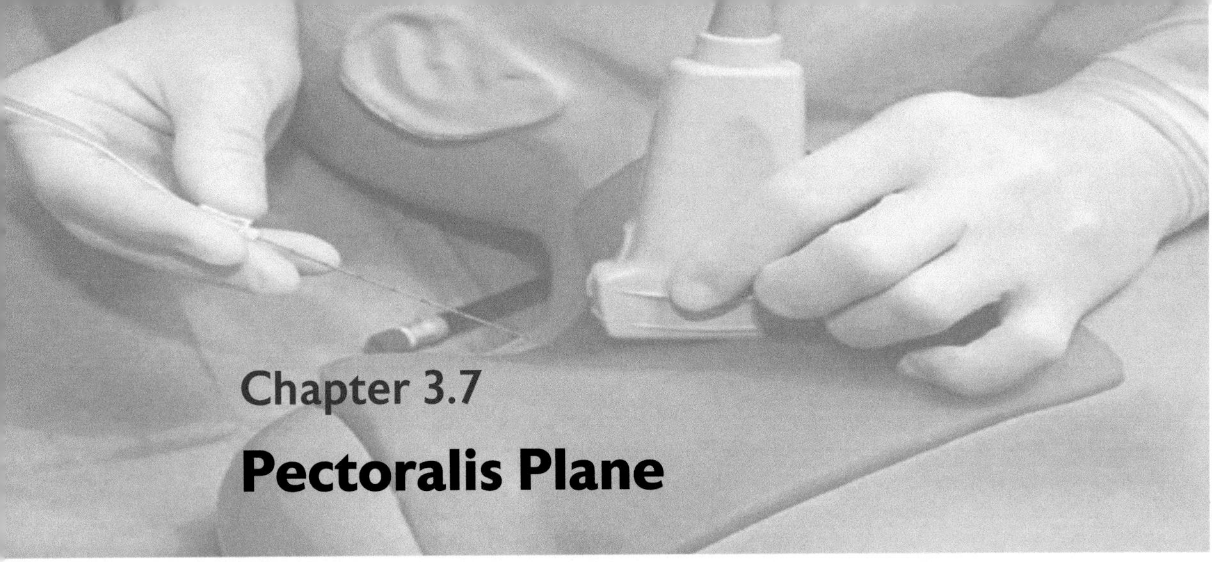

Chapter 3.7
Pectoralis Plane

Daniel Chun-suk Oh

Contents

Introduction

The use of ultrasonography to identify fascial layers has led to the development of several newer interfascial injection techniques for analgesia of the chest wall. These injections were developed as alternatives to thoracic epidural, paravertebral, intercostal, and intrapleural blocks. Generally, they are efficacious, relatively easy to perform, and have limited side-effect profiles.

The pectoralis plane (PECS) is a prime target for superficial and deep anterior/lateral chest wall pain. PECS blocks are similar to other plane blocks, such as transverse abdominus plane (TAP) and serratus blocks, in that they involve large volumes of injectate that spread to cover multiple nerves.[1] Compared to the serratus block, the PECS block covers a more superior and anterior portion of the chest wall. The indications for PECS blocks include acute perioperative pain and chronic pain of the chest wall. This includes breast surgery, port placement, thoracotomy incisions, axillary node dissections, chest wall tumor resections, postmastectomy pain syndrome, and post-thoracotomy pain syndrome.[2–4] Additionally, they may be used for perioperative pain management in breast surgery.[4–5]

The two main pectoralis plane injections include superficial PECS and the deep PECS blocks. The superficial PECS plane lies between the pectoralis major and minor muscles at the 2nd–3rd rib. The deep PECS plane lies between the pectoralis minor muscle and underlying rib. A PECS

I block targets the superficial PECS plane to block the lateral and medial pectoral nerves.[5] A PECS II block refers to targeting both the superficial and deep PECS planes. The PECS II block extends the blockade into the axilla, expanding its indications to axillary dissection, wide tumor excisions of the chest wall, and mastectomy.[6]

Critical Anatomy

The purpose of chest wall plane interventions is to target the innervation to the anterior and lateral chest wall between the various muscle plane layers of the pectoralis major/minor, serratus anterior, and transversus thoracis (Figures 3.7.1–2). The anterior chest wall is innervated by the medial and lateral pectoral nerves, T2–T6 spinal nerves, long thoracic nerve, and thoracodorsal nerve (Figure 3.7.3). The lateral pectoral nerve originates from C5–C7 and runs between the pectoralis major and minor to supply the pectoralis major. The medial pectoral nerve originates from C8–T1 and runs deep to the pectoralis minor to supply the pectoralis major and minor. The T2–T6 spinal nerves run in a plane between the intercostal muscles and give off lateral and anterior branches. The anterior branch innervates the medial breast. The lateral branch pierces the intercostal and serratus anterior muscles in the midaxillary line, and then gives off anterior and posterior cutaneous branches. The long thoracic nerve originates from C5–C7 and runs on the outer surface of the serratus anterior muscle to the axilla, where it supplies the serratus anterior muscle. The thoracodorsal nerve originates from C6–C8 and runs deep in the posterior axillary wall to supply the latissimus dorsi muscle.[4–6]

PECS I consists of a single injection between the pectoralis major and minor in an axial oblique plane at the level of the coracoid and the 2nd rib to block the lateral and medial pectoral nerves.[5] PECS II consists of an additional injection between pectoralis minor and serratus anterior or rib at the 3rd or 4th rib level. Our approach further subdivides the additional injection of the PECS II into the superficial lateral pectoralis plane (SL-PECS), between the pectoralis major and minor, and deep lateral pectoralis plane (DL-PECS), between the pectoralis minor and serratus anterior or rib. This injection blocks the lateral branch of the T2–T4 spinal nerves and may reach the anterior branch if sufficient injectate penetrates the external intercostal muscles.[6]

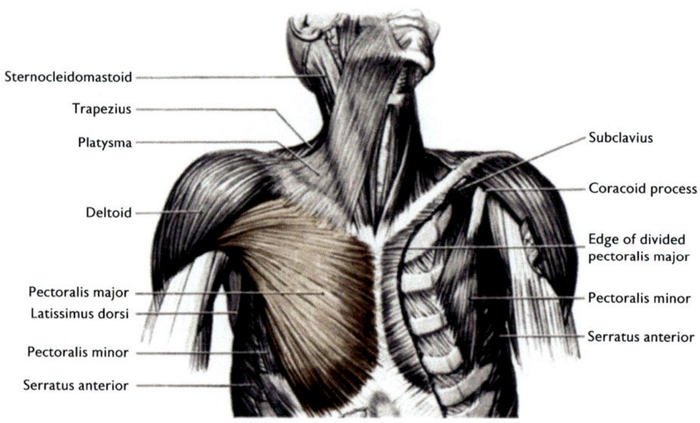

Figure 3.7.1 Muscles of the anterior wall of the trunk. On the anatomical left side, the pectoralis major is removed to show the pectoralis minor and serratus anterior. (Reprinted with permission from Cunningham's Manual of Practical Anatomy: Thorax and Abdomen, 16th Edition)

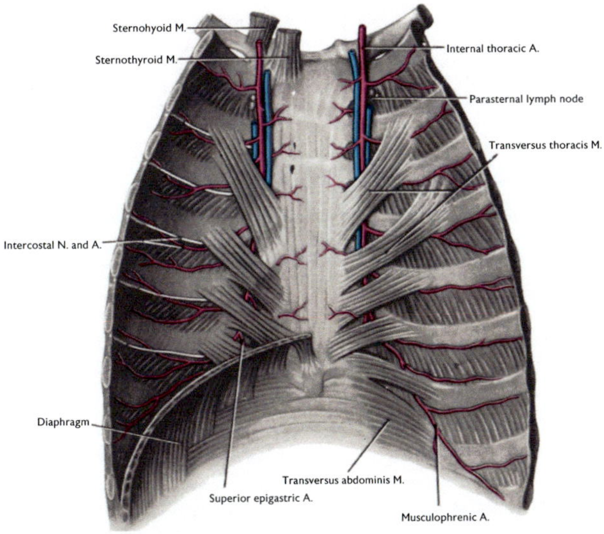

Figure 3.7.2 Posterior surface of the anterior thoracic wall revealing the transversus thoracis muscle. (Reprinted with permission from Cunningham's Manual of Practical Anatomy: Thorax and Abdomen, 16th Edition)

Equipment and Patient Preparation

1. Monitors and Sterility

a. No specific monitors are needed for this procedure, but emergency resuscitation equipment should be available immediately. This includes ACLS drugs, supplemental oxygen, airway adjuncts, and suction.

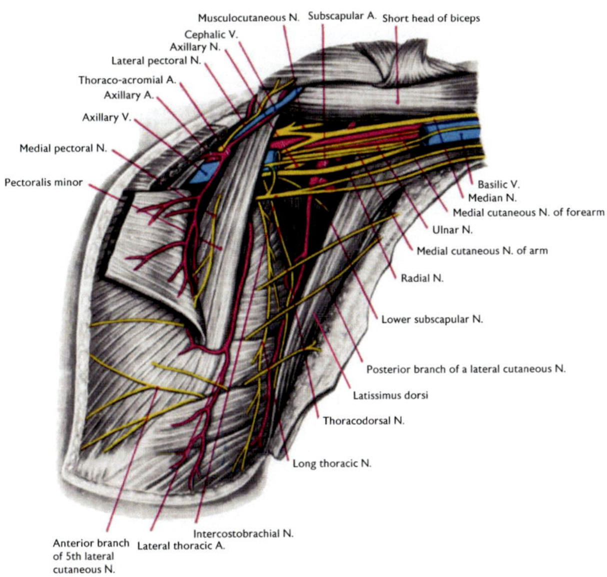

Figure 3.7.3 Contents of the axilla exposed by reflection of the pectoralis major revealing the various nerves and anterior chest wall innervations. (Reprinted with permission from Cunningham's Manual of Practical Anatomy: Thorax and Abdomen, 16th Edition)

b. Strict antiseptic technique should be observed including sterile probe cover, ultrasound gel, and sterile gloves. Chlorhexidine or other skin prep agent should be used to clean the skin prior to commencing the procedure.

2. **Equipment**
   a. Probe: High-frequency linear array transducer (8–12 MHz)
   b. Needle type: 22- or 25-gauge, 1.5- to 2-inch needle
   c. Local anesthetic (4–9 mL per plane): Lidocaine 1%–2%; ropivacaine 0.2%–0.5%; bupivacaine 0.25%–0.5%
   d. Adjuvant (0.25–1 mL per plane): Particulate or nonparticulate steroid
3. **Position**
   a. Supine

Procedure Technique

PECS I Approach

1. **Prepare equipment and supplies, position the patient supine, and sterilize the procedural area with antiseptic solution.** The patient may rest their arm by their chest or abduct the arm above their head.
2. **Place the ultrasound probe in an axial orientation and rotate the medial aspect of the ultrasound probe caudal.** The pectoralis major and minor muscles should be visualized (Figure 3.7.4). The axillary artery and the cords of the brachial plexus should be visible deep to the pectoralis minor.
3. **Inject local anesthetic subcutaneously for analgesia at the procedural site.**
4. **Insert the procedural needle with an in-plane approach from a lateral-to-medial direction.** Advance the needle through the pectoralis major muscle. Correct needle placement can be confirmed with hydrodissection between the pectoralis major and minor muscles.
5. **Inject the medication between the pectoralis major and minor muscles.** Remove the needle and apply a dressing.

Superficial (SL-PECS) and Deep (DL-PECS) Lateral Pectoralis Plane

1. **Prepare equipment and supplies, position the patient supine, and sterilize the procedural area with antiseptic solution.** The patient should abduct the arm above their head.
2. **Place the ultrasound probe in a sagittal oblique orientation at the level of the 3rd–4th ribs.** The pectoralis major, minor, and possibly the serratus anterior muscles should be visualized (Figure 3.7.5).
3. **Inject local anesthetic subcutaneously for analgesia at the procedural site.**
4. **Insert the procedural needle with an in-plane approach from a caudad-to-cephalad direction.** Advance the needle through the pectoralis major and minor muscles to either rib or superficial to the serratus anterior muscle. Correct needle placement can be confirmed with hydrodissection.
5. **For the DL-PECS, inject the medication between the pectoralis minor and rib or serratus anterior (Figure 3.7.5—needle #2).**
6. **For the SL-PECS, retract the needle to the layer between the pectoralis major and minor and inject the medication between these layers (Figure 3.7.5—needle #1).** Remove the needle and apply a dressing.

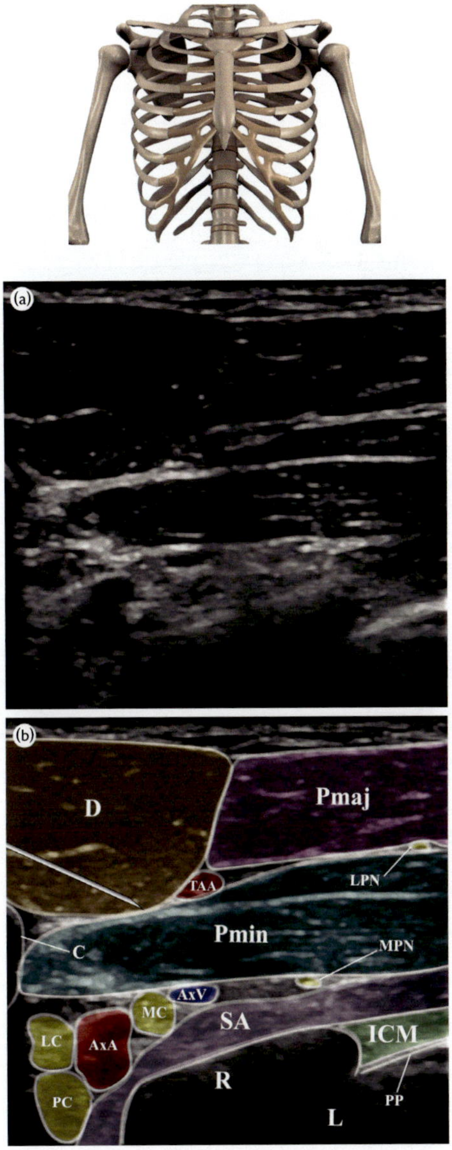

Figure 3.7.4 **a,** Ultrasound image of the anterior thorax at the level of the coracoid and 2nd rib in an axial oblique plane. **b,** Labeled ultrasound image of an in-plane needle placement for a PECS1 block. *D* deltoid, *Pmaj* pectoralis major, *TAA* pectoral branch of the thoracoacromial artery, *LPN* lateral pectoral nerve, *C* coracoid, *Pmin* pectoralis minor, *LC* lateral cord of brachial plexus, *PC* posterior cord of brachial plexus, *AxA* axillary artery, *MC* medial cord of brachial plexus, *AxV* axillary vein, *MPN* medial pectoral nerve, *SA* serratus anterior, *R* rib, *ICM* intercostal muscles, *PP* parietal pleura, *L* lung.

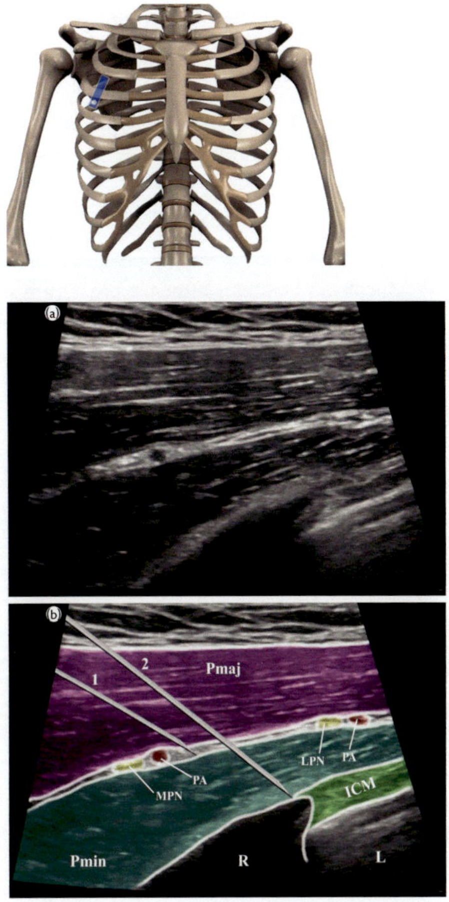

Figure 3.7.5 **a,** Ultrasound image of the anterior thorax at the level of the 3rd rib in a sagittal oblique plane. **b,** Labeled ultrasound image of approach 1 shows an in-plane needle placement for a superficial lateral pectoralis plane (SL-PECS) block, which targets the medial and lateral pectoral nerves. Approach 2 shows an in-plane needle placement for a deep lateral pectoralis plane (DL-PECS) block. *Pmaj* pectoralis major, *MPN* medial pectoral nerve, *LPN* lateral pectoral nerve, *PA* pectoral branch of the thoracoacromial artery, Pmin pectoralis minor, *ICM* intercostal muscles, *R* rib, *L* lung.

Tips and Safety Considerations

- Use doppler imaging to identify satellite vessels to avoid inadvertent puncture and intravascular injection.
- During the PECSI injection, avoid an approach deep to the pectoralis minor, which will puncture/target the axillary artery or cords of the brachial plexus.

Post-Op Management Considerations

Although the risk of developing pneumothorax is low after PECS I, SL-PECS, and DL-PECS blocks, any difficulty in breathing after the procedure should be evaluated by obtaining a bedside chest X-ray. Supplemental oxygen should be made available to the patient and if required, a chest tube can be inserted if pneumothorax is suspected.

Further Reading

- Valimahomed A, Zocca J, Gulati A. Chapter 9: Breast Cancer Pain: A Review of Pathology and Interventional Techniques in: Gulati A, Puttanniah V, Bruel BM, Rosenberg WS, Hung JC. *Essentials of Interventional Cancer Pain Management*. New York, NY: Springer; 2019:63–84.
- NYSORA. Blanco R, Barrington MJ. Pectoralis and Serratus Plane Blocks; 2023. https://www.nysora.com/regional-anesthesia-for-specific-surgical-procedures/thorax/pectoralis-serratus-plane-blocks/.

References

1. Wahba SS, Kamal SM. Thoracic paravertebral block versus pectoral nerve block for analgesia after breast surgery. Egyptian J Anaesth. 2014;30:129–135.
2. Madabushi R, Tewari S, Gautam SK, Agarwal A, Agarwal A. Serratus anterior plane block: a new analgesic technique for post-thoracotomy pain. Pain Physician. 2015;18:E421–424.
3. Kaushal B, Chauhan S, Saini K, Bhoi D, Bisoi AK, Sangdup T, Khan MA. Comparison of the efficacy of ultrasound-guided serratus anterior plane block, pectoral nerves II block, and intercostal nerve block for the management of postoperative thoracotomy pain after pediatric cardiac surgery. J Cardiothorac Vasc Anesth. 2019;33(2):418–425.
4. Blanco R, Parras T, McDonnell JG, Prats-Galino A: Serratus plane block: a novel ultrasound-guided thoracic wall nerve block. Anaesthesia. 2013;68:1107–1113.
5. Blanco R. The "pecs block": a novel technique for providing analgesia after breast surgery. Anaesthesia. 2011;66(9):847–848.
6. Blanco R, Fajardo M, Parras Maldonado T. Ultrasound description of Pecs II (modified Pecs I): a novel approach to breast surgery. Rev Esp Anestesiol Reanim. 2012;59(9):470–475.

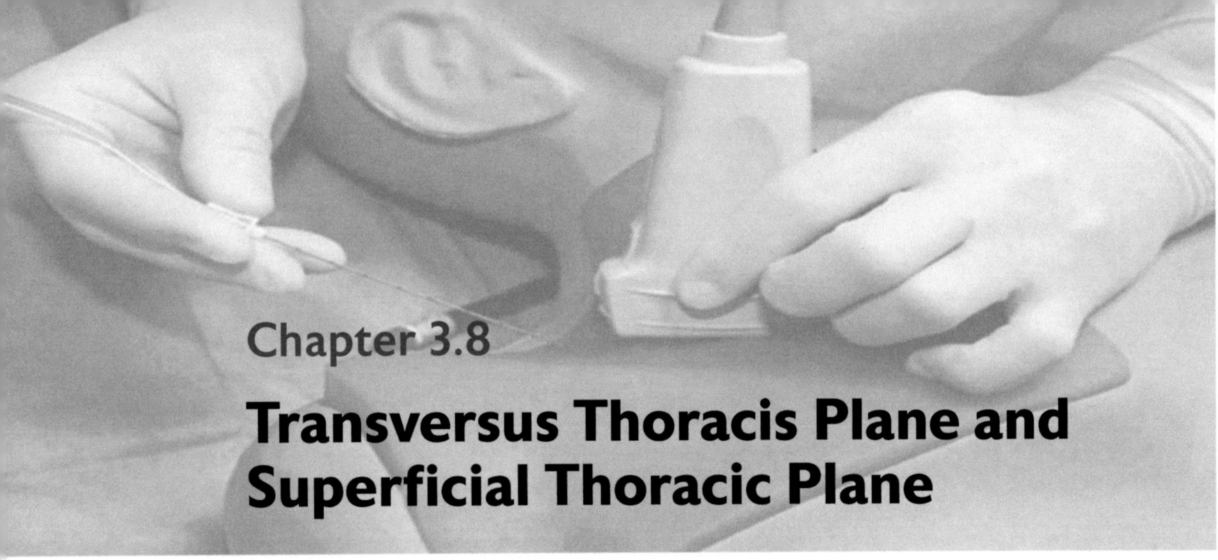

Chapter 3.8

Transversus Thoracis Plane and Superficial Thoracic Plane

Daniel Chun-suk Oh

Contents

Introduction

The transversus thoracis plane (TTP) and superficial thoracic plane (STP) are prime targets for superficial and deep anterior chest wall and sternal pain.[1] The TTP block targets the anterior branches of the T2–T6 anterior intercostal nerves, which lie between the internal intercostal and transversus thoracis muscles. The STP block targets the T1–T5 anterior intercostal nerves between the pectoralis and intercostal muscles. The STP block was developed as a less technically challenging alternative to the TTP block, which is often complicated by poor visualization of the transversus thoracis muscle and close proximity of the internal thoracic artery.[2–3]

Given the novelty of blocks, there are few clear indications. However, the available literature demonstrates the efficacy of TTP and STP blocks in relieving pain from in median sternotomy, thoracotomy, sternal fractures, sternal metastasis, medial rib fractures, breast surgery (usually in conjunction with pectoralis plane [PECS] blocks), defibrillator placement, post-thoracotomy pain syndrome, postmastectomy pain syndrome, breast tissue expander surgery, and metastatic disease.[4–11]

Critical Anatomy

Chest wall plane blocks target the innervation to the anterior and lateral chest wall between the various muscle plane layers of the pectoralis major/minor, serratus anterior, and transversus thoracis (Figures 3.8.1–2). The anterior chest wall is innervated by the medial and lateral pectoral nerves, T2–T6 spinal nerves, long thoracic nerve, and thoracodorsal nerve (Figure 3.8.3). The medial pectoral nerve originates from C8–T1 and runs deep to the pectoralis minor muscle to supply the pectoralis major and minor muscles. The lateral pectoral nerve originates from C5–C7 and runs between the pectoralis major and minor muscles to supply the pectoralis major muscle. The T2–T6 spinal nerves run between the intercostal muscles and give off the lateral and anterior branches. The lateral branch pierces the intercostal muscle and serratus anterior muscle in the midaxillary line to give off the anterior and posterior cutaneous branches. The anterior branch pierces the intercostal muscles and serratus anterior muscles anteriorly to supply the medial breast. The long thoracic nerve originates from C5–C7 and runs on the outer surface of the serratus anterior muscle, which it also innervates. The thoracodorsal nerve originates from C6–C8 and runs deep in the posterior axillary wall to supply the latissimus dorsi muscle.[2,4–6]

The TTP injection is the transversus thoracis muscle plane between the internal intercostal and transversus thoracis muscles at the level of the 3rd–5th ribs next to the manubrium and sternum. The target is the anterior branches of the T2–T6 intercostal nerves which innervate the internal mammary region.[2,4–6]

The STP injection is to the plane between the pectoralis major and intercostal muscles. This plane is superficial to the sternocostal junction. It targets the anterior cutaneous branches of the T1–T5 intercostal nerves, which provide sensation to the anterior chest wall. In our experience, since the injection plane is more superficial than the TTP, there is reduced risk of pleural puncture.

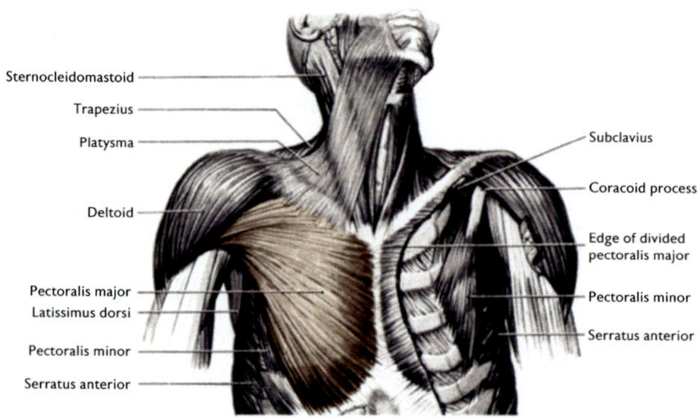

Figure 3.8.1 Muscles of the anterior wall of the trunk. On the anatomical left side, the pectoralis major is removed to show the pectoralis minor and serratus anterior. (Reprinted with permission from Cunningham's Manual of Practical Anatomy: Thorax and Abdomen, 16th Edition)

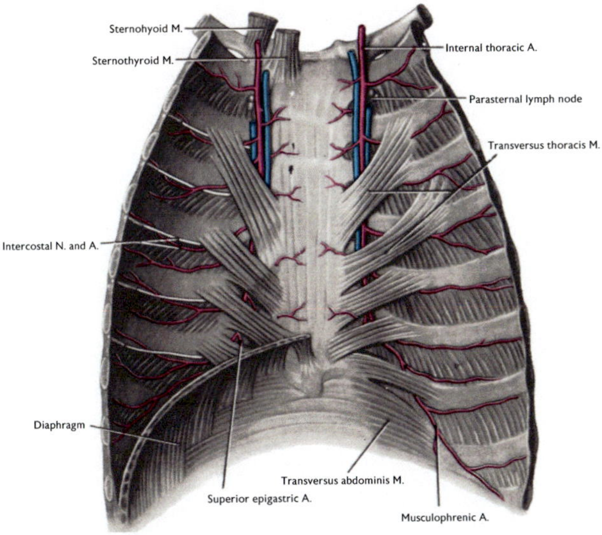

Figure 3.8.2 Posterior surface of the anterior thoracic wall revealing the transversus thoracis muscle. (Reprinted with permission from Cunningham's Manual of Practical Anatomy: Thorax and Abdomen, 16th Edition)

Equipment and Patient Preparation

1. Monitors and Sterility

a. No specific monitors are needed for this procedure, but emergency resuscitation equipment should be available immediately. This includes ACLS drugs, supplemental oxygen, airway adjuncts, and suction.

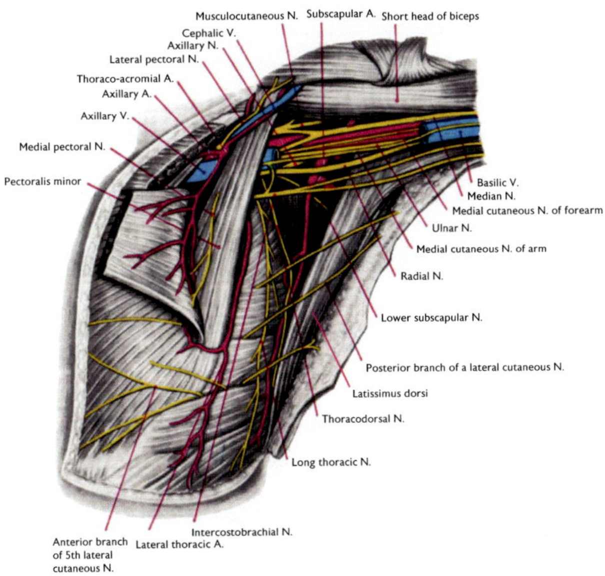

Figure 3.8.3 Contents of the axilla exposed by reflection of the pectoralis major revealing the various nerves and anterior chest wall innervations. (Reprinted with permission from Cunningham's Manual of Practical Anatomy: Thorax and Abdomen, 16th Edition)

b. Strict antiseptic technique should be observed including sterile probe cover, ultrasound gel, and sterile gloves. Chlorhexidine or other skin prep agent should be used to clean the skin prior to commencing the procedure.

2. **Equipment**
   a. Probe: High-frequency linear array transducer (8–12 MHz)
   b. Needle type: 25- or 30-gauge, 1- to 2-inch needle (ideally short bevel or blunt tip needle for safety)
   c. Local anesthetic (1–3 mL per TTP, 2–4 mL per STP): Lidocaine 1%–2%; ropivacaine 0.2%–0.5%; bupivacaine 0.25%–0.5%
   d. Adjuvant (0.5–1 mL per plane): Particulate or nonparticulate steroid
3. **Position**
   a. Supine

Procedure Technique

Transversus Thoracis Plane (TTP) Block

1. **Prepare equipment and supplies, position the patient supine, and sterilize the procedural area with antiseptic solution.**
2. **Identify the correct rib level by counting caudally from the 1st rib or cephalad from the 12th rib.** Take note that patients may have anatomic variations in their number of ribs.
3. **Place the ultrasound probe in a parasagittal position to visualize the T4–T5 intercostal space.** The probe should be just lateral to the sternal border and should visualize the costosternal joint.
4. **Visualize the target for TTP block (Figure 3.8.4)**. The nerves lie between the internal intercostal and transversus throracis muscles. Visualize pleura and ensure it is out of the anticipated path of the needle to avoid injury.
5. **Inject local anesthetic subcutaneously for analgesia at the procedural site.**
6. **Use the procedure needle and advance with an in-plane approach to deposit injectate in the TTP (Figure 3.8.4).**
7. **Repeat the procedure at various levels as required.**

Superficial Thoracic Plane (STP) Block

1. **Prepare equipment and supplies, position the patient supine, and sterilize the procedural area with antiseptic solution.**
2. **Place the ultrasound probe in a transverse position at the level of the pain along the sternum.** The probe should be moved laterally to visualize the costosternal joint.
3. **Visualize the target for STP block (Figure 3.8.5)**. The nerves lie between the pectoralis major muscle and the sternum. Visualize pleura and ensure it is out of the anticipated path of the needle to avoid injury.
4. **Inject local anesthetic subcutaneously for analgesia at the procedural site.**
5. **Use the procedure and advance with an in-plane approach to deposit injectate in the STP (Figure 3.8.5).**
6. **Repeat the procedure at various levels as required.**

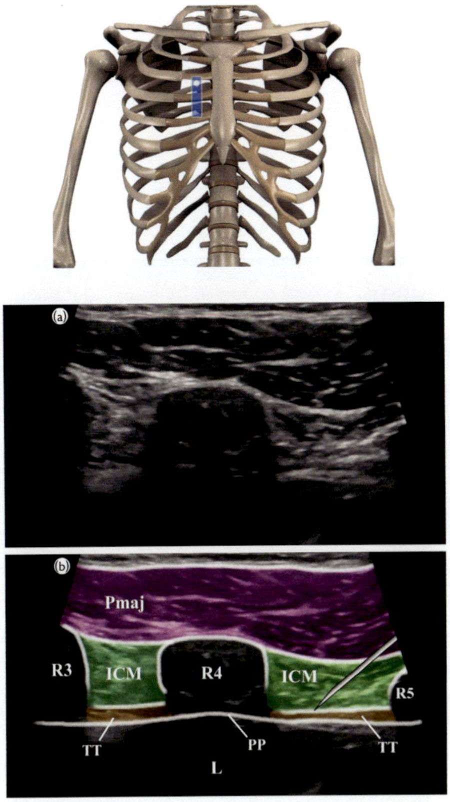

Figure 3.8.4 **a,** Ultrasound image of the anterior thorax at the level of the 4th–5th ribs in a parasternal sagittal plane. **b,** Labeled ultrasound image of in-plane needle placement for a transversus thoracis plane block in short-axis. *Pmaj* pectoralis major, *R3* 3rd rib, *R4* 4th rib, *R5* 5th rib, *ICM* intercostal muscle, *TT* transversus thoracis muscle, *PP* parietal pleura, *L* lung.

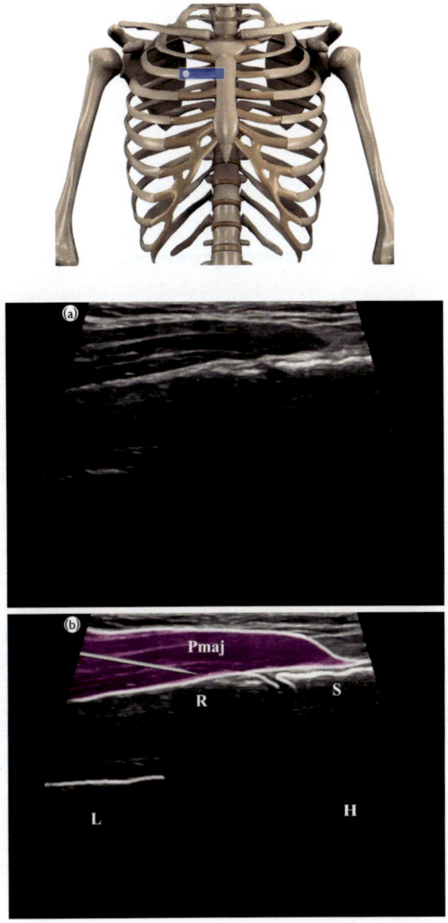

Figure 3.8.5 **a,** Ultrasound image of the anterior thorax at the level of the 3rd rib in an axial plane. **b,** Labeled ultrasound image of in-plane needle placement for a superficial thoracic plane block in short-axis. *Pmaj* pectoralis major, *R* 3rd rib, *S* sternum, *L* lung, *H* heart.

Tips and Safety Considerations

- Use doppler imaging to identify satellite vessels to avoid inadvertent puncture and intravascular injection.
- Avoid a steep TTP approach, to prevent puncture of the heart or lung tissue.

Post-Op Management Considerations

Although the risk of developing pneumothorax is low after an STP/TTP block, any difficulty in breathing after the procedure should be evaluated by obtaining a bedside chest X-ray. Supplemental oxygen should be made available to the patient and if required, a chest tube can be inserted if pneumothorax is suspected.

References

1. H. Ueshima and A. Kitamura, "Clinical experiences of ultrasound-guided transversus thoracic muscle plane block: a clinical experience," Journal of Clinical Anesthesia, vol. 27, no. 5, pp. 428–429, 2015.
2. Y. Ohgoshi, K. Ino, and M. Matsukawa, "Ultrasound-guided parasternal intercostal nerve block," Journal of Anesthesia and Clinical Research, vol. 30, no. 5, p. 916, 2016.
3. S. Fujii, D. Vissa, S. Ganapathy, M. Johnson, and J. Zhou, "Transversus thoracic muscle plane block on a cadaver with history of coronary artery bypass grafting," Regional Anesthesia and Pain Medicine, vol. 42, no. 4, pp. 535–537, 2017.
4. H. Ueshima and H. Otake, "Where is an appropriate injection point for an ultrasound-guided transversus thoracic muscle plane block?" Journal of Clinical Anesthesia, vol. 33, pp. 190–191, 2016.
5. R. Del Buono, F. Costa, and F. E. Agrò, "Parasternal, pecto-intercostal, pecs, and transverse thoracic muscle plane blocks: a rose by any other name would smell as sweet," Regional Anesthesia and Pain Medicine, vol. 41, no. 6, pp. 791–792, 2016.
6. E. Piraccini, G. Biondi, H. Byrne et al., "Ultrasound guided transversus thoracic plane block, parasternal block and fascial planes hydrodissection for internal mammary post thoracotomy pain syndrome," European Journal of Pain, vol. 22, no. 9, pp. 1673–1677, 2018.
7. D. M. Pöpping, N. Elia, E. Marret et al., "Protective effects of epidural analgesia on pulmonary complications after abdominal and thoracic surgery: a meta-analysis," Archives of Surgery, vol. 143, no. 10, pp. 990–999; discussion 1000, 2008.
8. L. Guimarães-Pereira, P. Reis, F. Abelha, L. F. Azevedo, and J. M. Castro-Lopes, "Persistent postoperative pain after cardiac surgery: a systematic review with meta-analysis regarding incidence and pain intensity," Pain, vol. 158, no. 10, pp. 1869–1885, 2017.
9. H. V. Bhatt, N. Hernandez, and A. Shariat, "Successful use of serratus and transversus thoracic plane blocks for subcutaneous implantable cardioverter-defibrillator placement," Journal of Cardiothoracic and Vascular Anesthesia, vol. 32, no. 1, pp. e22–e23, 2018.
10. E. Bignami, A. Castella, V. Pota et al., "Perioperative pain management in cardiac surgery: a systematic review," Minerva Anestesiologica, vol. 84, no. 4, pp. 488–503, 2018.
11. K. P. Thomas, S. Sainudeen, S. Jose, M. Y. Nadhari, and P. B. Macaire, "Ultrasound-guided parasternal block allows optimal pain relief and ventilation improvement after a sternal fracture," Pain and Therapy, vol. 5, no. 1, pp. 115–122, 2016.

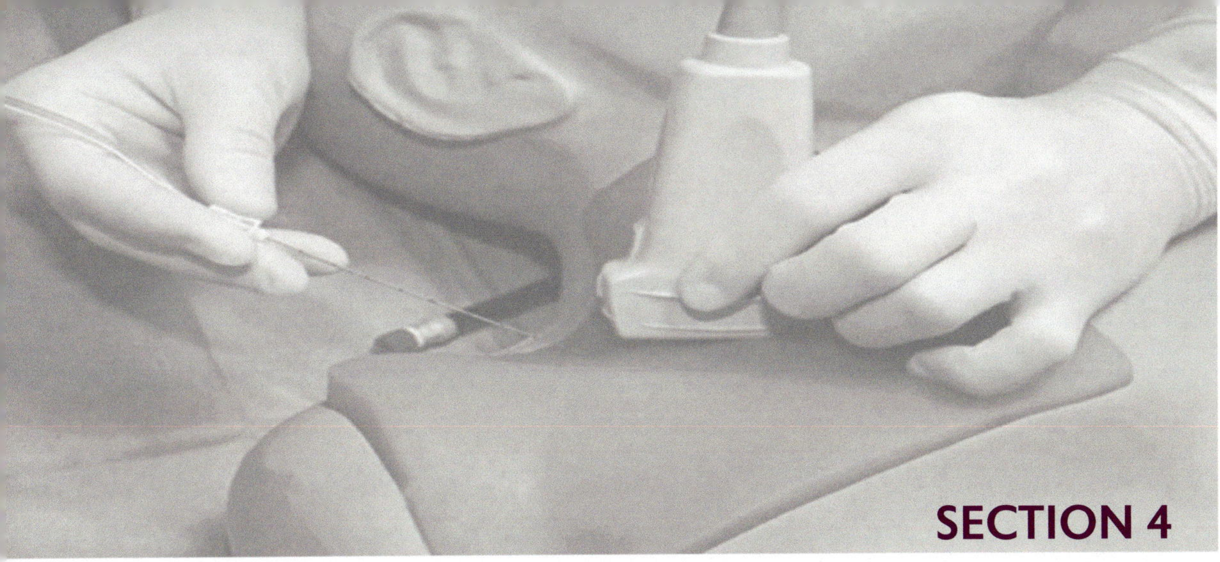

SECTION 4

ABDOMINOPELVIC SECTION

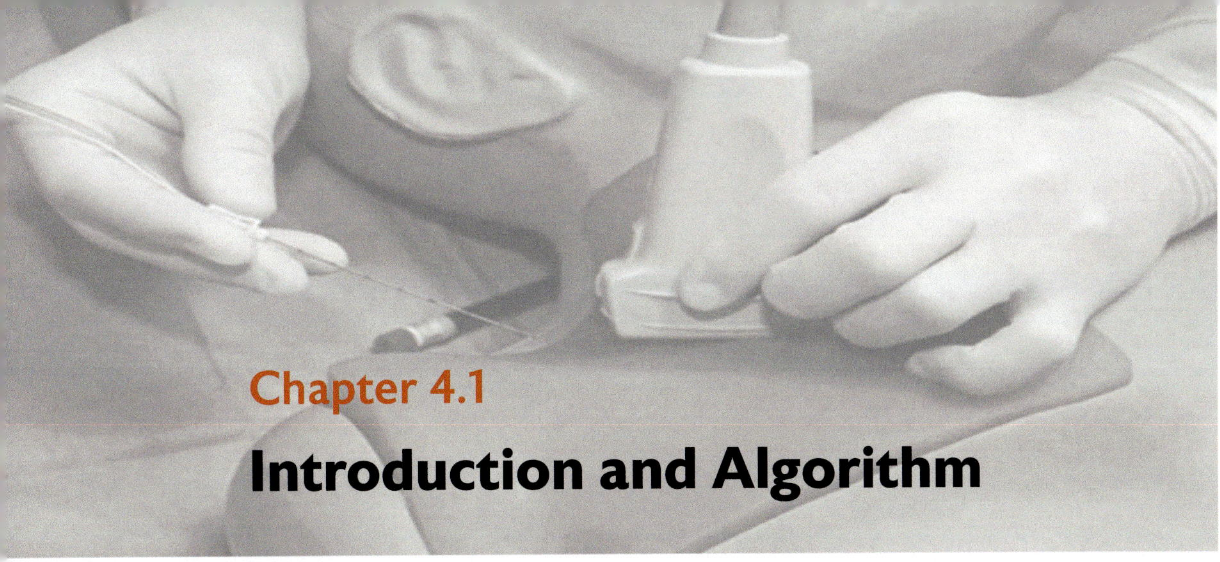

Chapter 4.1

Introduction and Algorithm

Amitabh Gulati

Contents

Introduction

During embryologic development, the gut is divided into three major divisions: the foregut, midgut, and hindgut. These are respectively supplied by branches of the celiac artery, the superior mesenteric artery, and the inferior mesenteric artery.[1] The major derivatives of each division are listed below in Table 4.1.1. Neural innervation to these organs follows the celiac, superior mesenteric, and inferior mesenteric plexuses, which can be targeted with interventional pain treatment strategies.[2,3]

Malignancy-Related Visceral Pain

Common cancers of the abdomen and pelvis include pancreatic, liver, colorectal, bladder, renal, prostate, and gynecologic (ovarian, uterine, and cervical) cancers. Many of these cancers present with visceral pain that is characterized as diffuse, poorly localized, and dull in nature, and may be related to capsular distention. This presentation is due to the location of afferent nerve fibers within the viscera and the convergence of sympathetic and parasympathetic inputs into the central nervous system.[4]

Table 4.1.1 Major Derivatives of the Primitive Gut during Embryonic Development

Foregut	Midgut	Hindgut
Trachea & respiratory tract	Lower duodenum	Distal 1/3 of transverse colon
Lungs	Jejunum	Descending colon
Esophagus	Ileum	Sigmoid colon
Stomach	Cecum	Rectum
Liver	Appendix	Upper anal canal
Gallbladder & bile ducts	Ascending colon	Urogenital sinus
Pancreas (dorsal & ventral)	Proximal 2/3 of transverse colon	
Upper duodenum		

Tumor infiltration of the pancreatic head results in pain that is localized to the epigastrium and radiates to the back. The upper abdominal organs such as the pancreas and stomach are innervated by the sympathetic preganglionic fibers from thoracic splanchnic nerves: the greater (T5–T10), lesser (T10–T11), and least (T12) splanchnic nerves. The celiac plexus is usually located at the level of the T12–L1 vertebral body. Hepatic cancer can present with pain due to infiltration of liver capsule, hepatic vessels, or the biliary tract.[2,3]

The liver parenchyma is innervated by the hepatic plexus, which carries both sympathetic and parasympathetic fibers (from the vagus nerve); whereas the liver capsule also carries innervation from the lower intercostal nerves (typically T7-T11). Hence, pain due to liver malignancy typically presents as a dull right subcostal pain. Distension of the liver can also place pressure on the diaphragm or biliary tract, resulting in referred pain transmitted via the phrenic nerve to the right supraclavicular region.

Gastric cancer patients can present with visceral epigastric pain due to the innervation of the stomach. Sympathetic innervation is provided from presynaptic sympathetic fibers of the greater thoracic splanchnic nerves from T6 to T10 segments.[2,3] Parasympathetic innervation comes from the vagus trunk.[2,3]

The small intestine and colon up to the splenic flexure receive parasympathetic innervation from the vagus nerve and sympathetic innervation from the greater (T5–T9) and lesser (T10–T11) thoracic splanchnic nerves. These nerves synapse via the celiac and superior mesenteric plexuses. Distal to the splenic flexure, the remainder of the gastrointestinal tract is innervated by sympathetic innervation from the lumbar splanchnic nerves (L1–L2) via the inferior mesenteric plexus. Retroperitoneal lymphadenopathy, bowel obstruction, ureteric obstruction, and peritoneal carcinomatosis can also cause visceral pain syndromes.[5]

Thirty to fifty percent of patients with prostate cancer also have pain.[6] These patients often present with rectal pain, perineal pain, and tenesmus. Renal cell cancer usually presents with flank pain but can also cause other pains as it often metastasizes to the Lymphatic system, lung, liver, bone, and adrenal glands. The kidney is innervated by sympathetic, parasympathetic, and afferent sensory fibers. Sympathetic fibers from T10–L1 form the renal plexus via synapses in aorticorenal ganglia, celiac ganglia, and lesser splanchnic nerves.[7] Gynecologic malignancies will often present with pelvic pain and pelvic floor dysfunction due to viscerosomatic convergence of the innervation within the pelvic organs. Dual projections from the thoracolumbar and sacral segments of the spinal cord play a role in innervation of the pelvic organs.[8]

Malignancy-Related Somatic Pain

Nociceptive somatic pain arising from gastrointestinal and genitourinary cancers presents as pelvic or abdominal wall pain. The perineal area can present with localized pain due to tumor involvement of the local musculature or neural invasion. Hepatic or colorectal malignancies can give rise to abdominal metastases with localized pain. Specific peripheral nerve blocks and fascial plane blocks can be utilized to alleviate pain arising from these localized areas.

Pain arising from metastatic bone disease is common in various malignancies, with prostate cancer being the most common.[9–11] Tumor infiltration of the bone causes pain, osteolysis, and bone sclerosis. This weakens bone, increasing the risk of pathologic fractures and leading to secondary pain issues. If the pain is due to metastatic disease in the spine, it can be treated interventionally with epidurals, medial branch blocks, and ablative techniques.[12]

Malignancy-Related Neuropathic Pain

Infiltration of tumor into neural structures causes neuropathic pain, sensory changes, and motor deficits in the specific neural territory. In addition, chemoradiation-induced fibrosis and damage to neural elements can also cause neuropathic pain. The distribution of pain and deficits depends on whether the tumor is infiltrating the central nervous system, nerve root, plexus, or peripheral nerve.

Radiculopathy can present with involvement of the nerve root by tumor or damage by therapy such as surgery and radiation. With gastrointestinal and urological malignancies, the presentation can be along the thoracic, lumbar, or sacral nerve roots.

Plexopathy is seen when pathology involves the plexus itself or the distal nerve roots. It often presents as poorly defined neurologic symptoms involving the lumbar or sacral plexuses and may be accompanied by autonomic changes as well. When the lumbar plexus is involved there is pathology around the psoas muscle which affects the L1–L4 nerve roots. The presentation will usually be pain in the proximal leg, thigh, and knee. Renal, gynecologic, and rectal cancers can affect the L4–S1 nerves along the plexus resulting in pain along the posterior leg, buttock, and foot. Perineal pain is a manifestation of the sacral plexus and nerve roots and can be associated with anal sphincter dysfunction.[13] Isolated mononeuropathies are uncommon in gastrointestinal and urological malignancies but can involve the intercostal, lateral femoral cutaneous, hypogastric, ilioinguinal, or pudendal nerves.

Treatment-Related Pain Syndromes

Treatment of gastrointestinal and urological malignancies may result in pain symptoms due to chemotherapy, surgery, and radiation. The platinum agents are a mainstay in treating urologic and gynecologic tumors, and these are a known cause of chemotherapy-induced peripheral neuropathy (CIPN).[14] Although transient for most patients, CIPN can persist as a chronic pain syndrome.

Surgical treatment is the mainstay of therapy for most gastrointestinal and genitourinary malignancies. Given the nature of the surgeries performed, various chronic pain syndromes can arise as complications from surgery. Entrapment of adjacent nerves and placements of abdominal drains can result in abdominal wall pain and visceral abdominopelvic pain.

Radiation treatment can cause nerve axon injury, tissue fibrosis, and vascular damage to nerves in the radiation field. Abdominal radiation treatment commonly results in lumbosacral plexopathy and as mentioned above, can present with weakness, sensory changes, and neuropathic pain in one or both legs. A common presentation in these malignancies is radiation-induced enteritis. Following tissue ischemia, neovascularization and fibrosis cause abdominal pain, bowel changes, and bloating.

Treatment Algorithm

Given the various pain syndromes that can arise within this anatomic area, it is critical to appreciate the neurologic structures that are involved in pain initiation and transmission. These specific foci can then be targeted using peripheral blocks, neuraxial blocks, neurolytic blocks, or intrathecal pump implantation. The embryologic distinction between foregut, midgut, and hindgut structures is important in targeting specific neuroanatomic structures for pain therapy. Specific plexus anatomy is involved in pain transmission for various organs and provides a roadmap for therapeutic targets (Figure 4.1.1a). Somatic and neuropathic pain localized to specific nerve targets can be targeted by peripheral nerve blocks. Depending on the response to these diagnostic blocks, more invasive strategies can be utilized for effective and longer lasting analgesia (Figure 4.1.1b).

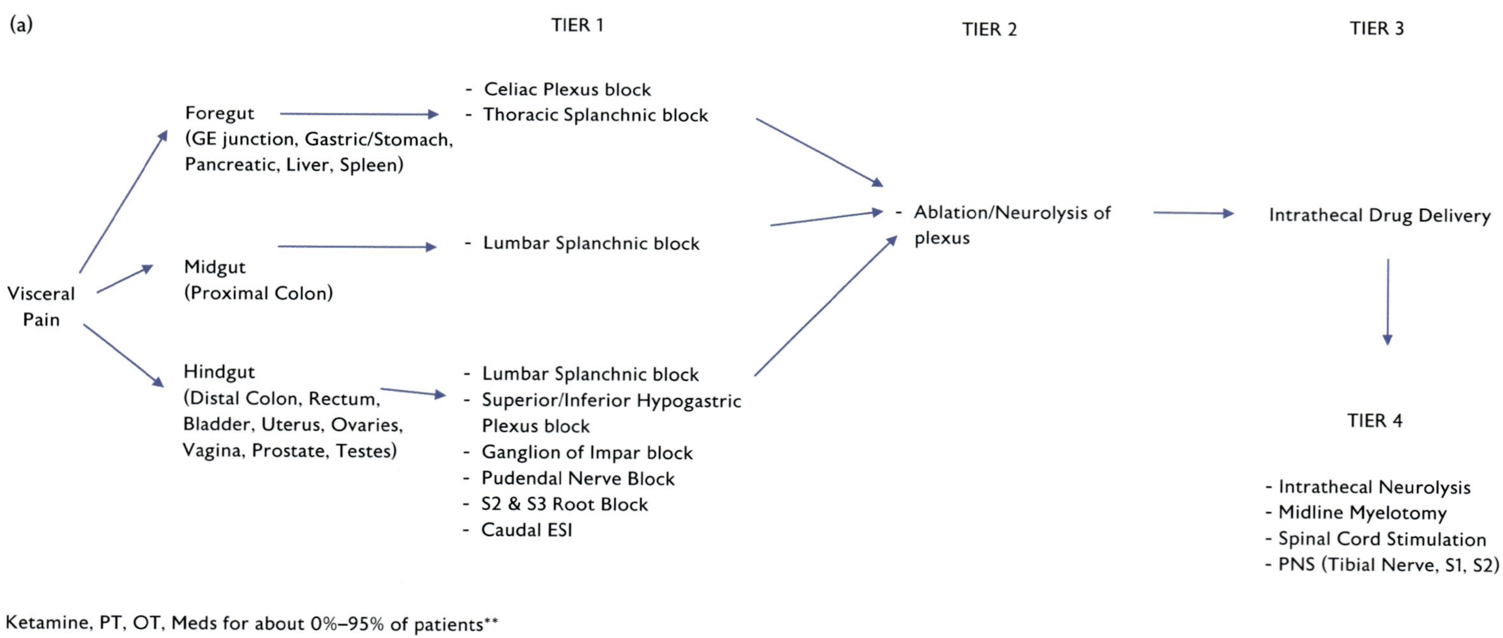

Figure 4.1.1 Interventional algorithm for abdominopelvic pain. **a,** Visceral abdominopelvic pain. **b,** Somatic/neuropathic abdominopelvic pain.

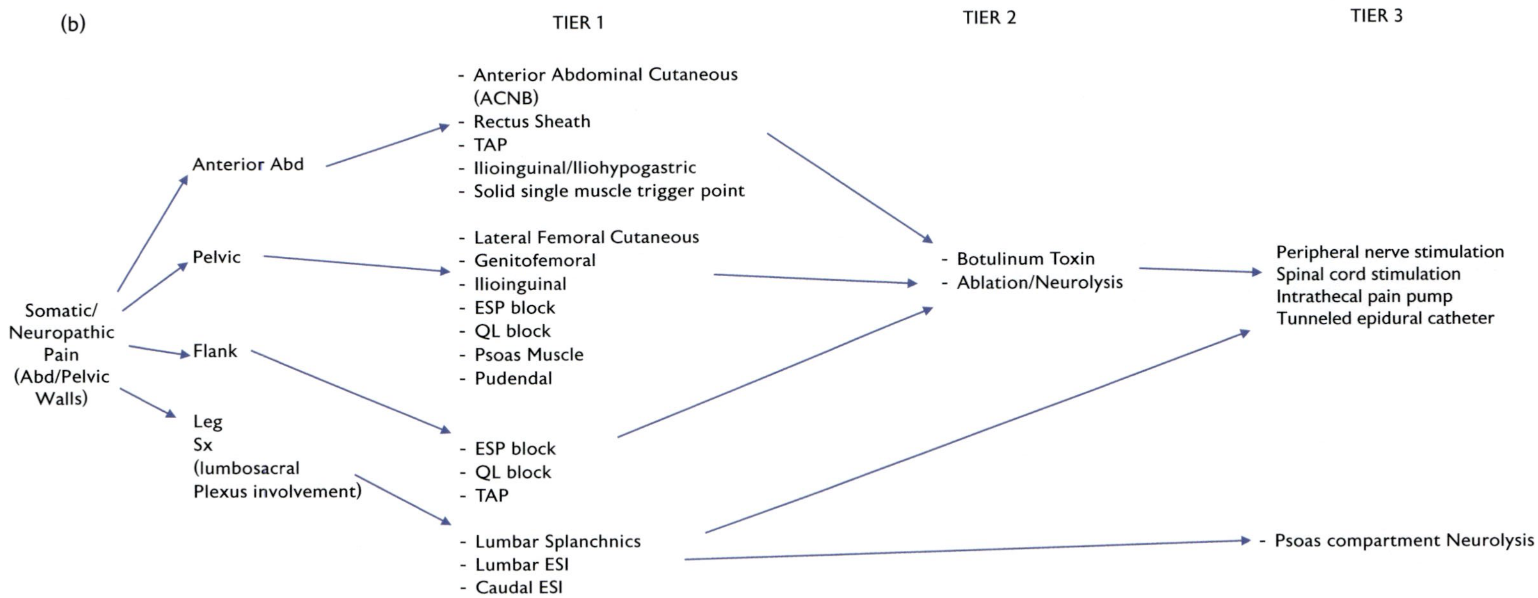

Figure 4.1.1 Continued

Table 4.1.2 Contraindications to Abdominopelvic Interventions

Contraindications	Related Types
Absolute	Patient refusal or inability to consent, active infection over site of injection
Special Consideration	Immunocompromised state, abnormal anatomy (postsurgical intervention), position tolerance
Relative	Abnormal coagulation profile, use of anticoagulants, local or uncontrolled systemic infection, allergy to local anesthetics or contrast

Contraindications

Patient refusal or inability to consent for the procedure are absolute contraindications. In the cancer population, consideration should be given to the immune status of the patient. Relative contraindications are active infection at the injection site, sepsis, coagulopathy, bleeding dyscrasia, allergy to local anesthetic medication, hemodynamic instability, and anatomical abnormalities. Patients undergoing chemotherapy and/or radiation therapy have an increased risk of infection from an invasive procedure while in an immunocompromised state. Additionally, the potential for acquired abnormal anatomy should be considered as patients with cancer may have regional invasion of disease or postsurgical changes (Table 4.1.2).

Special considerations in the cancer population also include positioning tolerance. Patients with large-volume ascites can have difficulty with prone positioning. Shared decision-making is important in all clinical settings, and especially with palliative care in cancer patients. The relief of refractory visceral pain outweighing the risks of a procedure must be considered if quality of life is a main objective.

Conclusions

Knowledge of the underlying neuroanatomy is important for devising patient-centered treatment plans based on clinical presentations. There are a wide variety of interventional targets in the abdomen and pelvis, which will be discussed in detail in the following chapters. The algorithm presented in this chapter serves as a step-by-step approach to managing pain in the oncologic population and is organized from the least invasive to most invasive strategies.

References

1. Sadler TW. Chapters 15 and 16. *Langman's Medical Embryology*. Wolters Kluwer; 2018.
2. Moore KL et al. *Clinically Oriented Anatomy*. Lippincott Williams & Wilkins; 2013.
3. Agur AMR et al. *Grant's Atlas of Anatomy*. Lippincott Williams & Wilkins; 2013.
4. *Cancer Pain: Assessment and Management*. Cambridge University Press; 2010.
5. Pak D et al. Chapter 11: Gastrointestinal Cancer Pain. Gulati A et al. (eds.). *Essentials of Interventional Cancer Pain Management*. 1st ed. Springer Nature; 2019: 97–106.
6. Siegel R et al. Cancer statistics, 2014. *CA: A Cancer Journal for Clinicians* 64.1 2014: 9–29.
7. Ali M et al. Anatomy of the pelvic plexus and innervation of the prostate gland. *Clinical Anatomy* 17.2 2004: 123–129.
8. Janing W et al. Pain Arising from the Urogenital Tract. Maggi CA (ed.). *Nervous Control of the Urogenital System*. Harwood Academic; 1998: 300–310.
9. Coleman RE. Metastatic bone disease: clinical features, pathophysiology and treatment strategies. *Cancer Treatment Reviews* 27.3 2001: 165–176.
10. Serafini AN. Therapy of metastatic bone pain. *Journal of Nuclear Medicine* 42.6 2001: 895–906.
11. Buga S et al. The management of pain in metastatic bone disease. *Cancer Control* 19.2 2012: 154–166.
12. Birthi P et al. Interventional treatment of refractory cancer pain. *Cancer Journal* 19.5 2013: 390–396.
13. Brejt N et al. Pelvic radiculopathies, lumbosacral plexopathies, and neuropathies in oncologic disease: a multidisciplinary approach to a diagnostic challenge. *Cancer Imaging* 13.4 2013: 591.
14. Quasthoff S et al. Chemotherapy-induced peripheral neuropathy. *Journal of Neurology* 249 2002: 9–17

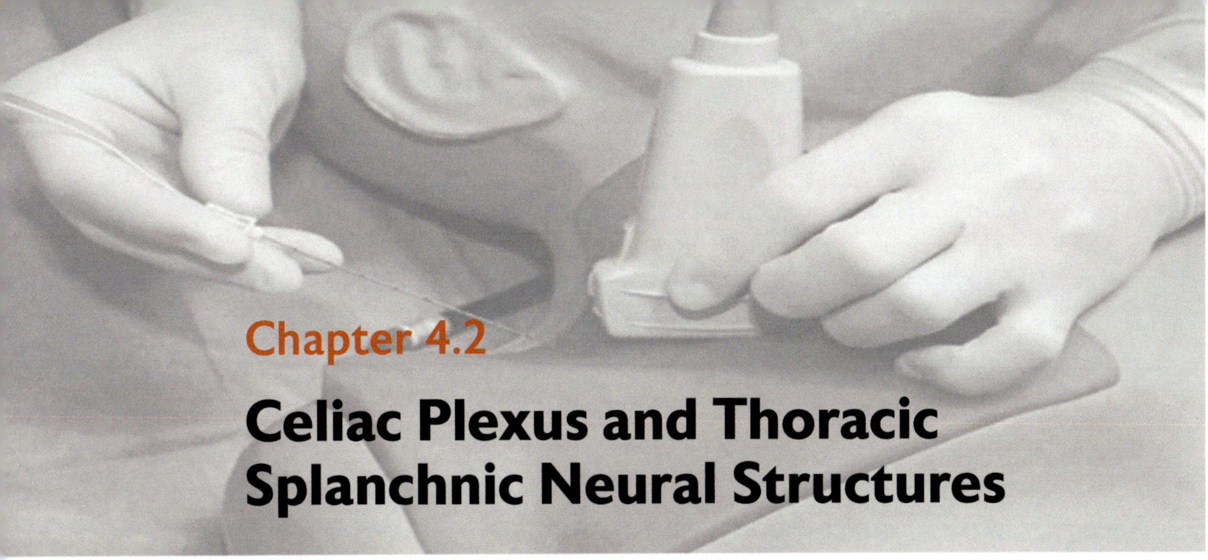

Chapter 4.2

Celiac Plexus and Thoracic Splanchnic Neural Structures

Lucas First

Contents

Introduction

Major intra-abdominal organs (embryologically, the foregut organs) such as the stomach, proximal small intestine, colon, pancreas, liver, and gallbladder can cause significant pain from a multitude of oncologic diseases. The autonomic innervation of these structures is via the celiac plexus, making the plexus a potential target for neurolysis in patients suffering from abdominal visceral pain. Up to 90% of patients with advanced stage pancreatic cancer report abdominal pain.[1,2] In a randomized controlled trial, Wong et al.[3] demonstrated the powerful analgesic effect of a neurolytic celiac plexus block (NCPB). They found that in pancreatic cancer, the block achieved significantly better pain control when compared to optimized systemic analgesic therapy. NCPB has been reported to provide effective pain relief in pancreatic cancer–related pain in up to 74% of patients.[4] There are two common approaches, a transcrural celiac plexus block and a retrocrural thoracic splanchnic block. Different techniques have been utilized to assist with needle guidance to the correct anatomic location, including fluoroscopy, computed tomography (CT), endoscopic ultrasound, and percutaneous ultrasound. We will detail the use of fluoroscopy, CT, and percutaneous ultrasound in this chapter.

Indications

Celiac plexus nerve block is indicated for intractable abdominal pain from malignant and chronic nonmalignant sources after failed adequate analgesia with more conservative measures. The leading indication for the block is pancreatic cancer, which was first described over a century ago by Kappis[5] (Table 4.2.1). Other benign and malignant cancers from the stomach, small intestine, liver, biliary tree, and colon (ascending through midtransverse) can be addressed with an NCPB.[6–10] The most common non-malignant indication is chronic pancreatitis, where it has been used with varying success. It has also been used in treatment for pain due to median arcuate ligament syndrome.[11–12]

Critical Anatomy

The celiac plexus consists of multiple large ganglia including the celiac, aorticorenal, and superior mesenteric ganglia (Figure 4.2.1). Part of the autonomic nervous system, it is responsible for the relay of both sympathetic and parasympathetic efferent signals. Additionally, the celiac plexus transmits sensory afferent signals from visceral abdominal organs.

The thoracic splanchnic nerves are made up of the greater (T5–T9), lesser (T10–T11), and least (T12) splanchnic nerves, which carry presynaptic sympathetic fibers originating from the thoracic sympathetic chain and synapse within the ganglia of the celiac plexus. The anatomic distinction between the thoracic splanchnic nerves and the celiac plexus is important. The splanchnic nerves are located superior to the diaphragm and travel inferiorly before piercing the crus of the diaphragm and reaching the celiac plexus. The celiac plexus is located inferior to the diaphragm, sitting anterolaterally to the aorta, at approximately the L1 vertebral level.[11–12] Parasympathetic fibers synapsing in the plexus originate from the vagus nerve.

Nociceptive sensory afferent fibers carry pain signals from the pancreas, stomach, small intestine, liver, biliary tree, and colon (ascending through midtransverse). Pain from the omentum and mesentery may also be transmitted in these fibers, potentially as the result of diffuse metastatic disease to these structures.

Equipment and Patient Preparation

1. **Monitors and Sterility**
   a. No specific monitors are needed for this procedure, but emergency resuscitation equipment should be available immediately. This includes ACLS drugs, supplemental oxygen, airway adjuncts, and suction.

Table 4.2.1 Indications for Celiac Plexus or Thoracic Splanchnic Block

Indications	Celiac Plexus and Thoracic Splanchnic Block Mechanism
Diagnostic Nerve Block	Initial single injection block with local anesthetic to determine efficacy of temporary pain relief. If successful, proceed with a subsequent neurolytic block, usually with a chemical neurolytic.
Pancreatic Cancer	Relieves pain secondary to pancreatic cancer. May be more effective if tumor burden is located in the head of pancreas as opposed to the tail.
Other Intra-abdominal Cancers	Relieves pain arising from a variety of cancers including stomach, small intestine, liver, biliary tree, and colon (ascending through midtransverse).
Chronic Pancreatitis	Manages abdominal pain secondary to chronic pancreatitis. Evidence remains marginal when compared to use in pancreatic cancer.

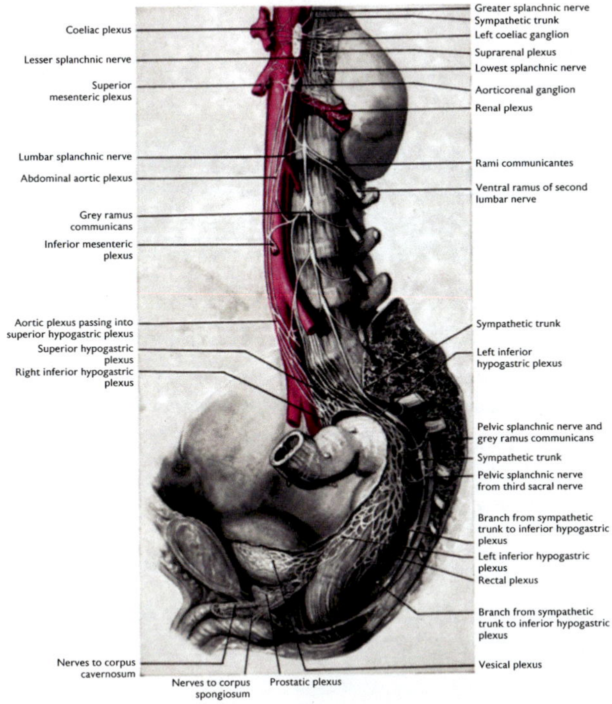

Figure 4.2.1 Anatomical representation of the celiac plexus. (Reprinted with permission from Cunningham's Manual of Practical Anatomy: Thorax and Abdomen, 16th Edition)

b. Strict antiseptic technique should be observed including sterile probe cover, ultrasound gel, and sterile gloves. Chlorhexidine or other skin prep agent should be used to clean the skin prior to commencing the procedure.

2. Equipment

a. Imaging:
   i. CT-guided intervention: Conventional computerized X-ray imaging/tomography (CT) machine
   ii. Fluoroscopy-guided intervention: Conventional fluoroscope with C-arm capability
   iii. Ultrasound-guided intervention: Low-frequency (2–5 MHz) curvilinear array ultrasound probe

b. Needle type:
   i. CT/Fluoroscopy: 22- or 25-gauge, 5- to 7-inch needle
   ii. Ultrasound: 22- or 25-gauge, 5-inch spinal needle

c. Local anesthetic (retrocrural—9 mL each side; transcrural—15–20 mL): Lidocaine 1%–2%; ropivacaine 0.2%–0.5%; bupivacaine 0.25%–0.5%

d. Adjuvant (1 mL): Nonparticulate or particulate steroid

e. Neurolysis (retrocrural—10–15 mL; transcrural—15–20 mL): 10% phenol or 50%–100% ethanol[2]

3. Position

a. Prone (CT/fluoroscopy)

b. Supine (ultrasound)

Step-by-Step Technique

CT Approach (Figure 4.2.2)

1. Once the patient is positioned, area prepped, and prescan CT has been complete, start by using local anesthetic for skin wheal; bilaterally at the predetermined paravertebral region.

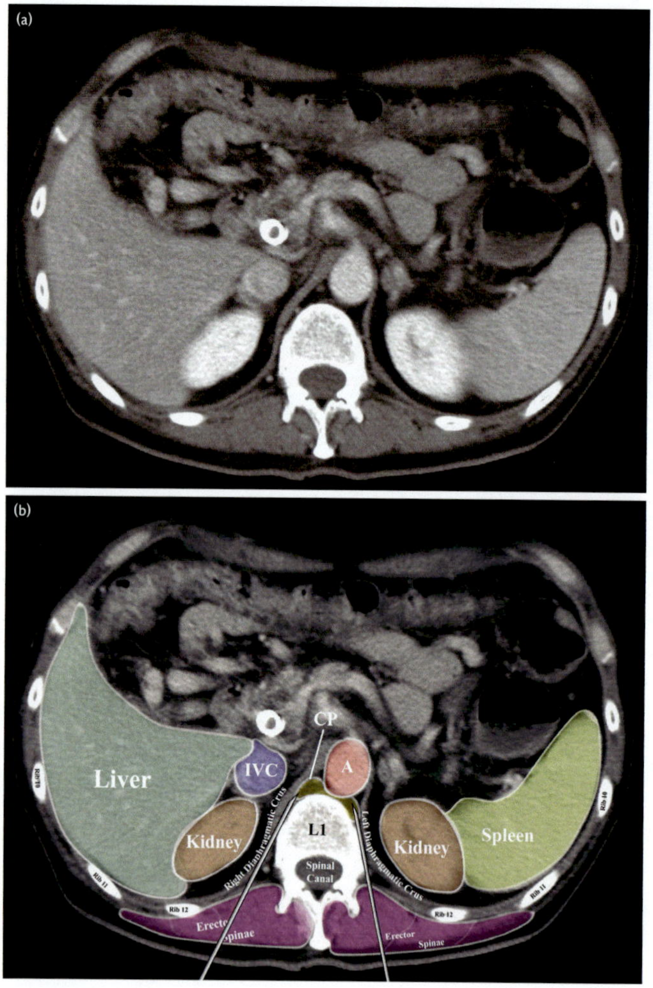

Figure 4.2.2 a/b, Axial CT image at the L1 level above the transverse process illustrating the bilateral retrocrural approach for a celiac plexus injection. *CP* Typical celiac plexus target area, *IVC* inferior vena cava, *A* aorta.

In order to familiarize the proceduralist to the anatomy, CT prescanning is critical. Normal anatomy may be distorted by abdominal malignancy.

2. **Initial advancement of the needle.** During planning, the initial angle and depth of the needle insertion are measured for a safe trajectory. Precise planning enables the proceduralist to avoid vital structures and easily access the correct anatomical region without encountering osseous structures such as the rib and transverse process.[7]
3. **Continue needle advancement in stepwise fashion as planned during simulation with periodic rescanning with CT.**
4. **Final needle positioning.** In the retrocrural approach, the needle tip will be posteromedial to the crus of the diaphragm and posterior to the pancreas and aorta at the level of T12 or L1. In relation to surrounding vasculature, ideal positioning is around the celiac trunk and the root of the superior mesenteric artery.[7]
5. **Contrast administration.** Deposit 1–2 mL of contrast.

6. **Confirmation.** CT scanning is now reperformed to confirm appropriate localization and spread of contrast. Posterior spread of contrast toward the neuroforamina must be ruled out before proceeding to neurolysis.
7. **Neurolysis.** Once an appropriate contrast pattern is confirmed, the neurolytic agent is injected.
8. **Repeat steps 2–7 on the contralateral side.**
9. **Ensure the patient has no motor or sensory changes in the lower extremities after the procedure.**

Fluoroscopy—Thoracic Splanchnic Block (Retrocrural Approach)

1. **Once the patient is positioned, area prepped, and equipment is ready, start by using local anesthetic for a skin wheal, superficial to the T12/L1 vertebral body and 6–8 cm from midline (Figure 4.2.3) bilaterally.** This approach requires targeting the thoracic splanchnic nerves bilaterally. The needles remain posterior to the crura of the diaphragm, hence the retrocrural approach. The C-arm is positioned obliquely 20–30 degrees toward the side of needle insertion (Figure 4.2.4). An additional 20–30 degrees of cephalad angulation is needed for visual optimization of the T12/L1 vertebral body.[8]
2. **Initial advancement of the needle.** The spinal needle is guided inferior to the 12th rib, superior to the transverse process of L1, and directly toward the anterolateral surface of the T12/L1 vertebral body. Repeated images are obtained to ensure accurate needle advancement.
3. **Lateral view.** The needle is then advanced 1–2 cm anteriorly to the anterior third of the T12/L1 vertebral body using a lateral safety view to assess depth (Figure 4.2.5).
4. **AP view.** The final needle position should be visualized medial to the lateral border of the T12/L1 vertebral body.
5. **Contrast administration.** The contrast pattern should be visualized over the anterolateral surface of the L1 vertebral body (Figures 4.2.6–7).

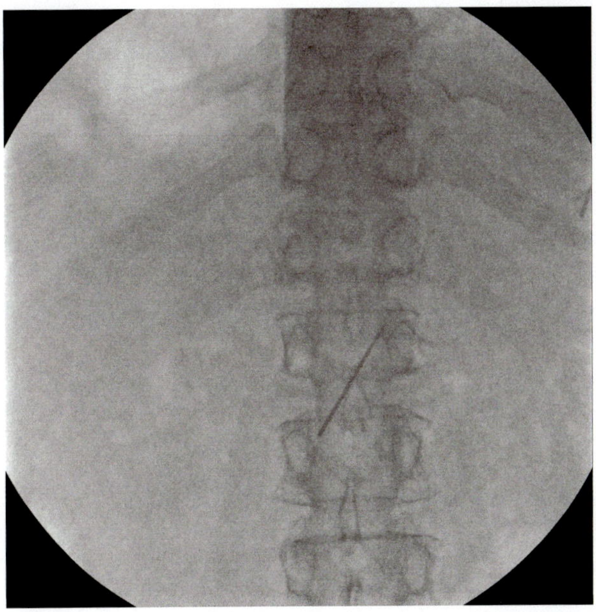

Figure 4.2.3 A-P fluoroscopic image with the upper tip of the needle marking the L1 level.

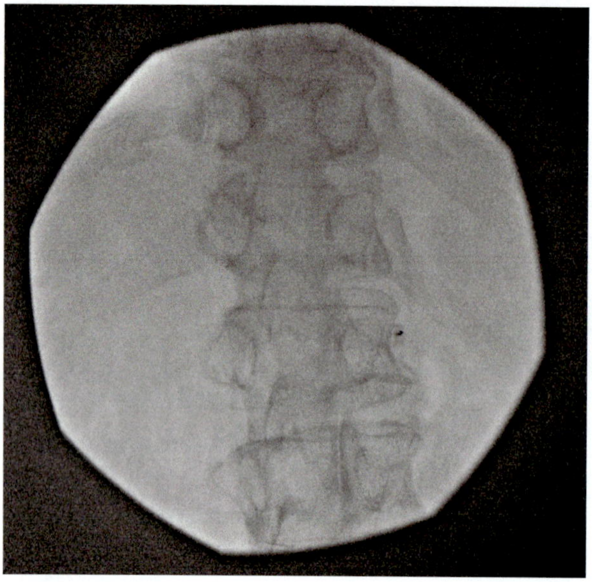

Figure 4.2.4 Fluoroscopic image with 20 degrees of obliquity toward the right side and a needle placed coaxially just superior the L1 transverse process and lateral to the vertebral body.

6. **Neurolysis.** Once an appropriate contrast pattern is confirmed, the neurolytic agent is injected.
7. **Repeat steps 2–6 on the contralateral side.**
8. **Ensure the patient has no motor or sensory changes in the lower extremities after the procedure.**

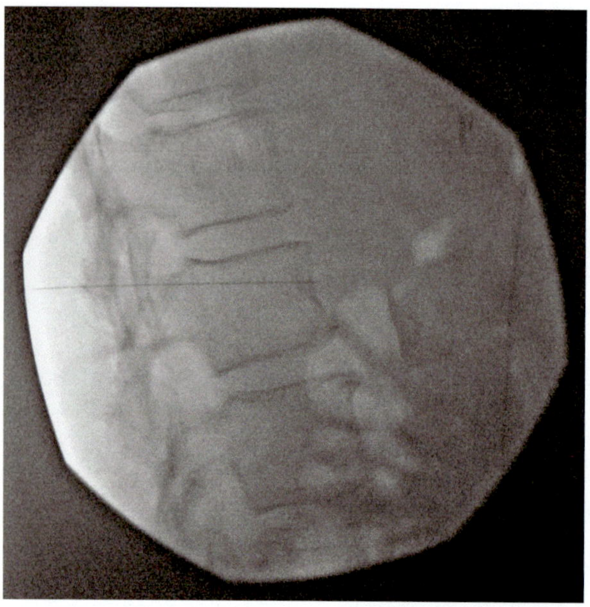

Figure 4.2.5 Lateral fluoroscopic image with the needle advanced just anteriorly to the anterior third of the L1 vertebral body for a retrocrural celiac plexus approach.

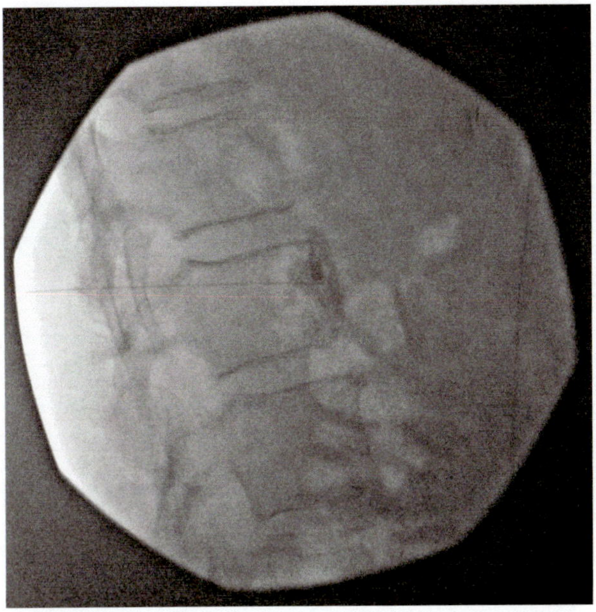

Figure 4.2.6 Lateral fluoroscopic image with contrast visualized over the anterolateral surface of the L1 vertebral body for a retrocrural celiac plexus approach.

Fluoroscopy—Transaortic/Transcrural Approach

1. **Once the patient is positioned, area prepped, and equipment is ready, start by using local anesthetic for a skin wheal, superficial to the superior margin of the L1 vertebral body, 6–8 cm from midline to the left.** The C-arm is positioned obliquely 20–30 degrees, optimizing

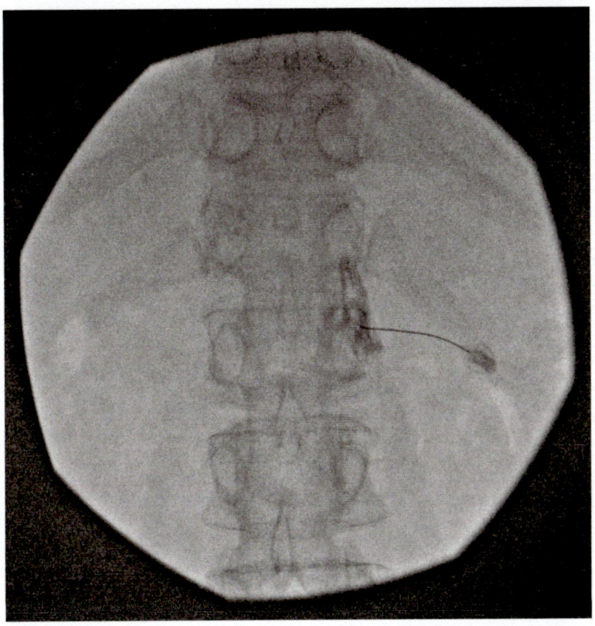

Figure 4.2.7 A-P fluoroscopic image with contrast visualized spreading medial to the lateral border of the L1 vertebral body and pedicle for a retrocrural celiac plexus approach.

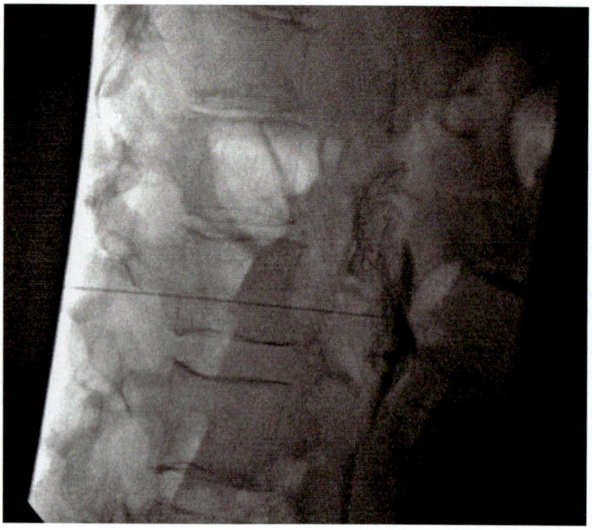

Figure 4.2.8 Lateral fluoroscopic image with contrast visualized over the anterior surface of the aorta at the L1 vertebral level for a transaortic/transcrural celiac plexus approach.

the view of the tip of the transverse process of L1 over the anterolateral margin of the L1 vertebral body.[8]

2. **Initial advancement of the needle.** The spinal needle is guided inferior to the 12th rib, superior to the transverse process of L1, and directly toward the anterolateral surface of the L1 vertebral body. Repeated images are obtained to ensure accurate needle advancement.
3. **Lateral view.** Once the needle has reached the anterolateral surface of the L1 vertebral body, the C-arm is repositioned into a lateral safety view before further needle advancement. The needle is then advanced until anterior to the L1 vertebral body. Careful aspiration should be performed with each minor advancement, as blood return may signal penetration of the aorta. If this occurs, continue to advance anteriorly until piercing the anterior wall of the aorta and no blood is returned with aspiration.
4. **AP view.** The final needle positioned should be visualized medial to the lateral border of the L1 vertebral body.
5. **Contrast administration.** Returning to a lateral view, 1–2 mL of contrast should be injected under live fluoroscopy. A pulsatile pattern as the contrast rests on the anterior surface of the aorta should be observed (Figure 4.2.8). Returning to an AP view, the contrast should be spread on both sides of midline (Figure 4.2.9).
6. **Neurolysis.** Once an appropriate contrast pattern is confirmed, the neurolytic agent is injected.
7. **Ensure the patient has no motor or sensory changes in the lower extremities after the procedure.**

Ultrasound Approach

1. **Once the patient is positioned, area prepped, and a prescan of the area is complete; start by using local anesthetic for a skin wheal.** The initial starting position of the ultrasound transducer is just caudal to the xiphoid process over the epigastrium.
2. **Identify the celiac trunk and superior mesenteric artery in short-axis and long-axis views.** The celiac trunk is the first major artery that comes off the abdominal aorta at this location (Figure 4.2.10), corresponding approximately to the T12 vertebral body. Moving caudally, the next artery to arise is the superior mesenteric artery at approximately L1.

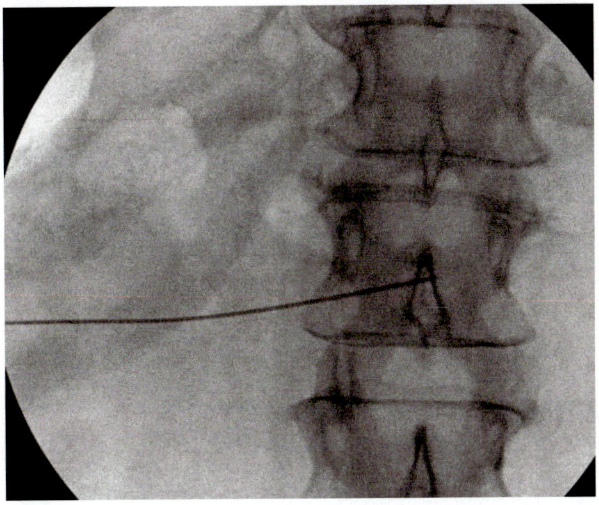

Figure 4.2.9 A-P fluoroscopic image with contrast visualized spread on both sides of midline at the L1 vertebral level for a transaortic/transcrural celiac plexus approach.

3. **Initial advancement of the needle.** The spinal needle is guided with real-time in-plane visualization as it enters the anterior abdominal wall. Advancement of the needle is performed in a short-axis view after the needle is introduced laterally to the ultrasound transducer.[5]
4. **Continue needle advancement.** Several critical structures will be in view during needle advancement, including the liver, pancreas, stomach, and superior mesenteric vein. Duplex mode is utilized to identify the ram-horn-like celiac trunk as it arises from the abdominal aorta.
5. **Final needle positioning.** The needle tip should be positioned just cephalad to the celiac artery trunk where the celiac plexus is located (Figure 4.2.10). Of note, the celiac plexus itself is not clearly visualized even by high-resolution ultrasound.
6. **Final safety measures.** Negative aspiration and a negative test dose should be completed to decrease the risk of intravascular injections.
7. **Neurolysis.** Once proper safety measures are complete, the neurolytic agent is injected in real time under direct visualization.
8. **Ensure the patient has no motor or sensory changes in the lower extremities after the procedure.**

Postprocedure Management

Transient diarrhea is the most common adverse event following an NCPB, previously reported in 44% of patients.[9] Orthostatic hypotension is the second most common adverse event, previously reported in 38% of patients.[9] It is critical to ensure the patient is properly hydrated before and after the procedure. Oral hydration is often sufficient; however, IV fluids may be necessary. Both orthostatic hypotension and diarrhea result from unopposed parasympathetic activity after the block, resulting in vasodilation and increased peristalsis respectively.

Other potential major complications include intravascular injection, pneumothorax, spinal cord injury, paralysis, retroperitoneal hematoma or abscess formation, and hematuria (if the kidney is incidentally punctured). These major complications have been reported in < 1% of cases.

The use of repeat NCPB in pancreatic cancer patients was investigated in a pilot study by McGreevy et al.[10] They reported the success rate of an initial NCPB as high as 67%, with the mean duration of pain relief approximately 3 months. On repeat NCPB, the success rate decreased to 29%. The authors postulated this decrease in efficacy was due to progression of disease, as supported by imaging.

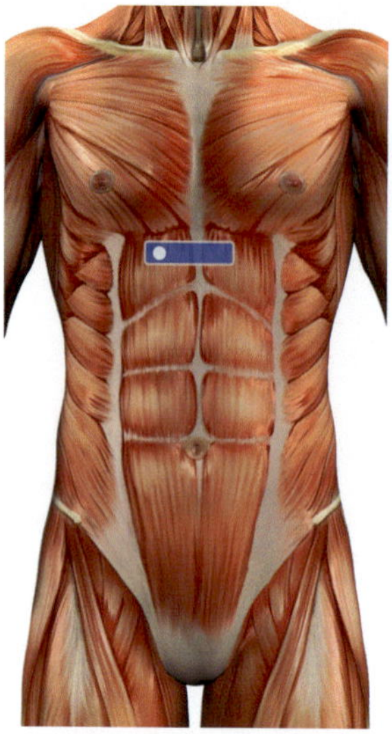

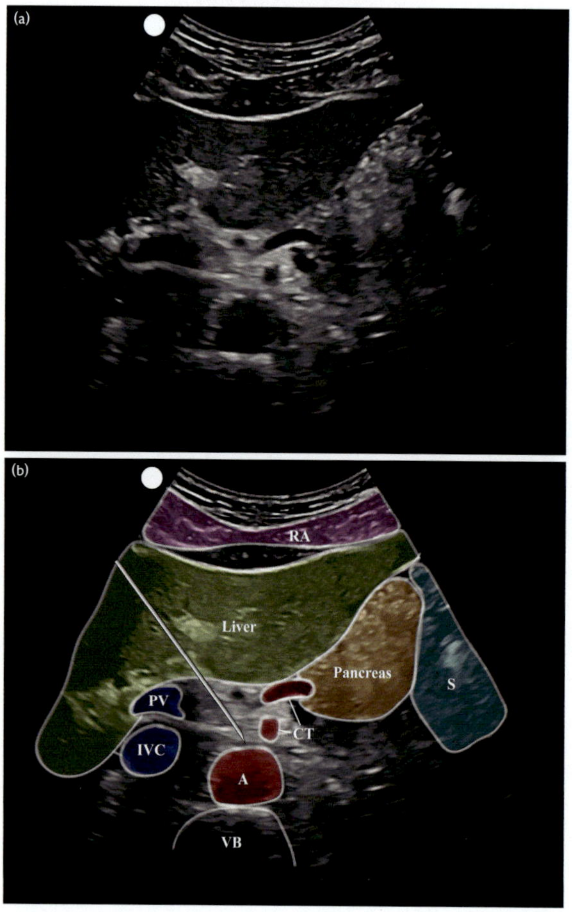

Figure 4.2.10 **a,** Ultrasound image of the right upper anterior abdomen in an axial plane. **b,** Labeled ultrasound image of in-plane needle placement for a celiac plexus block. *RA* rectus abdominis, *S* stomach, *PV* portal vein, *CT* celiac trunk, *IVC* inferior vena cava, *A* aorta, *VB* vertebral body.

References

1. Sachdev AH, Gress FG. Celiac plexus block and neurolysis: a review. Gastrointest Endosc Clin N Am. 2018;28(4):579–586.
2. Caraceni A, Portenoy RK. Pain management in patients with pancreatic carcinoma. Cancer. 1996;78(3 Suppl):639–653.
3. Wong GY, Schroeder DR, Carns PE, Wilson JL, Martin DP, Kinney MO, Mantilla CB, Warner DO. Effect of neurolytic celiac plexus block on pain relief, quality of life, and survival in patients with unresectable pancreatic cancer: a randomized controlled trial. JAMA. 2004;291(9):1092–1099.
4. Lohse I, Brothers SP. Pathogenesis and treatment of pancreatic cancer related pain. Anticancer Res. 2020;40(4):1789–1796.
5. Narouze SN. *Atlas of Ultrasound-Guided Procedures in Interventional Pain Management*. New York, NY: Springer, 2011. Print.
6. Pope JE, Deer TR. *Treatment of Chronic Pain Conditions: A Comprehensive Handbook*. New York, NY: Springer, 2017. Print.
7. Narouze, SN. *Multimodality Imaging Guidance in Interventional Pain Management*. New York, NY: Oxford, 2017. Print.
8. Rathmell JP. *Atlas of Image-Guided Intervention in Regional Anesthesia and Pain Medicine*. Philadelphia: Wolters Kluwer Health, 2015. Print.
9. Eisenberg E, Carr DB, Chalmers TC. Neurolytic celiac plexus block for treatment of cancer pain: a meta-analysis. Anesth Analg. 1995;80(2):290–295.
10. McGreevy K, Hurley RW, Erdek MA, Aner MM, Li S, Cohen SP. The effectiveness of repeat celiac plexus neurolysis for pancreatic cancer: a pilot study. Pain Pract. 2013;13(2):89–95.
11. Mercadante, Sebastiano, Nicosia, Francesco. Celiac plexus block: a reappraisal. Reg Anesth Pain Med. 1998;23(1):37–48.
12. Kambadakone A, Thabet A, Gervais DA, Mueller PR, Arellano RS. CT-guided celiac plexus neurolysis: a review of anatomy, indications, technique, and tips for successful treatment. *Radiographics*. 2011;31(6):1599–1621.

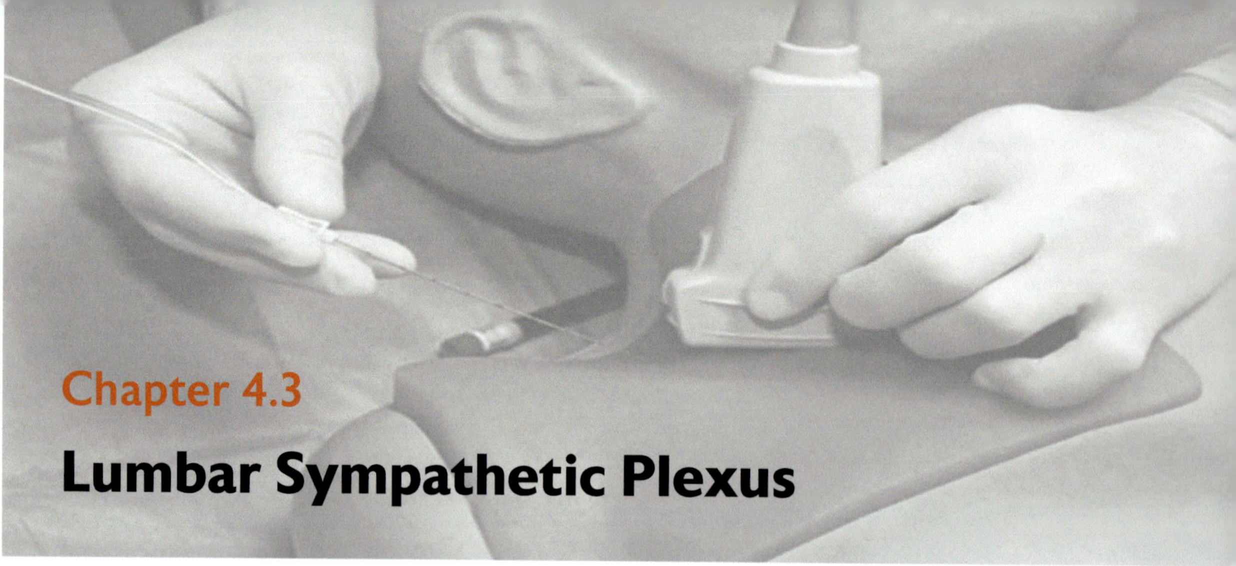

Chapter 4.3

Lumbar Sympathetic Plexus

Paul Ryan Haffey

Contents

Introduction

The sympathetic nervous system has been implicated in a variety of painful conditions that are difficult to treat. Pain in the cancer population arises from central and peripheral tumors, surgical resection, complex regional pain syndrome (CRPS), and postchemotherapy or postradiation treatment. Interventions targeting the lumbar sympathetic chain have proven to be beneficial in relieving sympathetically mediated pain related to the abdominal compartment, low back, and lower extremities. This is best achieved for the lower extremities by performing a lumbar sympathetic block (LSB).[1]

Indications

Cancer patients suffering from cancer-related back pain, abdominopelvic and lower extremity tumors, surgical resection, phantom limb, and invasion or compression of the lumbar plexus often obtain relief though a LSB. Active oncologic pain of both the pelvis and lower extremity may improve with a LSB. Radiation and surgery may create neuropathic pain syndromes, which improve with an LSB.

Relevant Anatomy

The lumbar sympathetic chain comprises paired ganglia that reside on the anterolateral aspect of the first through fourth lumbar vertebrae (Figure 4.3.1).[1] Preganglionic fibers exit the spinal canal alongside the ventral roots of the lumbar spinal nerves at each level to join the sympathetic chain as the white rami communicantes, which then synapse with the corresponding ganglion. These postganglionic fibers subsequently exit the chain to join the spinal nerves that form the lumbar and lumbosacral plexuses or meet to form the vascular plexus surrounding the iliac and femoral arteries via the gray rami communicantes. Sympathetic innervation to the lower extremities travels with most of the nerves that supply this region. The largest segment of the lumbar sympathetic ganglia resides at the level of the second and third lumbar vertebrae, which makes this region a favorable target for interventions.[1]

Equipment and Patient Preparation

1. **Monitors and Sterility**
   a. No specific monitors are needed for this procedure, but emergency resuscitation equipment should be available immediately. This includes ACLS drugs, supplemental oxygen, airway adjuncts, and suction.
   b. Strict antiseptic technique should be observed including sterile probe cover, ultrasound gel, and sterile gloves. Chlorhexidine or other skin prep agent should be used to clean the skin prior to commencing the procedure.
2. **Equipment**
   a. Fluoroscopy: Conventional fluoroscope with C-arm capability
   b. Needle type: 22- or 25-gauge, 3.5- to 7-inch needle

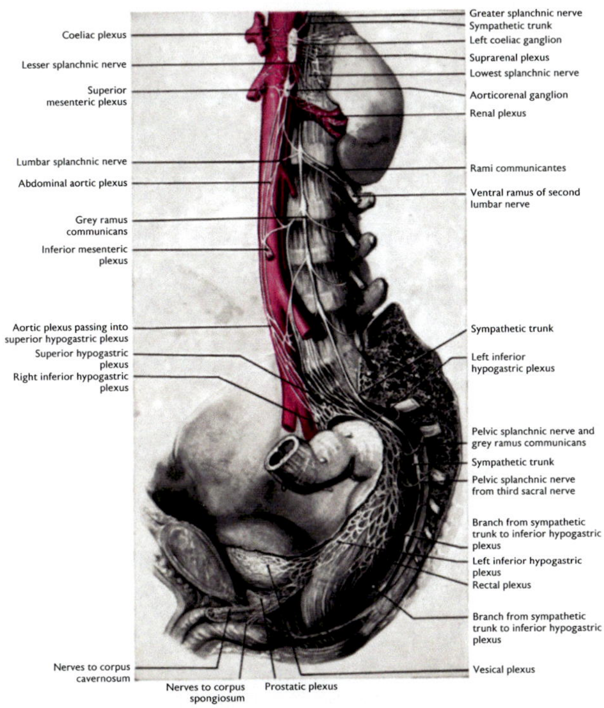

Figure 4.3.1 Anatomical representation of the lumbar sympathetic plexus. (Reprinted with permission from Cunningham's Manual of Practical Anatomy: Thorax and Abdomen, 16th Edition)

c. Local anesthetic (9 mL each side): Lidocaine 1%–2%; ropivacaine 0.2%–0.5%; bupivacaine 0.25%–0.5%
d. Adjuvant (1 mL each side): Nonparticulate or particulate steroid
e. Neurolysis (10–15 mL each side): 10% phenol or 50%–100% ethanol[2]

3. Position

a. Prone (fluoroscopy)

Step-by-Step Technique

CT Planning for Fluoroscopic Approach

Prior CT imaging can be used to determine the adequate obliquity required to perform the block under fluoroscopy and avoid any vital structures. Figure 4.3.2.[2] This demonstrates that creating a needle path line between a point on the transverse process (TP) and the anterolateral border of the vertebral body can help simulate the best approach to the lumbar splanchnics. The TP can be split into 0%, which is the most medial portion of the TP as it connects to the pedicle, to 100%, which is the most lateral portion of the TP. It is important to consider when simulating a path that at 0% of the TP the needle may not have enough of an angle to reach the anteromedial portion of the vertebral body where the lumbar sympathetic chain classically exists. However, at 100% of the TP the needle may pass through vital structures such as pleura or kidney. Thus, this approach allows you to determine the ideal obliquity based on the overlap percentage of the TP with the anterolateral border of the vertebral body to perform the procedure safely and effectively.

Fluoroscopic Approach

1. **Once the patient is positioned, area prepped, and equipment is ready; start by using local anesthetic for a skin wheal, superficial to the L2 or L3 vertebral body, 6–8 cm from midline (Figure 4.3.3).[3] bilaterally.** The C-arm can be positioned obliquely degrees toward the side of needle insertion (Figure 4.3.4).[4]
2. **Initial advancement of the needle.** The spinal needle is guided superior to the transverse process of L2/3 (Figure 4.3.5),[5] directly toward the anterolateral surface of the L2/3 vertebral body. Repetitive images are obtained to ensure accurate needle advancement.
3. **Lateral view.** The needle is then advanced 1–2 cm anteriorly to the anterior third of the L2/3 vertebral body (Figure 4.3.6).[6]
4. **AP view.** The final needle position should be visualized medial to the lateral border of the L2/3 vertebral body.
5. **Contrast administration.** Perform an aspiration to ensure that the needle has not pierced any vascular structures or the cerebrospinal fluid. Contrast media is then introduced with ideal spread to the anterior aspects of the first through fourth lumbar vertebrae (Figure 4.3.7–8).[7]
6. **Injectate administration.** Injectate is then administered incrementally while intermittently aspirating to check for inadvertently vascular uptake.
7. **Repeat steps 2–6 on the contralateral side for bilateral symptoms.**
8. **Ensure the patient has no motor or sensory changes in the lower extremities.**

Tips

- The target for LSB is the lumbar sympathetic chain or splanchnic nerves residing on the anterolateral aspect of the body of the second and third lumbar vertebra. Most interventionists make this the primary target for final needle placement, as proper positioning and contrast confirmation will ensure adequate flow of medication to superior and inferior sympathetic ganglia.

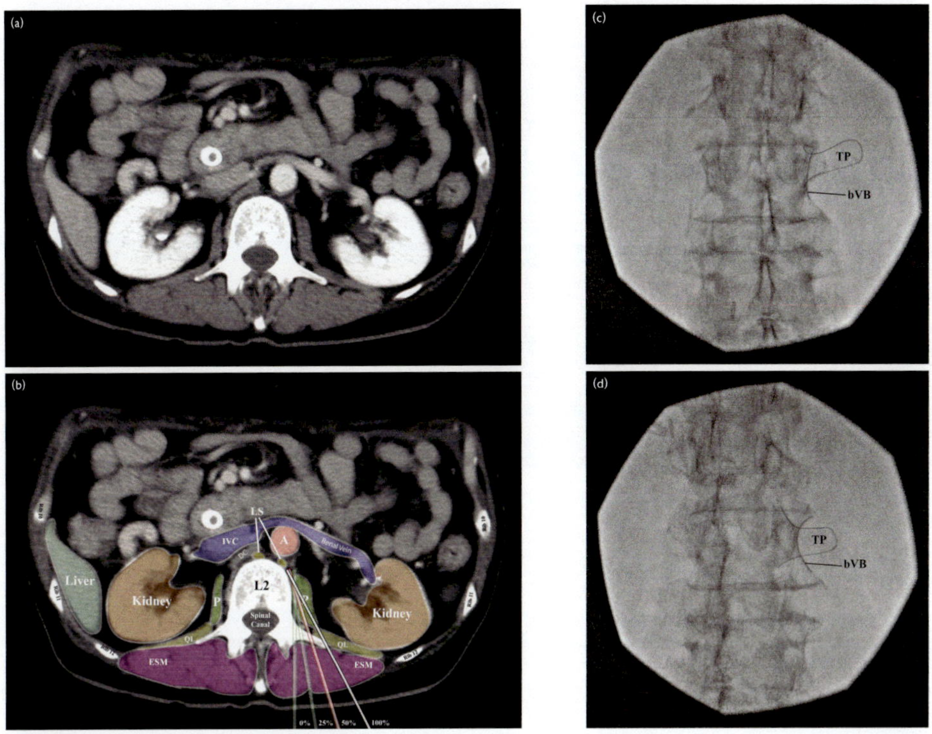

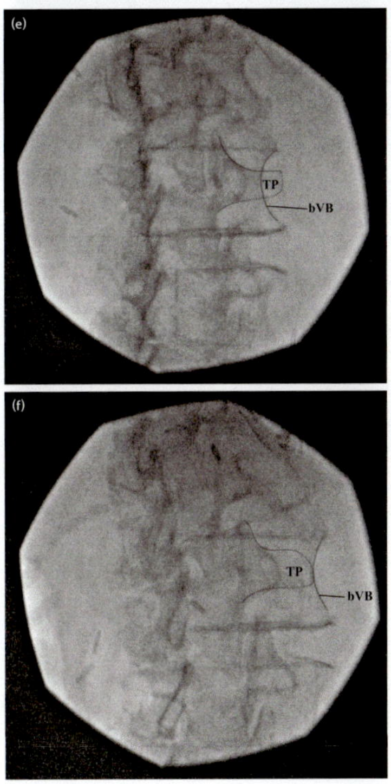

Figure 4.3.2 a/b, Axial CT image at the L1 level demonstrating the approach of the needle placement in relation to the percentage of the transverse process (TP) overlapping with the anterolateral border of the vertebral body (bVB). **c,** A-P fluoroscopic image demonstrating 0-degrees obliquity correlating with 0% overlap. **d,** Fluoroscopic image demonstrating 10-degrees obliquity correlating with 25% overlap. **e,** Fluoroscopic image demonstrating 20-degrees obliquity correlating with 50% overlap. **f,** Fluoroscopic image demonstrating 30-degrees obliquity correlating with 100% overlap. *LS* lumbar splanchnics, *IVC* inferior vena cava, *A* aorta, *DC* diaphragmatic crus, *P* psoas muscle, *QL* quadratus lumborum, *ESM* erector spinae muscles.

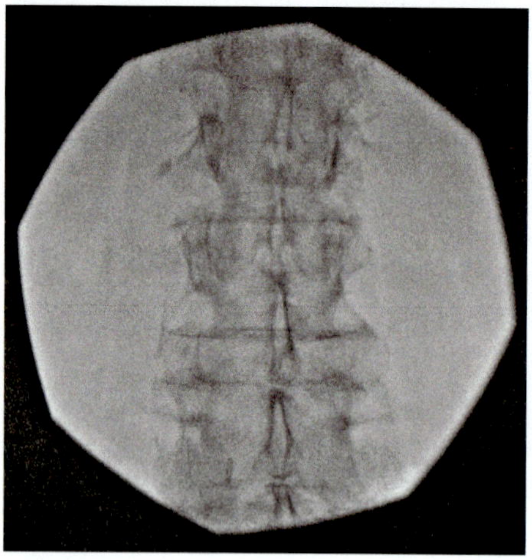

Figure 4.3.3 A-P fluoroscopic image showing the L1–3 levels.

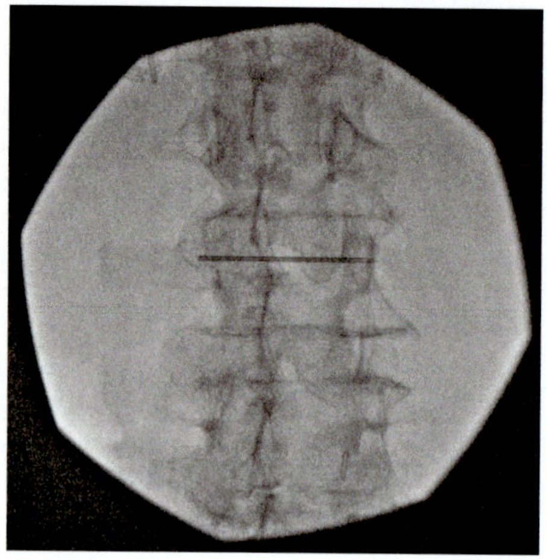

Figure 4.3.4 Fluoroscopic image with 10 degrees of obliquity or 25% overlap of the transverse process with the lateral boarder of the vertebral body. The needle is placed over the L2 level.

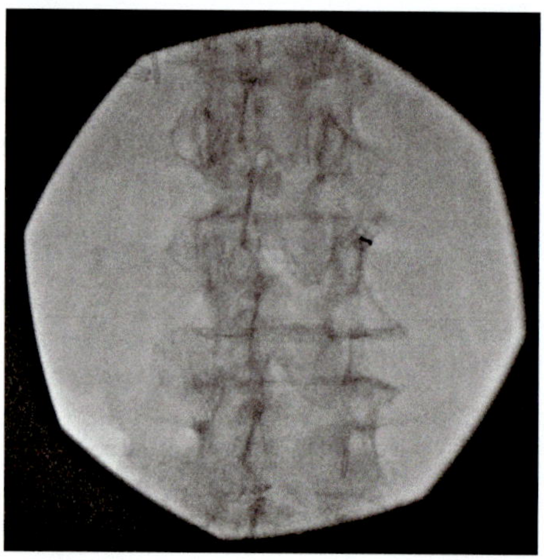

Figure 4.3.5 Fluoroscopic image with 10 degrees of obliquity toward the right side and a needle placed coaxially just superior the L2 transverse process and lateral to the vertebral body.

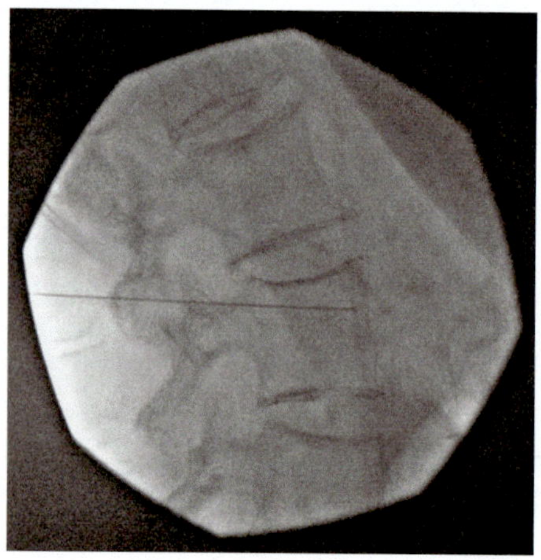

Figure 4.3.6 Lateral fluoroscopic image with the needle advanced just anteriorly to the anterior third of the L2 vertebral body for a lumbar sympathetic approach.

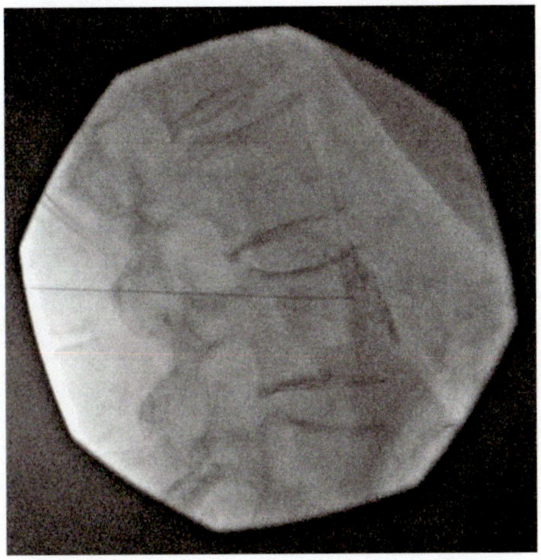

Figure 4.3.7 Lateral fluoroscopic image with contrast visualized over the anterolateral surface of the L2 vertebral body for a lumbar sympathetic approach.

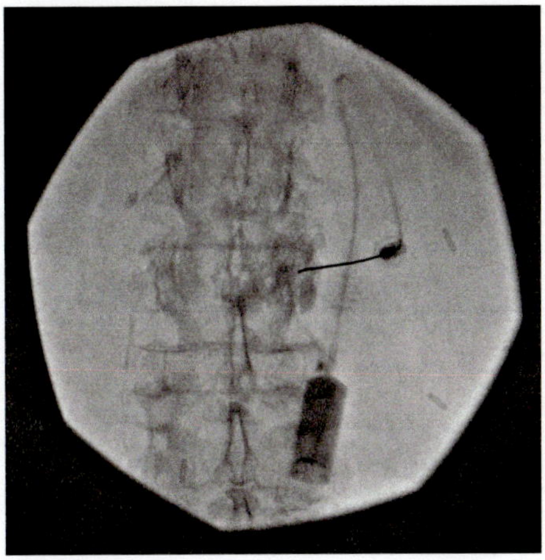

Figure 4.3.8 A-P fluoroscopic image with contrast visualized spreading medial to the lateral boarder of the L2 vertebral body and pedicle for a lumbar sympathetic approach.

Safety Consideration

- Great care must be taken to avoid piercing the exiting spinal nerve. This is best achieved by placing the needle superolateral to the L2 or L3 transverse process.

Postprocedure Management

Successful LSB can be determined by monitoring for skin temperature changes of between 1°C–2°C, evidence of vasodilatation, and pain relief is reported by the patient. Patients should also be counseled on and monitored for potential complications such as vascular injury leading to hematoma formation (within the retroperitoneal space), local anesthetic toxicity, infection, nerve injury, and peritoneal perforation.

References

1. Baig S, Moon JY, Shankar H. Review of sympathetic blocks: Anatomy, sonoanatomy, evidence, and techniques. Reg Anesth Pain Med. 2017;42(3):377–391.
2. de Oliveira R, dos Reis MP, Prado WA. The effects of early or late neurolytic sympathetic plexus block on the management of abdominal or pelvic cancer pain: Pain. 2004;110(1):400–408.
3. Furman MB, Berkwits L, Cohen I, Goodman BS, Kirschner JS, Lee TS, Lin PS (Ed). Atlas of Image-Guided Interventional Spinal Procedures, 2nd ed. Philadelphia: Elsevier, 2018.
4. Royle JP. A history of sympathectomy. Aust N Z J Surg. 1999 Apr;69(4):302–307. doi:10.1046/j.1440-1622.1999.01566.x. PMID: 10327122.
5. Rathmell J. Atlas of Image-Guided Intervention in Regional Anesthesia and Pain Medicine. Wolters Kluwer/Lippincott Williams & Williams, Philadelphia, 2012.
6. Spiegel MA, Hingula L, Chen GH, Legler A, Puttanniah V, Gulati A. The Use of L2 and L3 Lumbar Sympathetic Blockade for Cancer-Related Pain, an Experience and Recommendation in the Oncologic Population. Pain Med. 2020;21(1):176–184.
7. Zechlinski JJ, Hieb RA. Lumbar sympathetic neurolysis: How to and when to use? Tech Vasc Interv Radiol. 2016;19(2):163–168.

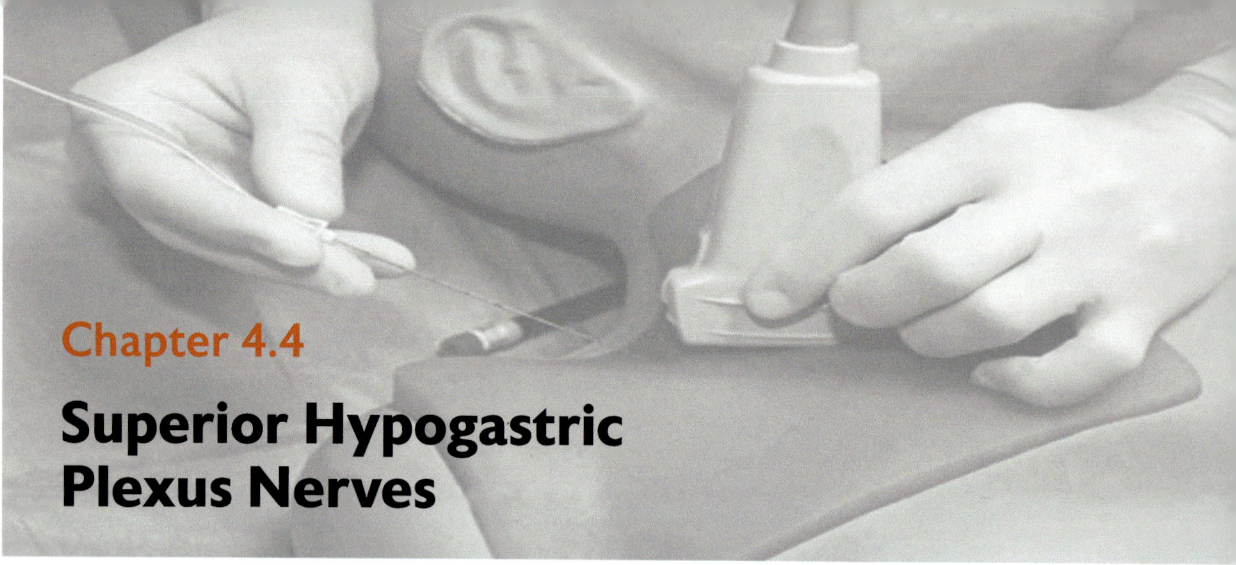

Chapter 4.4

Superior Hypogastric Plexus Nerves

Lee Hingula, B. Carolina Hernández-Porras, Ricardo Plancarte, Angel Manuel Juárez-Lemus, Marcela Sámano-García, Rocío Guillén-Nuñez, Ale Ismael García-Cazares, and Dustin Liebling

Contents

Introduction

The superior hypogastric plexus is a single midline structure formed by the combination of the sympathetic chains. It contains afferent and sympathetic efferent fibers innervating the pelvic organs. Plancarte first described a technique to block the plexus in 1990 on 28 patients with either cancer or radiation injury.[1-5] He found it to be efficacious in relieving pain without complications.[6] The technique is performed as originally described, fluoroscopically, utilizing either local anesthetic or neurolytic agents. Since it was first performed, multiple studies have confirmed its safety and efficacy.[4,5]

Indications

Superior hypogastric plexus blockade can be used for pelvic pain from malignant or benign sources. Early studies demonstrated that visual analogue pain scores were decreased in 70% of patients with cancer.[5] There was a mean drop in opioid reduction of 22% more in the successfully treated group than in the failure group.[5] Most of the patients in this study had cervical cancer. The data suggests it to be highly effective for bladder cancer pain as well, with some evidence suggesting it to be more effective in adults above age 59 than in younger individuals. Superior hypogastric plexus blockade may be less effective for benign conditions.[4]

Contraindications and Complications

Complications of the superior hypogastric plexus block are rare. Severe nerve injury is not nearly as likely as with more cephalad sympathetic blocks since blood supply to the anterior spinal cord is unlikely to be compromised at this level. Bilateral neurolysis should not be performed in men due to the possibility of sexual dysfunction. Inadvertent subarachnoid or epidural injection, somatic nerve injury, ureteral damage or renal puncture are possible as well.[2]

Critical Anatomy

The superior hypogastric plexus is a retroperitoneal structure. It lies inferior to the aortic bifurcation and anterior to the lower L5 and upper S1 vertebral bodies (Figure 4.4.1). It contains postganglionic sympathetic fibers, which innervate the organs of the pelvis except the ovaries and fallopian tubes. These fibers receive contribution from the inferior mesenteric ganglion and from the lumbar splanchnic nerves that travel with the aorta.[2] Biochemical analyses suggest there may

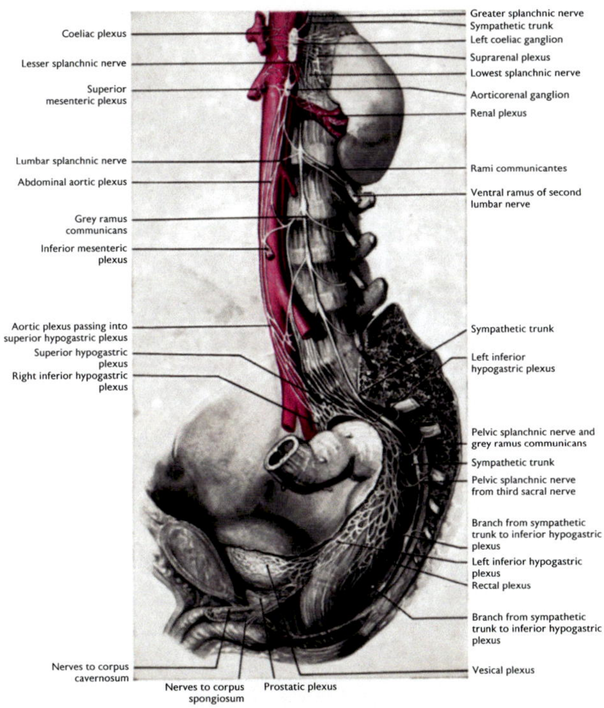

Figure 4.4.1 Anatomical representation of the superior hypogastric plexus. (Reprinted with permission from Cunningham's Manual of Practical Anatomy: Thorax and Abdomen, 16th Edition)

be preganglionic parasympathetic fibers in the plexus as well.[1] Visceral afferent fibers travel through the superior hypogastric plexus from pelvic organs and enter the spinal cord via the lumbar or sacral nerve roots.[2]

Equipment and Patient Preparation

1. **Monitors and Sterility**
   a. No specific monitors are needed for this procedure, but emergency resuscitation equipment should be available immediately. This includes ACLS drugs, supplemental oxygen, airway adjuncts, and suction.
   b. Strict antiseptic technique should be observed including sterile probe cover, ultrasound gel, and sterile gloves. Chlorhexidine or other skin prep agent should be used to clean the skin prior to commencing the procedure.
2. **Special Patient Preparation**
   a. Transdiscal Approach
      i. Antibiotic prophylaxis with 1 gram cefazolin or 1 gram vancomycin.
3. **Equipment**
   a. Imaging
      i. Fluoroscopy: Conventional fluoroscope with C-arm capability
      ii. Probe: Low-frequency linear array transducer (2–5 MHz)
   b. Needle type: 22- or 25-gauge, 5- to 7-inch needle
   c. Local anesthetic (9 mL each side): Lidocaine 1%–2%; ropivacaine 0.2%–0.5%; bupivacaine 0.25%–0.5%
   d. Adjuvant (1 mL each side): Nonparticulate or particulate steroid
   e. Neurolysis (8–10 mL): 10% phenol or 50%–100% ethanol[2]
4. **Position**
   a. Prone (fluoroscopy)
   b. Supine (ultrasound)

Step-by-Step Technique

Fluoroscopy-Guided Approach

A. Classic or Posterolateral Approach[6]

1. **Prepare equipment and supplies, position the patient supine, and sterilize the procedural area with antiseptic solution.** A pillow can be placed under the lower abdomen, to reduce lumbar lordosis.
2. **In an anteroposterior view, square the lower L5 and upper S1 endplates.** At 10 to 15 cm lateral to the spinous process, the L5 the transverse process is located.
3. **The two 7-inch, 22-gauge needles entry point is lateral to the right and left transverse process (**Figure 4.4.2**).**
4. **Both needles must be inserted 30-degree cephalad to caudad (off the medial sagittal plane) and 45-degree medial (off the coronal plane) (**Figure 4.4.3**).**
5. **Contact the lower border of the outer third of the transverse process, remove the needle by approximately 30 mm, and redirect it in a more caudal position**
6. **Take a lateral view to verify needle depth is still at the vertebral body (**Figure 4.4.4**)**
7. **Keep the path medially but avoid entering the intervertebral disc (**Figure 4.4.5**).**

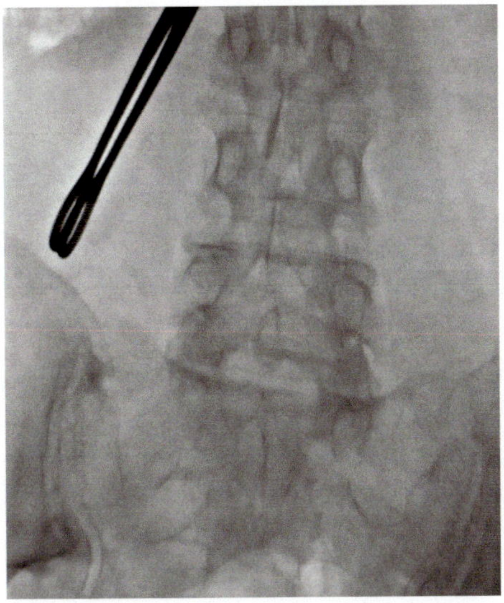

Figure 4.4.2 A-P fluoroscopic image of the lumbar spine marking the entry point is lateral to the L5 transverse process.

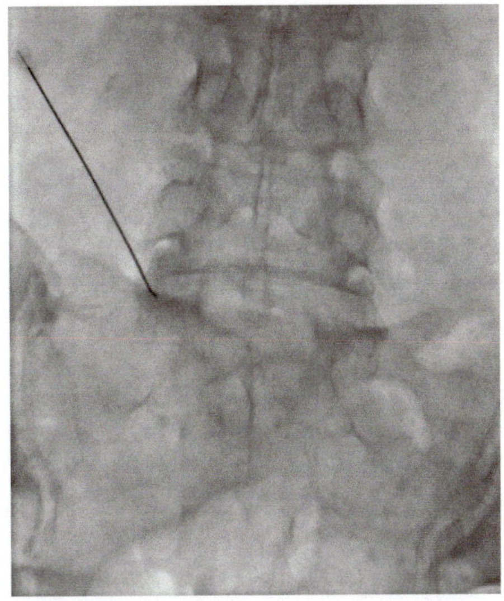

Figure 4.4.3 A-P fluoroscopic image of the lumbar spine showing the spinal needle inserted at the L5/S1 interdiscal space at an angle of 30-degrees caudad and 45-degrees medial.

8. **Advance in a perfect lateral position and 1 to 2 millimeters before the intervertebral disc ends**. Consider connecting a 3- or 5-mL syringe for loss of resistance, which may occur after passing the psoas and paravertebral space.
9. **Reverify in an anteroposterior view for accurate needle path.**

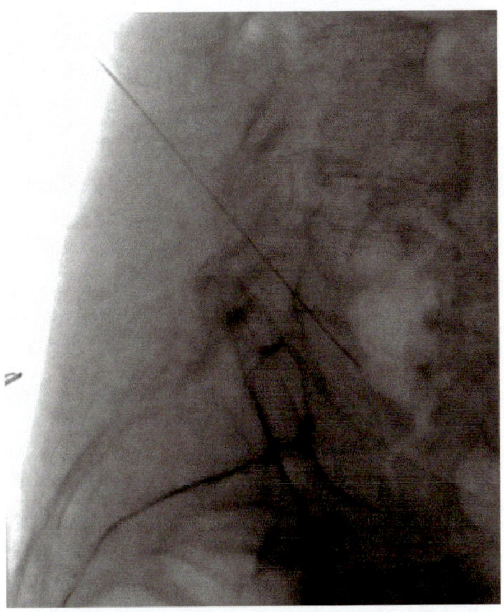

Figure 4.4.4 Lateral fluoroscopic image of the lumbar spine verifying needle depth is not beyond the vertebral body.

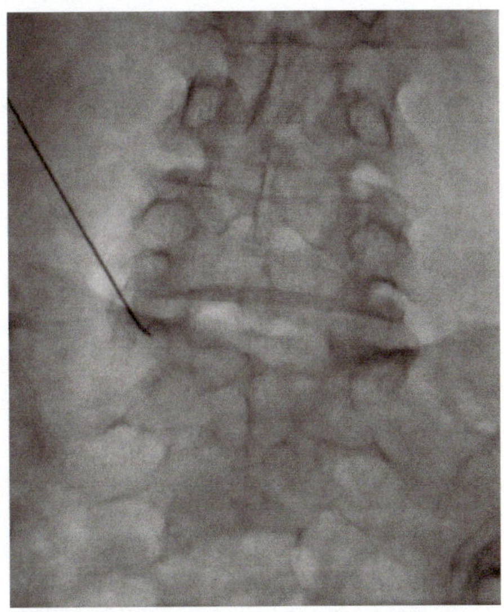

Figure 4.4.5 A-P fluoroscopic image of the lumbar spine showing the spinal needle path medially but avoiding entry into the intervertebral disc.

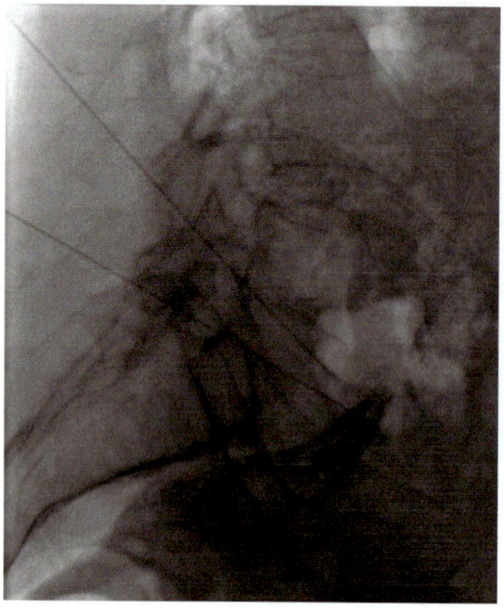

Figure 4.4.6 Lateral fluoroscopic image of the lumbar spine verifying accurate needle path and contrast spread without vascular uptake.

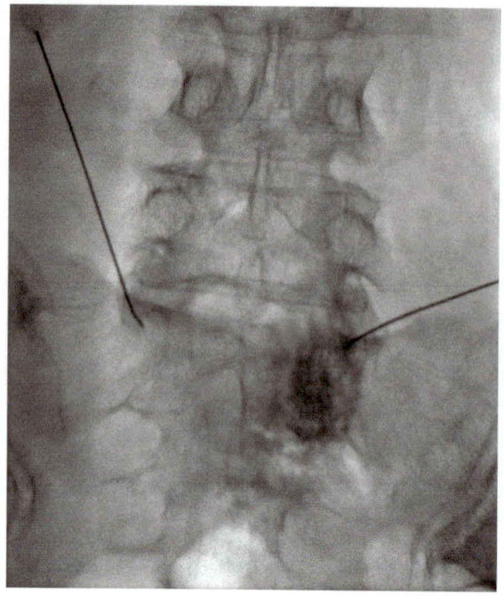

Figure 4.4.7 A-P fluoroscopic image of the lumbar spine verifying accurate needle path and contrast spread without vascular uptake.

10. **Apply 2–3 mL of non-ionic contrast in dynamic lateral fluoroscopy to verify accurate placement of the needles and to rule out intravascular injection (Figure 4.4.6**). Consider applying 3 to 8 mL of air in each needle for further verification (Figure 4.4.7).
11. **In case of L5 mega-apophysis or Bertolotti's syndrome the approach can be at performed at L4/L5 intervertebral space (**Figure 4.4.8**).**
12. **Take an anteroposterior radiograph for visualization of contrast spread at retroperitoneum, right and left sided (**Figure 4.4.9**).**
13. **For neurolysis, 8 to 10 mL of 10% phenol must be used on each side. For diagnostic block 0.25% bupivacaine must be used.**

B. **Transdiscal Approach[7]**

1. **Prepare equipment and supplies, position the patient prone, and sterilize the procedural area with antiseptic solution.** A pillow can be placed under the lower abdomen, to reduce lumbar lordosis.
2. **Square off the lower L5 and upper S1 endplates in an anteroposterior view, place the spinous process at the middle of the image (**Figure 4.4.10**).**
3. **Move to an oblique view until the superior articular process of S1 is seen.**
4. **Introduce a 22-gauge spinal needle through this view in the lower part of the intervertebral disc (**Figure 4.4.11**).**
5. **Advance 3 to 5 cm (depends in the anatomical characteristics of the patient) and take a lateral view**. A true lateral view is very important while advancing the needle through the disc. In the true lateral view, the L5 inferior and S1 superior endplates are "squared off" and L5/S1 intervertebral foramen is seen as one unique rounded image (Figure 4.4.12).
6. **If the patient complains while advancing the needle, you may have touched the L5 root**. Please retract the needle 5 mm and take a lateral view in order to confirm the needle at the entry of the foramina. Turn the needle tip up or down to avoid the nerve root. In the case

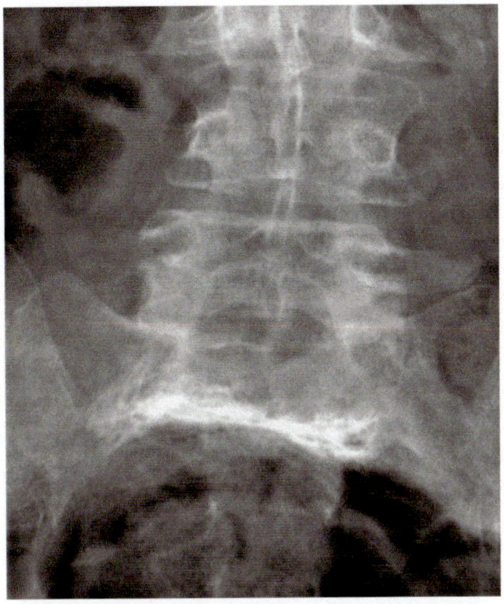

Figure 4.4.8 A-P fluoroscopic image of the lumbar spine demonstrating a patient with Bertolotti's syndrome where the approach can be performed at the L4/L5 intervertebral space.

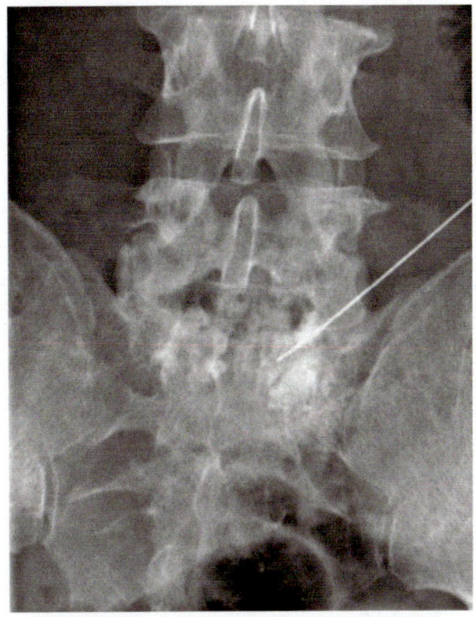

Figure 4.4.9 A-P fluoroscopic image of the lumbar spine demonstrating bilateral contrast spread retroperitoneally.

that the needle is at the intervertebral disc, the patient is likely experiencing discogenic pain. Place 0.5 mm lidocaine and continue advancing the needle.

7. **Advance the needle to the lateral third or at the middle of the disc, connect a 3 or 5 mL syringe for loss of resistance to air or liquid (Figure 4.4.12).** Loss of resistance indicates the needle reached retroperitoneum. If you do not lose resistance after advancing 3 cm, take a lateral view to confirm the needle passed within the disc. This view verifies that needle does not pass too anterior, which means potential bowel punction.

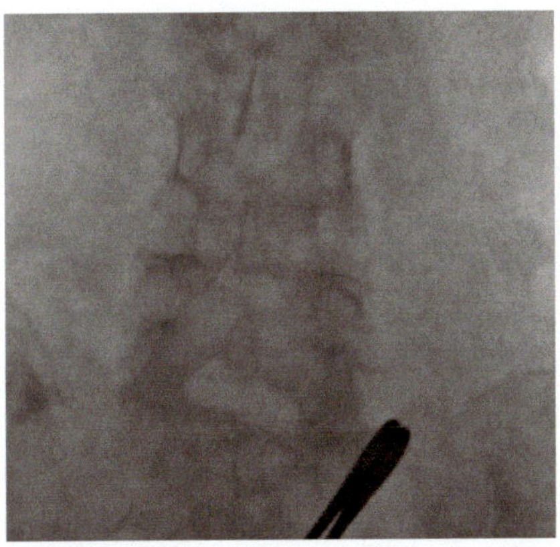

Figure 4.4.10 A-P fluoroscopic image of the lumbar spine with the lower L5 and upper S1 endplates squared and marking the entry point is lateral to the L5/S1 disc.

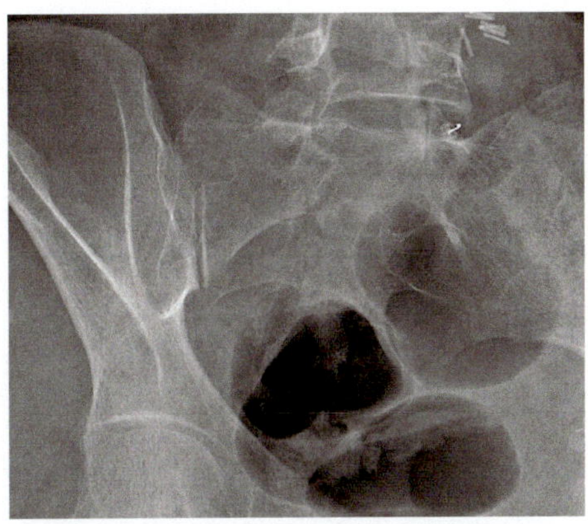

Figure 4.4.11 Oblique fluoroscopic image of the lumbar spine the spinal needle entering just lateral to the superior articular process of S1 and eventually through the lower part of the intervertebral disc.

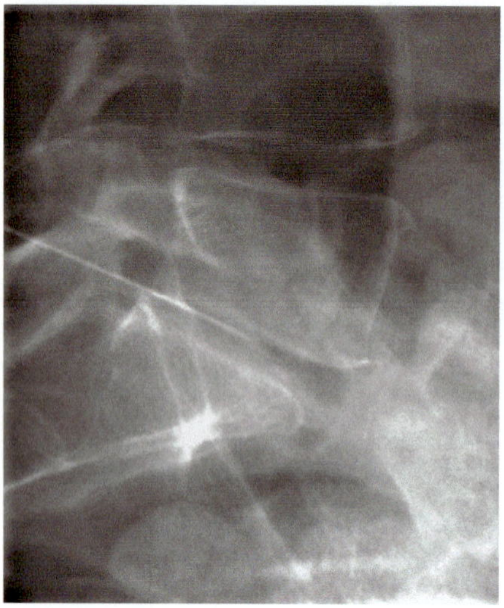

Figure 4.4.12 True lateral fluoroscopic image of the lumbar spine with the L5 inferior and S1 superior endplates are squared off showing the spinal needle traversing intradiscally to the middle third of the disc.

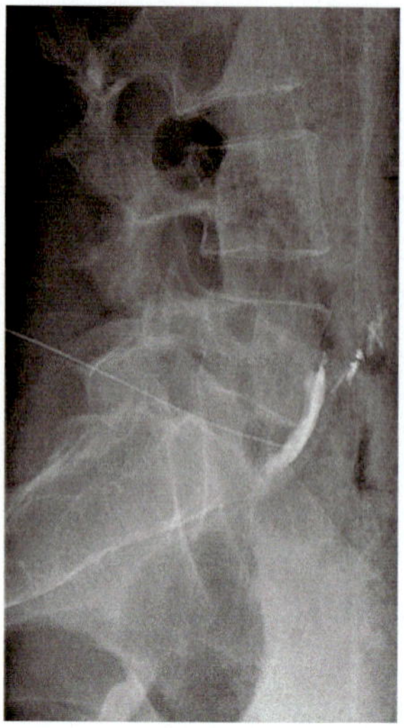

Figure 4.4.13 True lateral fluoroscopic image of the lumbar spine demonstrating contrast spread anterior to the L5–S1 disc in a linear fashion over the anterior surface of the intervertebral disc.

8. **Apply 1 to 2 mL of nonionic contrast medium.** It should demonstrate spread anterior to the L5–S1 disc, a linear fashion over the anterior surface of the intervertebral disc (Figure 4.4.13).
9. **Also in lateral, if there is correct spread of contrast medium, you can apply 5 to 10 mL of air.** Air can be visualized along the anterior sacrum body (Figure 4.4.13).
10. **Take an anteroposterior radiograph for visualization of contrast spread at retroperitoneum.** If the spread is not bilateral, apply 5 mL of air and 2 mL of contrast medium (Figure 4.4.14).

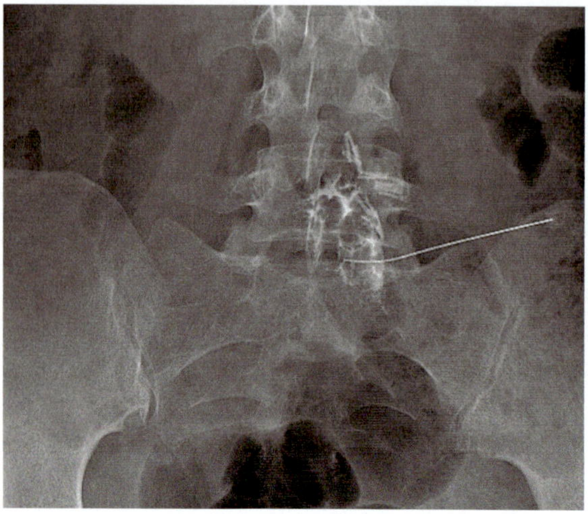

Figure 4.4.14 A-P fluoroscopic image of the lumbar spine to assess for bilateral contrast spread. In this case, spread is mainly unilateral (favoring the right side). If the spread is not bilateral, you can apply 5 mL of air and 2 mL of contrast medium to assess further spread.

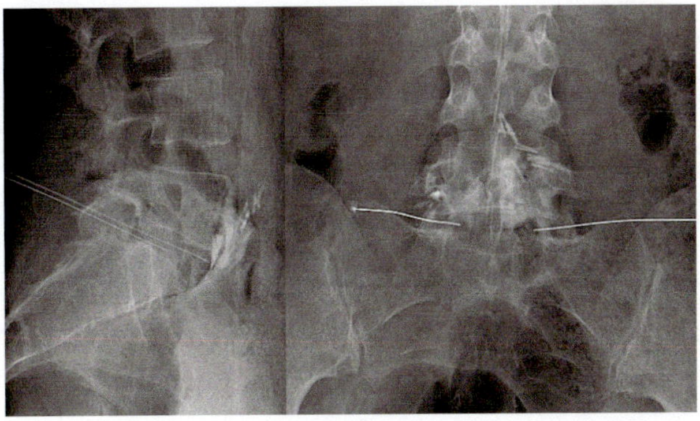

Figure 4.4.15 Lateral (left) and A-P (right) fluoroscopic image of the lumbar spine demonstrating a two transdiscal needle approach to ensure bilateral spread for a superior hypogastric plexus block.

11. **In diagnostic blocks, unilateral spread will likely result in partial response or unilateral response**. In the neurolytic block, a more oblique approach may be necessary, which requires obliquing up to 20 degrees more than the diagnostic block so needle tip can follow a more medial pathway. If unable to reach a more medial distribution with a more pronounced oblique view, two transdiscal needles can be used (Figure 4.4.15).
12. **Apply 15 mL of bupivacaine 0.35% in diagnostic block and 10 to 15 mL of 10% phenol for neurolysis in a unilateral approach.** In case of bilateral transdiscal approach 8 to 10 mL of 10% phenol or alcohol in each needle.

CT-Guided Approach

1. **Prepare equipment and supplies, position the patient prone, and sterilize the procedural area with antiseptic solution.** A pillow can be placed under the lower abdomen, to reduce lumbar lordosis.

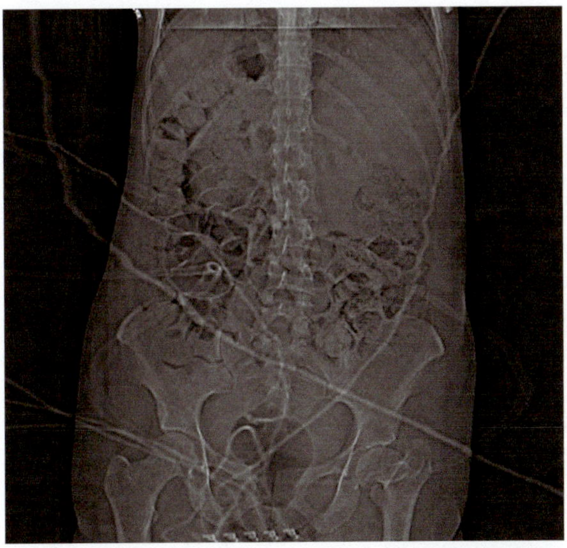

Figure 4.4.16 CT scout image or topogram of the lumbosacral region.

2. **Some CT machines have software to help plan the needle path. If this is not the case, take a scout image/topogram of the lumbosacral region (Figure 4.4.16)**. Once the L5 level is identified, an axial image can then be taken as illustrated by Figure 4.4.17.
3. **Plan the needle insertion site and needle trajectory.** In the sagittal plane with a CT ruler, measure the distance and angulation from the skin to the inferior border of the transverse process (Figure 4.4.18a). In the axial plane, measure paravertebral distance from the anterolateral margin of the L5 vertebral body and the adjacent major psoas (Figure 4.4.18b). Measure the distance

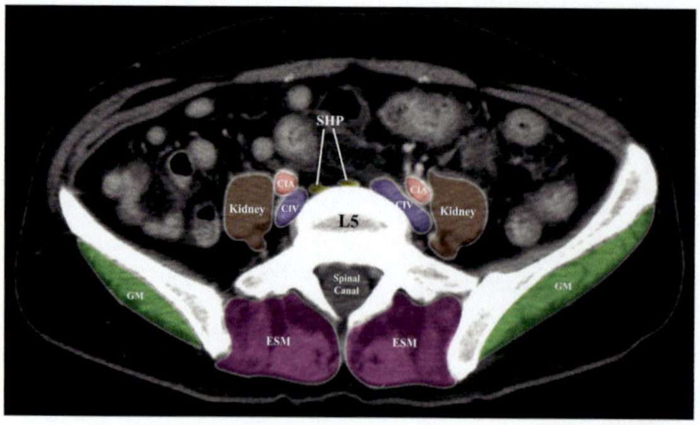

Figure 4.4.17 Labeled axial CT image at the L5 level. *CIA* common iliac artery, *CIV* common iliac vein, *SHP* superior hypogastric plexus, *GM* gluteus musculature, *ESM* erector spinae musculature.

between L5 spinous process and distance b (Figure 4.4.18c). Turn on the external laser beam at the skin needle entrance point. Remember laser will only give you the skin entrance needle point, but neither the distance from the spinous process (Figure 4.4.18c) nor the angulation of the needle (Figure 4.4.18a).

4. **Keeping the direction planned, introduce both needles.** Several low X-ray dose CT can be taken in order to confirm adequate direction and depth (Figure 4.4.19).
5. **As soon as the tip of the needles are in the anterior vertebral body of the sacrum or L5 (depends on the degree of the angulation), apply contrast and air (**Figure 4.4.20**).**
6. **Make sure air or contrast is not at any foramina level.** Advance the needle tip a few millimeters, apply contrast medium and make sure spread is at the retroperitoneum. If this is not the case, do not apply phenol in that needle.
7. **After verifying placement of both needles into the retroperitoneum (Figure 4.4.21), apply 8 to 10 mL of 10% phenol in each needle for neurolysis or local anesthetic for temporary blockade.** In some centers, you can apply 10 to 20 mL of alcohol for this procedure. Take a final reconstruction and visualize contrast-air-lytic agent distribution (Figure 4.4.22).

Tips

- Phenol is costly and its high viscosity makes it difficult to inject. As an alternative, 8–10 mL of 50%–100% Ethanol may be used for neurolysis as well.
- If the iliac wing is obstructing the view, increase the cephalad tilt.
- A 5-inch needle may be too short, particularly in obese patients, given the amount of caudal and lateral tilt needed.

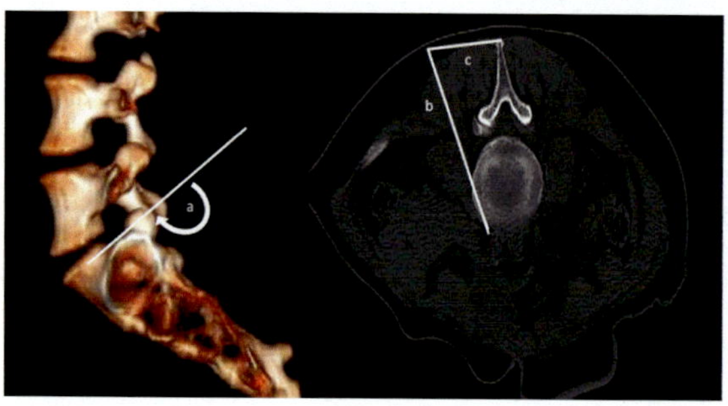

Figure 4.4.18 (Left) Sagittal CT image illustrating the measured distance and angulation from the skin to the inferior border of the lumbar transverse process. (Right) Axial CT image at the L5 level illustrating the measured paravertebral distance from the anterolateral margin of the L5 vertebral body and the adjacent major psoas (b) and the distance between L5 spinous process and distance b (c).

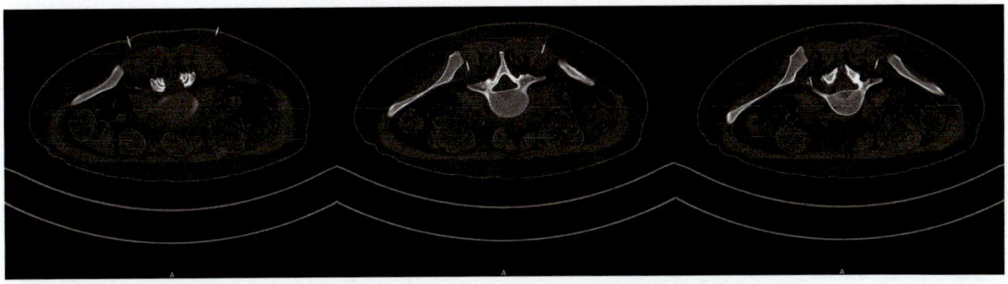

Figure 4.4.19 Sequential axial CT image at the L5 level taken as the needle is being advanced bilaterally to confirm adequate direction and depth.

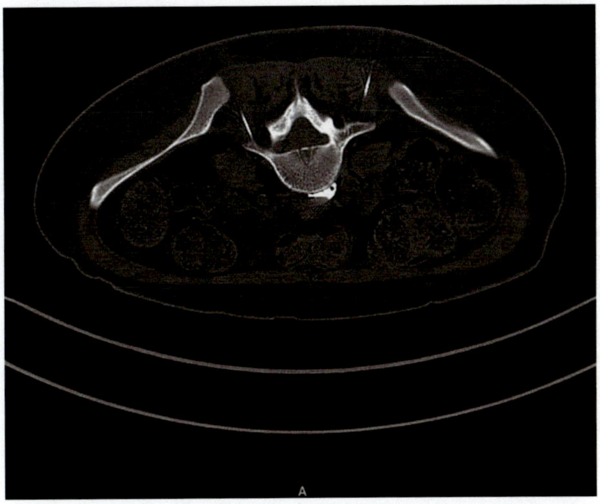

Figure 4.4.20 Axial CT image at the L5 level demonstrating contrast spread just anterior to the vertebral body.

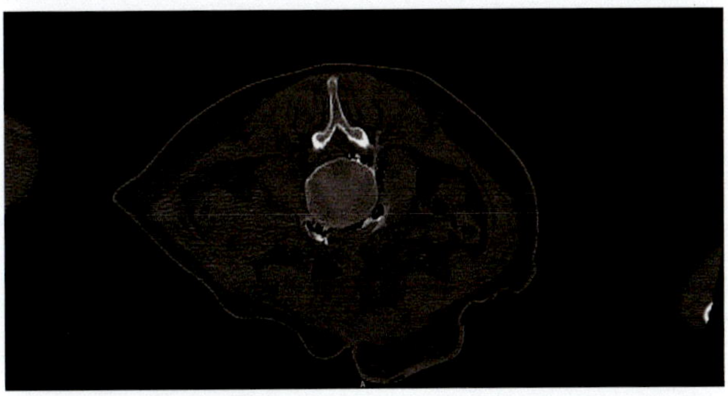

Figure 4.4.21 Axial CT image at the L5 level demonstrating a spread bilaterally just anterior the intervertebral disc.

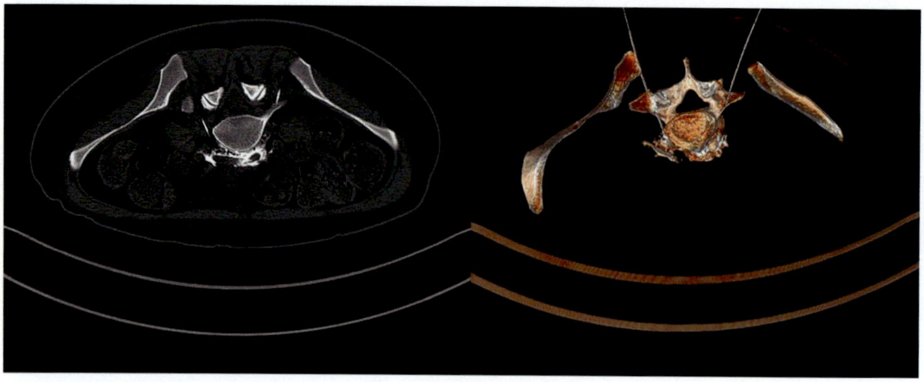

Figure 4.4.22 Axial CT image at the L5 level demonstrating a continued spread bilaterally just anterior the intervertebral disc after neurolytic was administered.

Ultrasound-Guided Approach

1. **Prepare equipment and supplies, position the patient supine, and sterilize the procedural area with antiseptic solution.**
2. **Place the ultrasound transducer transversely midline below the umbilicus** to locate the paired rectus abdominis and aorta/inferior vena cava.
3. **Translate caudally to identify to the bifurcation of the aorta and inferior vena cava.** The transducer will be approximately around the L5 and S1 level when the bifurcation of either of the vessels occur.
4. **The target is superficial to the aorta/inferior vena cava just cephalad to bifurcation or superficial to the L5/S1 vertebral bodies just caudad to the bifurcation of the vessels (**Figure 4.4.23**).**
5. **Inject local anesthetic subcutaneously for analgesia at the procedural site.**
6. **Insert the procedural needle with an in-plane approach from a lateral-to-medial direction.** The needle will traverse subcutaneous tissue, the rectus muscle, and the peritoneal cavity.
7. **Inject the medication around the plexus.** The injectate should be seen to push the peritoneal cavity upward. Remove the needle and apply a dressing.

Tips and Safety Considerations

- The anterior approach requires penetration of the peritoneal cavity. Typically, penetration of the bladder or any other vascular structures does not lead to significant complications. However, a thorough scan identifying the intestines/bowel should be done in order to avoid penetration of the viscera.

Radiofrequency Lesioning

There is a case report of SHP pulsed radiofrequency (PRF)[8–10] being used to treat a woman with interstitial cystitis. The authors performed two sessions at a 6-month interval of PRF treatment of the superior hypogastric plexus. They used a pulse frequency of 2 Hz and a pulse width of 20 ms for 120 seconds twice per session to maintain the tissue temperature near the electrode at 42°C. They reported the patient had pain relief for 2 years and 6 months.

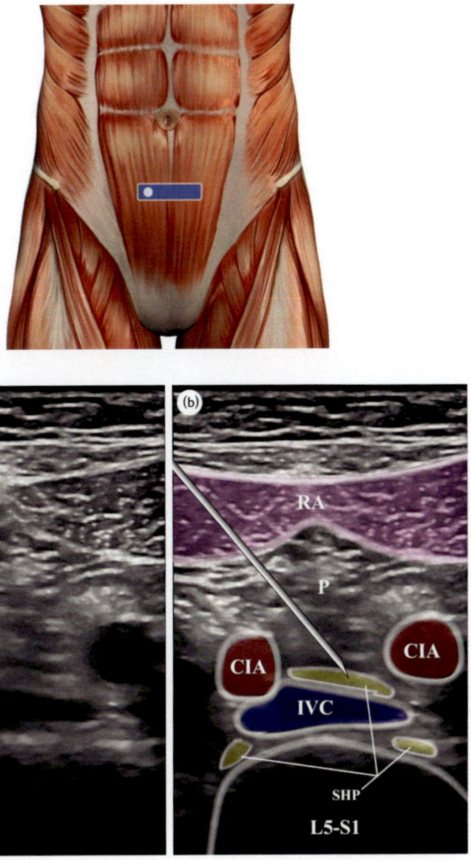

Figure 4.4.23 **a,** Ultrasound image of the anterior abdomen in a transverse axial plane at the L5–S1 level. **b,** Labeled ultrasound image of in-plane needle placement for a superior hypogastric plexus block. *RA* rectus abdominis, *AV* abdominal viscera, *P* peritoneal cavity, *CIA* common iliac artery, *IVC* inferior vena cava, *SHP* superior hypogastric plexus.

Few more cases of radiofrequency ablation are reported. In both radiofrequency models, they performed the classic technique and used 20-gauge, 10 cm radiofrequency needles with 10 mm active tips.

Limited high-quality data exist to support the use of radiofrequency ablation/PRF in the sympathetic nervous system, especially at the superior hypogastric plexus. Since SHPB is a large plexus and radiofrequency ablation lesions are millimetric in scale, ablations are unlikely to fully treat the entire SHPB. Further studies and cadaveric studies must be performed to confirm the feasibility of radiofrequency ablations of this area.

References

1. Kraima AC, van Schaik J, Susan S, van de Velde CJ, Hamming JF, Lakke EA, DeRuiter MC. New insights in the neuroanatomy of the human adult superior hypogastric plexus and hypogastric nerves. Auton Neurosci. 2015;189:60–67. doi: 10.1016/j.autneu.2015.02.001. Epub 2015 Feb 14. PMID: 25704391.
2. Warfield CA, Bajwa ZH. Principles and Practice of Pain Medicine. 2nd Edition. 2004. McGraw-Hill, New York.
3. Choi JW, Kim WH, Lee CJ, Sim WS, Park S, Chae HB. The optimal approach for a superior hypogastric plexus block. Pain Pract. 2018;18:314–321.

4. Kroll CE, Schartz B, Gonzalez-Fernandez M, Gordon AH, Babade M, Erdek MA, Mekhail N, Cohen SP. Factors associated with outcome after superior hypogastric plexus neurolysis in cancer patients. Clin J of Pain. 2014;30(1):55–62. doi: 10.1097/AJP.0b013e3182869d68.
5. de Leon-Casasola OA. Critical evaluation of chemical neurolysis of the sympathetic axis for cancer pain. Cancer Control. 2000;7(2):142–148. doi: 10.1177/107327480000700204. PMID: 10783818.
6. Plancarte R, Amescia C, Patt R, Aldrete JA. Superior hypogastric plexus block for pelvic cancer pain. Anesthesiology 1990;73(2):236–239.
7. Stogicza AR. Superior hypogastric plexus block: transdiscal approach. In: Stogicza AR, Mansano AM, Trescot AM, Staats PS (eds.), Interventional Pain. Springer, Cham; 2020: 171–176.
8. Kim JH, Kim E, Kim BI. Pulsed radiofrequency treatment of the superior hypogastric plexus in an interstitial cystitis patient with chronic pain and symptoms refractory to oral and intravesical medications and bladder hydrodistension: A case report. Medicine (Baltimore). 2016;95(49):e5549.
9. Noor NA, Urits I, Viswanath O, Alexandre L, Kaye AD. Radiofrequency ablation of the splanchnic nerve and superior hypogastric plexus for chronic abdominal pain status post-abdominal surgery. Cureus. 2020;12(12):e12189.
10. Zacharias NA, Karri J, Garcia C., et al. Interventional radiofrequency treatment for the sympathetic nervous system: a review article. Pain Ther. 2021 Jun;10(1):115–141.

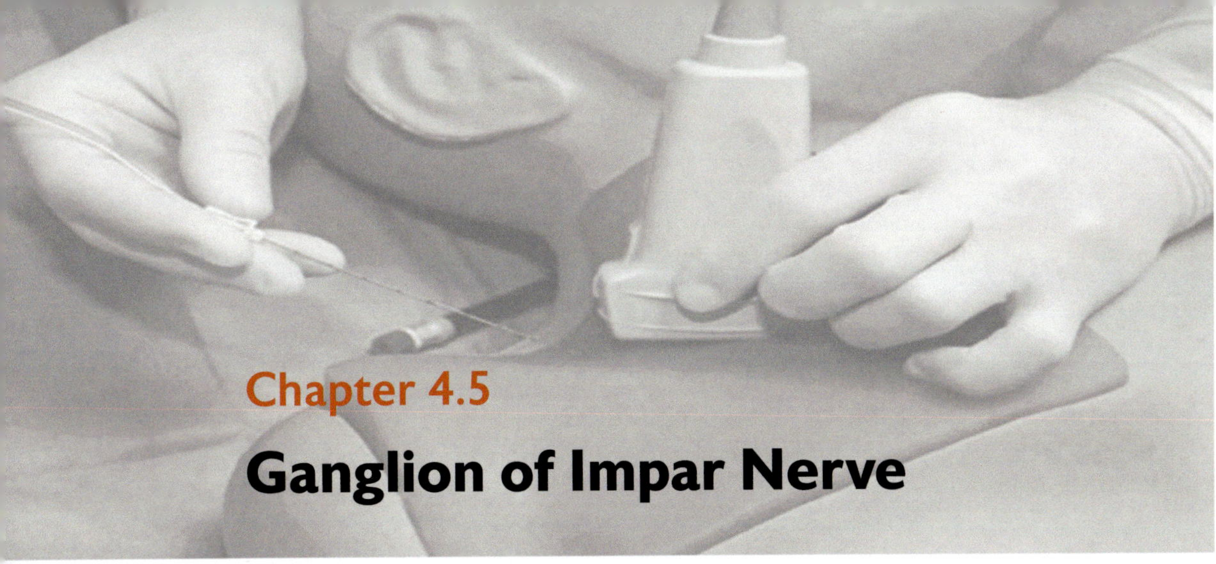

Chapter 4.5

Ganglion of Impar Nerve

Cameran Vakassi and Dustin Liebling

Contents

Introduction

The ganglion of impar is the terminal ganglion of the sympathetic chain, providing innervation to the lower pelvic structures.[1–2] It is formed by the paired paravertebral sympathetic chains fusing as a solitary ganglion in the retroperitoneum at the level of the sacrococcygeal junction.[3] It provides sympathetic and visceral innervation to the lower third of the rectum, vagina, vulva, urethra, and coccyx. Tumor-related perirectal or perineal pain can be worsened by defecation, and is often exacerbated by opiate-induced constipation, often placing these patients in a vicious cycle.[4] Pain from these structures is mediated by the sympathetic nervous system through the ganglion of impar, making it a useful target for relief. Visceral pain originating in these structures travels via sympathetic nerve fibers to the ganglion of impar, then to the sympathetic trunk, then to sacral nerve roots via the gray rami communicantes, next into the spinal cord, and finally terminates in the brain.[5]

Indications

The ganglion of impar block can be used for perineal or coccygeal pain, resulting from tumors an postradiation or postsurgical changes of the rectum, vagina, vulva, distal urethra, prostate, and coccyx.[6] It has also been described to provide relief in radiation-induced prostatitis or proctitis.[4]

Tumors of other nearby pelvic structure such as ovarian, colon, or bladder carcinoma can also cause compression on the rectum or perineum, resulting in discomfort. The block is also indicated for coccydynia, resulting from degenerative changes, traumatic fracture, or infection.[7] Other nonmalignant indications include postherpetic neuralgia, rectal tenesmus, perineal hyperhidrosis, vulvodynia, cystitis, and idiopathic perineal or coccygeal pain.[7–9]

Critical Anatomy

The ganglion of impar is a solitary 4–5 mm ganglion located in the retroperitoneum at the level of the sacrococcygeal junction. It is a midline structure, lying directly anterior to the coccyx and posterior to the rectum. The location of the ganglion may vary from the level of the sacrococcygeal junction to the second coccygeal vertebrae.[10]

Equipment and Patient Preparation

1. **Monitors and Sterility**
   a. No specific monitors are needed for this procedure, but emergency resuscitation equipment should be available immediately. This includes ACLS drugs, supplemental oxygen, airway adjuncts, and suction.
   b. Strict antiseptic technique should be observed including sterile probe cover, ultrasound gel, and sterile gloves. Chlorhexidine or other skin prep agent should be used to clean the skin prior to commencing the procedure.
2. **Equipment**
   a. Imaging
      i. CT-guided intervention: Conventional computerized X-ray imaging/tomography (CT) machine
      ii. Fluoroscopy-guided intervention: Conventional fluoroscope with C-arm capability
   b. Needle type: 22- or 25-gauge, 1.5- to 3.5-inch needle
   c. Local anesthetic (1–3 mL): Lidocaine 1%–2%; ropivacaine 0.2%–0.5%; bupivacaine 0.25%–0.5%
   d. Adjuvant (1–2 mL): Nonparticulate or particulate steroid
   e. Neurolysis (5–7 mL): 10% phenol or 50%–100% ethanol[2]
3. **Position**
   a. Prone (fluoroscopy)

Step-by-Step Technique

Fluoroscopy-Guided Approach

1. **Prepare equipment and supplies, position the patient prone, and sterilize the procedural area with antiseptic solution.** Place a pillow under the hips to reduce the lumbar lordosis.
2. **Identify the junction of S5 and coccyx with fluoroscopy in the anteroposterior and lateral views.**
3. **Using a midline entry point in the space identified via fluoroscopy, inject local anesthetic** in **the skin overlying the sacrococcygeal junction**.
4. **In the lateral view, insert the needle and advance under fluoroscopic guidance to the sacrococcygeal disc.**
5. **Advance the needle through the sacrococcygeal disc until the tip is anterior to the ventral sacrococcygeal ligament**

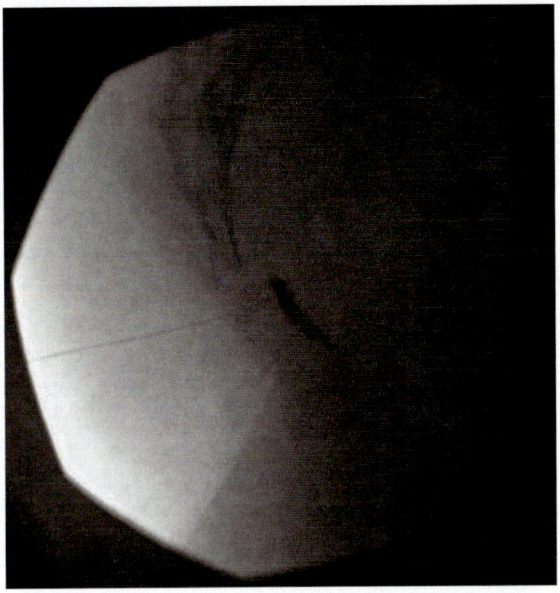

Figure 4.5.1 Lateral fluoroscopic image illustrating the needle traversing through the sacrococcygeal ligament and the classic contrast spread pattern of a "reverse comma" in the space of the Ganglion of Impar.

6. **Confirm needle tip position by injecting 1–2 mL of radio-opaque contrast into the retroperitoneal space.** The correct placement and spread of contrast will produce a "reverse comma" appearance on lateral view, and is confirmed to be midline in the anteroposterior view with no vascular or epidural spread (Figure 4.5.1).
7. **Prior to injecting the injectate, carefully aspirate for heme and CSF.**
8. **Inject the medication with periodic aspirations every 3–5 mL.** Remove the needle and apply a dressing.

CT-Guided Approach

A parasagittal CT-guided approach may be used in cases where rectal gas or stool obscure the view of the sacrococcygeal junction, and to help prevent inadvertent rectal puncture. This technique may also be mimicked under fluoroscopy.

1. The procedure is performed in an axial CT section of the sacrococcygeal disc.
2. A needle trajectory is planned off midline from both sides of the sacrum, to anterior to the sacrococcygeal junction.[11]

Tips

- A loss of resistance may be felt after traversing the sacrococcygeal ligament.
- Chemical ablation, pulsed radiofrequency, or cryoablation may be considered for longer-term relief.
- The sacrococcygeal disc may occasionally be calcified or fused, preventing access. In these cases, the anococcygeal or intracoccygeal approach may be used. The needle is inserted through the anococcygeal ligament and advanced against the anterior concavity of the inferior sacrum and coccyx to contact the ventral coccyx. This approach may increase the risk of infection as well as rectal perforation.[4]

Safety Considerations

- Rectal perforation is possible due to its close proximity to the ganglion. Care must be taken not to advance too far from the anterior surface of the coccyx.[12]
- Needle breakage is possible due to use of a small-bore needle while traversing the rigid disc.
- Rarely, sacral nerve roots may be in close proximity to the ganglion of impar, so care must be taken to avoid inadvertent damage in the case of ablation. This can be identified with motor testing identifying gluteus spasm.[13]

Postprocedure Management

Patients should be counseled on the expected results of the ganglion impar block and pertinent potential complications, which may include: rectal perforation, bleeding, infection, nerve injury, discitis with the trans-sacrococcygeal technique, and possible epidural spread of injectate. It is also possible to denervate parasympathetic fibers near the anterior sacrum as the injectate may spread cephalad along the anterior sacrum.[13]

References

1. Marker DR, U-Thainual P, Ungi T, Flammang AJ, Fichtinger G. MR-guided perineural injection of the ganglion impar: technical considerations and feasibility. *Skeletal Radiology*. 2016;45:591–597.
2. Sir E, Eksert S. Comparison of block and pulsed radiofrequency of the ganglion impar in coccygodynia. *Turk J Med Sci*. 2019;49(5):1555–1559. doi:10.3906/sag-1906-51
3. Oh CS, Chung IH, Ji HJ, et al. Clinical implications of topographic anatomy on the ganglion impar. *Anesthesiology*. 2004;101(1):249–250.
4. Khosla A, Adeyefa O, Nasir S. Successful treatment of radiation-induced proctitis pain by blockade of the ganglion impar in an elderly patient with prostate cancer: a case report. *Pain Medicine*. 2013;14(5):662–666. https://doi.org/10.1111/pme.12065
5. Le Clerc QC, Riant T, Levesque A, Labat JJ, Ploteau S, Robert R, Perrouin-Verbe MA, Rigaud J. Repeated ganglion impar block in a cohort of 83 patients with chronic pelvic and perineal pain. *Pain Physician*. 2017;20(6):E823–E828.
6. Plancarte R, Amescua C, Patt RB. Presacral blockade of the ganglion of Walther (ganglion impar). *Anesthesiology*. 1990;73:A751.
7. Sir E, Eksert S. Comparison of block and pulsed radiofrequency of the ganglion impar in coccygodynia. *Turk J Med Sci*. 2019;49(5):1555–1559. doi:10.3906/sag-1906-51
8. Malec-Milewska M, Horosz B, Kolęda I, et al. Neurolytic block of ganglion of Walther for the management of chronic pelvic pain. *Wideochir Inne Tech Maloinwazyjne*. 2014;9(3):458–462. doi:10.5114/wiitm.2014.43079
9. Kim SK, Ahn CS, Cho YR, Lim SY, Shin KM, Hong SY, et al. Ganglion impar block in the management of rectal tenesmoid pain. *Korean J Pain*. 1996;9:226–228.
10. Eker HE, Cok OY, Kocum A, et al. Transsacrococcygeal approach to ganglion impar for pelvic cancer pain: a report of 3 cases. *Reg Anesth Pain Med*. 2008;33:381–382.
11. Datir A, Connell D. CT-guided injection for ganglion impar blockade: a radiological approach to the management of coccydynia. *Clin Radiol*. 2010;65:21–25.
12. Malec-Milewska M, Horosz B, Kolęda I, et al. Neurolytic block of ganglion of Walther for the management of chronic pelvic pain. *Wideochir Inne Tech Maloinwazyjne*. 2014;9(3):458–462. doi:10.5114/wiitm.2014.43079
13. Oh CS Chung IH Ji HJ Yoon DM Clinical implications of topographic anatomy on the ganglion impar. *Anesthesiology*. 2004;101:249–250.
14. Lim SJ, Park HJ, Lee SH, Moon DE. Ganglion impar block with botulinum toxin type A for chronic perineal pain: a case report. *Korean J Pain*. 2010;23:65–69. https://doi.org/10.3344/kjp.2010.23.1.65

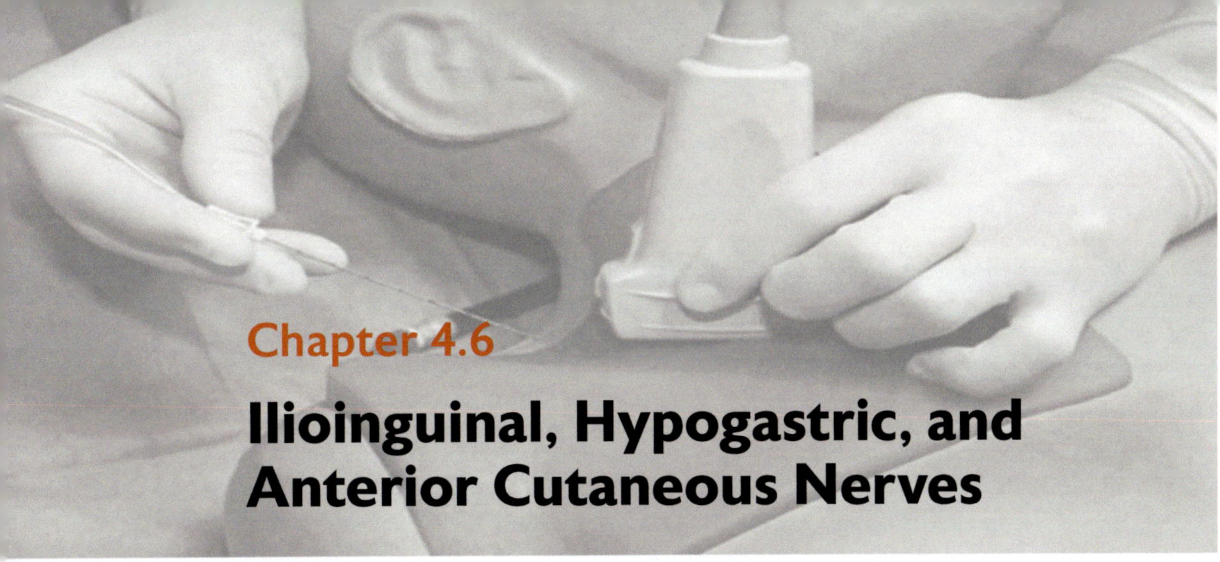

Chapter 4.6

Ilioinguinal, Hypogastric, and Anterior Cutaneous Nerves

Akshat Gargya

Contents

Introduction

Ilioinguinal and iliohypogastric nerves are frequently targeted in cancer patients scheduled for lower abdominal and pelvic surgery. These interventions are also used for chronic pain from lower abdominal, inguinal, and pelvic somatic cancer pain syndromes. Both the ilioinguinal and iliohypogastric nerves emerge from the lumbar plexus. The ventral primary rami of the T12 and L1 spinal nerves combine to form the ilioinguinal and iliohypogastric nerves.[1] Anterior cutaneous nerves are branches of the thoracoabdominal (T7–11) and subcostal (T12) plexuses and pass through neurovascular rings in the rectus muscle to supply the anterior abdominal wall. Anterior cutaneous nerves can become entrapped in these rings and are often the cause of chronic postsurgical abdominal pain.[2] Injections and ablations of these nerves can improve pain resulting from gastrostomy, anterior nephrostomy and jejunostomy tube placements, and various cancer pain syndromes.

Indications

Ilioinguinal and iliohypogastric nerves blocks provide postoperative analgesia for abdominal and pelvic surgeries for testicular cancer surgery, groin surgeries, orchidopexy repair, varicocele and hydrocele repair, and inguinal hernia repair.[3] They can also be utilized for chronic pain from chemotherapy-induced or radiation-induced neuropathies as well as soft tissue tumor resections within the superficial abdominopelvic musculature. A diagnostic block can differentiate pelvic pain originating from these somatic nerves from other neuralgias (e.g., pudendal neuralgia) and visceral pain.[4] Injecting local anesthetic in the oval shaped aponeurotic openings for anterior cutaneous nerves in the rectus muscle rings can diagnose anterior cutaneous nerve entrapment syndrome. Targeting these anterior cutaneous nerves may improve postsurgical pain and pain associated with chronic catheters, such as gastrostomy and jejunostomy tubes.

Critical Anatomy

Both the ilioinguinal and iliohypogastric nerves emerge from the lumbar plexus and travel to the lateral border of the psoas muscle. They then pass anterior to the quadratus lumborum muscle, reaching the iliac crest. Throughout its course, the ilioinguinal nerve runs inferior and parallel to the iliohypogastric nerve. At the level of iliac crest, the nerves then penetrate the transversus abdominis muscle to travel between transversus abdominis and internal oblique muscles (Figure 4.6.1). Both nerves provide motor innervation to transversus abdominis and internal oblique muscles. The ilioinguinal nerve then passes along the spermatic cord in males or round ligament in females to provide sensory innervation to the pubic symphysis, anterior scrotal surface, root of the penis in males, and labia majora in females. The iliohypogastric nerve divides into a lateral cutaneous branch and anterior (or medial) cutaneous branch. The lateral cutaneous branch lies between internal oblique and external oblique muscles and provides sensory innervation to the fascia and skin of superolateral gluteal region. The anterior (or medial) cutaneous branch lies between transversus abdominis and internal oblique muscles and supplies the skin of the inguinal area.[5]

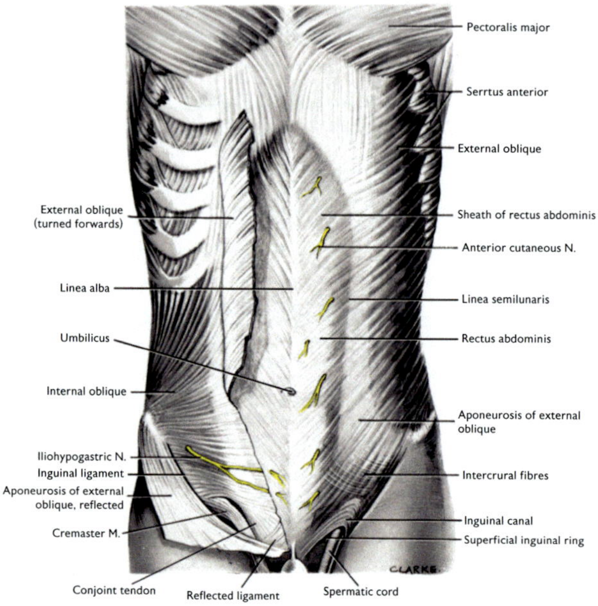

Figure 4.6.1 Anterior abdominal wall revealing the iliohypogastric and anterior cutaneous nerves. The external oblique muscle has been reflected on the right side of the body. (Reprinted with permission from Cunningham's Manual of Practical Anatomy: Thorax and Abdomen, 16th Edition)

Equipment and Patient Preparation

1. **Monitors and Sterility**
   a. No specific monitors are needed for this procedure, but emergency resuscitation equipment should be available immediately. This includes ACLS drugs, supplemental oxygen, airway adjuncts, and suction.
   b. Strict antiseptic technique should be observed including sterile probe cover, ultrasound gel, and sterile gloves. Chlorhexidine or other skin prep agent should be used to clean the skin prior to commencing the procedure.
2. **Equipment**
   a. Probe: High-frequency linear array transducer (8–12 MHz)
   b. Needle type: 22- or 25-gauge, 1.5- to 3.5-inch needle
   c. Local anesthetic (1–4 mL): Lidocaine 1%–2%; ropivacaine 0.2%–0.5%; bupivacaine 0.25%–0.5%
   d. Adjuvant (1 mL): Nonparticulate or particulate steroid
3. **Position**
   a. Supine

Step-by-Step Technique

Ilioinguinal and Iliohypogastric Nerves Approach (Figure 4.6.2)

1. **Prepare equipment and supplies, position the patient supine, and sterilize the procedural area with antiseptic solution.**
2. **Place the ultrasound probe in a transverse orientation just medial to the anterior superior iliac spine (ASIS).** Rotate the ultrasound probe so the medial aspect is directed toward the umbilicus.
3. **Identify the plane between the internal oblique and transversus abdominis muscles**. It is also critical to identify the peritoneal cavity and bowel just deep to the muscle layer.
4. **In case of difficult anatomy, color doppler can be utilized to identify pulsations of the deep circumflex iliac artery.** The artery runs parallel to the ilioinguinal nerve in the same plane and thus can be a useful guide to nerve location (which on ultrasound is seen as hypoechoic structure). Medial to the ilioinguinal nerve is the iliohypogastric nerve.
5. **Confirm the correct nerves have been identified by following them proximally to the ASIS.**
6. **Inject local anesthetic subcutaneously for analgesia at the procedural site.**
7. **Insert the procedural needle with an in-plane approach from a lateral-to-medial direction.** Use a 22- or 25-gauge needle. Advance the needle through the external oblique and internal oblique muscles to the targeted nerve.
8. **Inject the medication around the targeted nerve.** Remove the needle and apply a dressing.

Tips and Safety Considerations

- Use doppler imaging to identify the deep circumflex iliac artery to avoid vascular puncture and intravascular injection.
- Avoid an overly steep needle trajectory to prevent inadvertent peritoneal cavity perforation.
- Consider tracing the nerves cephalad in order to move the ASIS out of the way, allowing a shallower angle and avoiding pain from bony contact. Alternatively, translate the lateral aspect of the probe cephalad while keeping the target fascial plane in view.

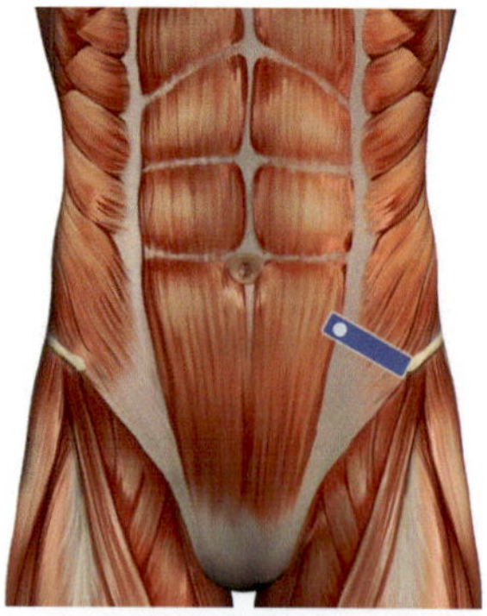

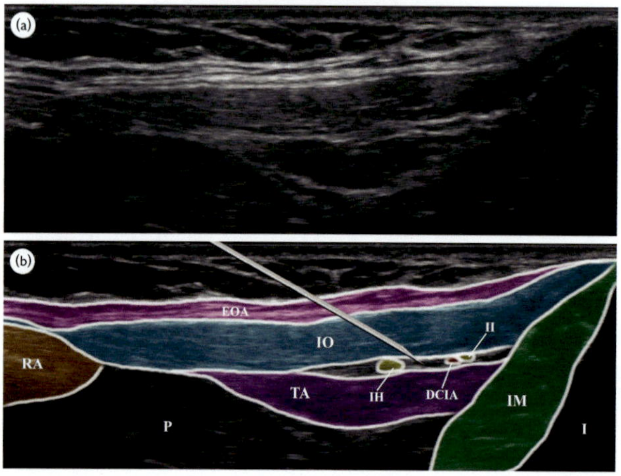

Figure 4.6.2 a, Ultrasound image of the anterior abdomen in a transverse axial oblique plane. **b,** Labeled ultrasound image of in-plane needle placement for an ilioinguinal and hypogastric nerve block in short-axis. *EOA* external oblique aponeurosis, *IO* internal oblique, *IM* iliacus muscle, *I* iliac bone, *RA* rectus abdominis, *TA* transversus abdominis, *IH* iliohypogastric nerve, *DCIA* deep circumflex iliac artery, *II* ilioinguinal nerve, *P* peritoneal cavity.

Anterior Cutaneous Nerve Approach (Figure 4.6.3)

1. **Prepare equipment and supplies, position the patient supine, and sterilize the procedural area with antiseptic solution.**
2. **Place the ultrasound probe in a transverse orientation just medial to the corresponding painful dermatomal level in the anterior abdominal wall.**
3. **Identify the plane between the rectus abdominis and oblique musculature (transversus abdominis, internal/external obliques).** Locate the lateral border of the rectus abdominis muscle (seen as a hypoechoic structure on ultrasound). The linea semilunaris (hyperechoic) is then visualized separating the rectus abdominis from the oblique musculature. The target nerve is localized in the region between the oblique musculature and the rectus abdominis as a hyperechoic honeycomb-like structure.
4. **Inject local anesthetic subcutaneously for analgesia at the procedural site.** The target nerves are located in the plane between the internal oblique and transversus abdominis muscles.
5. **Insert the procedural needle with an in-plane approach from a lateral-to-medial direction.** Use a 22- or 25-gauge needle. Advance the needle through the external oblique and internal oblique muscles to the targeted nerve.
6. **Inject the medication around the targeted nerve.** Remove the needle and apply a dressing.

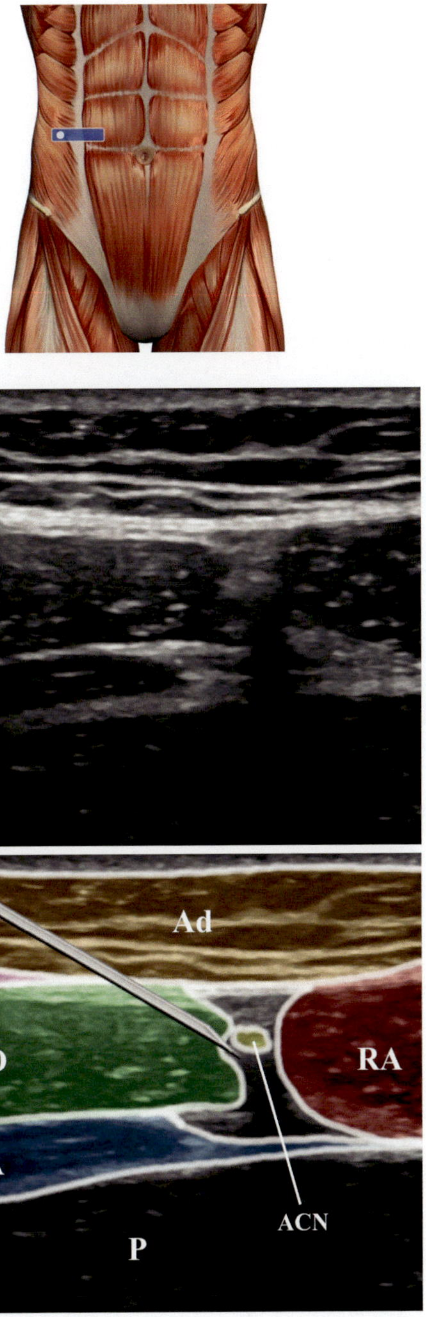

Figure 4.6.3 **a,** Ultrasound image of the anterior abdomen in a transverse axial plane. **b,** Labeled ultrasound image of in-plane needle placement for an anterior abdominal cutaneous nerve block in short-axis. *Ad* adipose, *EO* external oblique, *IO* internal oblique, *ACN* anterior cutaneous nerve (common location), *RA* rectus abdominis, *TA* transversus abdominis, *P* peritoneal cavity.

Tips and Safety Considerations

- Use doppler imaging to identify the satellite vessels to avoid inadvertent puncture and intravascular injection.
- Avoid an overly steep needle trajectory to prevent inadvertent peritoneal cavity perforation.

- Consider using a higher gauge/thinner needle for patient comfort.
- Aspirate before injection and consider hydrodissection with needle advancement.

Postprocedure Management

It is critical to perform a lower extremity neurological examination to rule out an unintended femoral cutaneous or femoral nerve blockade. Patients should be made aware of the potential of an ineffective block. Patients should also be counseled on potential complications such as vascular injury leading to hematoma formation, local anesthetic toxicity (rare), infection, nerve injury, and peritoneal perforation causing small or large bowel perforation (especially in patients with thin abdominal walls). There is also a risk for unintended femoral cutaneous or femoral nerve blockade due to tracking down of local anesthetic medications and hence patients should be counseled about potential fall risk.[6]

References

1. Puntillo F, Bertini L, Bosco M, Tedesco M, Baciarello M. US-guided nerve blocks: procedure technique. In: Silvestri E, Martino F, Puntillo F (eds.), Ultrasound-Guided Peripheral Nerve Blocks. Springer, Cham; 2018: 105–42
2. Clarke S, Kanakarajan S. Abdominal cutaneous nerve entrapment syndrome. Cont Edu in Anaes Crit Care. 2015;15(2):60–63. https://doi.org/10.1093/bjaceaccp/mku016
3. Eichenberger U, Greher M, Kirchmair L, Curatolo M, Moriggl B. Ultrasound-guided blocks of the ilioinguinal and iliohypogastric nerve: accuracy of a selective new technique confirmed by anatomical dissection. Br J Anaesth. 2006;97(2):238–243.
4. Peng PW, Tumber PS. Ultrasound-guided interventional procedures for patients with chronic pelvic pain: a description of techniques and review of literature. Pain Physician. 2008;11(2):215–224.
5. Sehgal N. Ilioinguinal Nerve. In: Abd-Elsayed A. (ed.), Pain. Springer, Cham; 2019: 533–536.
6. Udo I, Umeh K, Eyo C. Transient femoral nerve palsy following ilioinguinal nerve block for inguinal hernioplasty. Nig J of Surg. 2018;24(1):23.

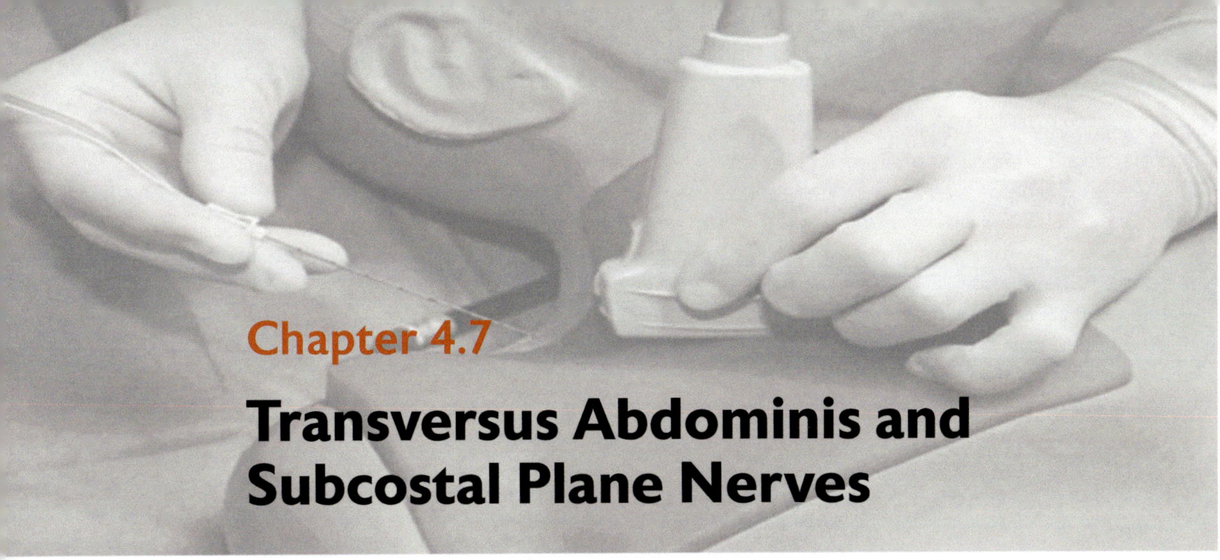

Chapter 4.7

Transversus Abdominis and Subcostal Plane Nerves

Akshat Gargya

Contents

Introduction

The transverse abdominis plane (TAP) block is a frequently performed regional, perioperative, field block done to provide analgesia for anterior abdominal surgeries.[1] Using ultrasound is considered the gold standard for performing this block, although it was first described as a blind landmark-based technique by Rafi.[2] The location to deposit local anesthetic medication differentiates the TAP block from the subcostal TAP (SCTAP) block. In the SCTAP block, medication is injected in the same muscle plane inferiorly and parallel to the costal margin, which is more cephalad to the TAP.[3]

Indications

TAP blocks are indicated in cancer patients for three particular reasons: (1) acute pain from palliative or curative anterior abdominal, gynecological, and urological surgeries; (2) chronic pain stemming from interventions such as ostomy placements or gastrostomy and jejunostomy tubes; and (3) chronic pain related to cancer and cancer treatments. TAP blocks often help pain related to laparoscopic or robotic hysterectomy, lower (uterine) segment Caesarean section with Pfannenstiel incision, nephrectomy, adrenalectomy, prostatectomy, and open umbilical/inguinal hernia repairs.[4] TAP blocks usually cover the abdominal wall from the T9 to L1 dermatomes. Additionally, neurolysis of the plane can help provide longer relief for those suffering from chronic pain.

In many abdominal surgeries or tube/drain placements where the incision extends cephalad above the umbilicus, the SCTAP block is useful. The SCTAP block provides blockade of sensory innervation to the anterior abdominal wall up to the T6 dermatome.[3] Both the TAP and SCTAP blocks can be offered to patients to reduce postoperative analgesic medication requirements where neuraxial anesthesia is contraindicated.

Critical Anatomy

The thoracolumbar nerves (T6–L1) are responsible for sensory innervation to the anterolateral abdominal wall. They divide to form anterior primary rami, which travel anteriorly out of the vertebral foramen (Figure 4.7.1). These anterior primary rami further divide into anterior and lateral cutaneous branches to supply the abdominal wall. The lateral cutaneous branches are located near the angles of ribs, while the anterior cutaneous branches communicate to form a plexus anterolaterally.[5]

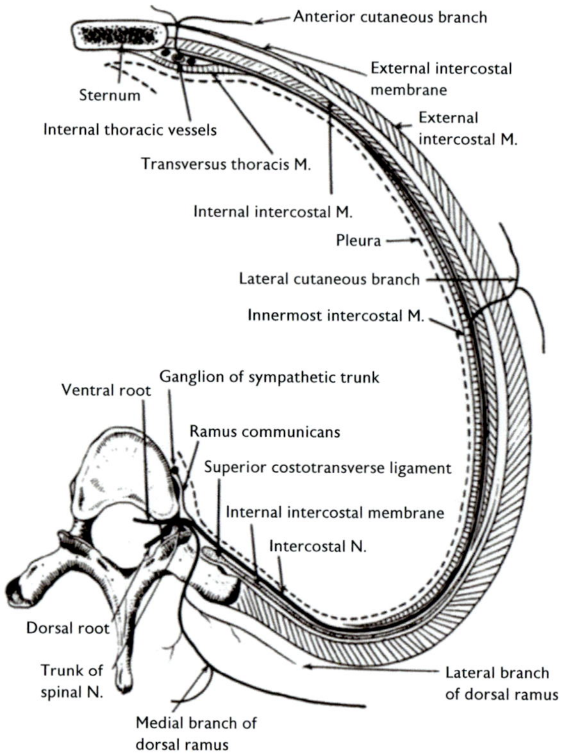

Figure 4.7.1 A diagram of the upper thoracic spinal nerve in an intercostal space. (Reprinted with permission from Cunningham's Manual of Practical Anatomy: Thorax and Abdomen, 16th Edition)

Equipment and Patient Preparation

1. **Monitors and Sterility**
   a. No specific monitors are needed for this procedure, but emergency resuscitation equipment should be available immediately. This includes ACLS drugs, supplemental oxygen, airway adjuncts, and suction.
   b. Strict antiseptic technique should be observed including sterile probe cover, ultrasound gel, and sterile gloves. Chlorhexidine or other skin prep agent should be used to clean the skin prior to commencing the procedure.
2. **Equipment**
   a. Probe: High-frequency linear array transducer (8–12 MHz)
   b. Needle type: 22- or 25-gauge, 1.5- to 3.5-inch needle
   c. Local anesthetic (4–9 mL each side): Lidocaine 1%–2%; ropivacaine 0.2%–0.5%; bupivacaine 0.25%–0.5%
   d. Adjuvant (1 mL each side): Nonparticulate or particulate steroid
3. **Position**
   a. Supine (preferred) or lateral decubitus

Procedure Technique

TAP Block (Figure 4.7.2)

1. **Prepare equipment and supplies, position the patient supine, and sterilize the procedural area with antiseptic solution.**
2. **Place the ultrasound probe in a transverse orientation plane in the lateral clavicular to midaxillary line, between the lower costal margin and iliac crest.**
3. **Identify the plane between the internal oblique and transverse abdominis muscles.** It is also critical to identify the peritoneal cavity and bowel just deep to the muscle layer. **Inject local anesthetic subcutaneously for analgesia at the procedural site. The target nerves are located in the plane between the internal oblique and transversus abdominis muscles.**
4. **Insert the procedural needle with an in-plane approach from a lateral-to-medial direction.** Use a 22- or 25-gauge needle. Advance the needle through the external oblique and internal oblique muscles to the plane above the transverse abdominis muscle.
5. **Inject the medication between the internal oblique and transversus abdominis muscles.** Remove the needle and apply a dressing.

Tips and Safety Considerations

- Use doppler imaging to identify the satellite arteries to avoid vascular puncture and intravascular injection.
- Avoid a needle trajectory that is too steep, to prevent perforation of the peritoneal cavity.

SCTAP Block (Figure 4.7.3)

1. **Prepare equipment and supplies, position the patient supine, and sterilize the procedural area with antiseptic solution.**
2. **Place the ultrasound probe in a transverse orientation midline below the xiphoid process.** Locate the paired rectus abdominis muscles.

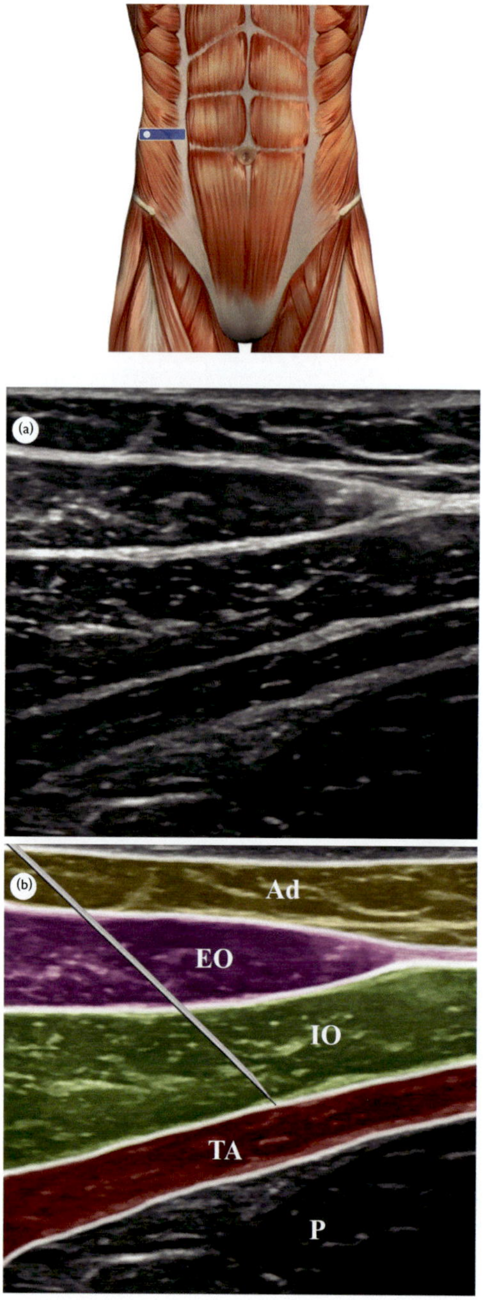

Figure 4.7.2 a, Ultrasound image of the anterior abdomen in an axial plane. **b,** Labeled ultrasound image of in-plane needle placement for a transversus abdominis plane block in short-axis. *Ad* adipose, *EO* external oblique, *IO* internal oblique, *TA* transversus abdominis, *P* peritoneal cavity.

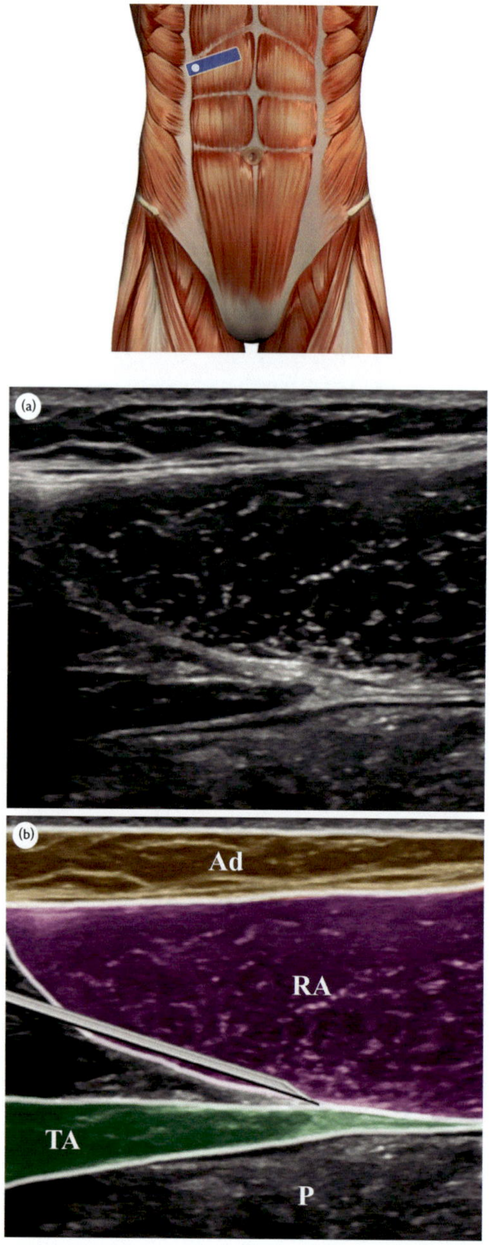

Figure 4.7.3 a, Ultrasound image of the anterior abdomen in an axial oblique plane. **b,** Labeled ultrasound image of in-plane needle placement for a subcostal plane block in short-axis. *Ad* adipose, *RA* rectus abdominis, *TA* transversus abdominis, *P* peritoneal cavity.

3. **Translate the ultrasound probe laterally to find the transversus abdominis below the rectus muscle.** The probe can also be moved obliquely to get a sharper picture.
4. **Translate further laterally and caudally to locate hyperechoic aponeurosis of the linea-semilunaris.**
5. **Identify the plane between the rectus and transversus abdominis muscles, which is the target plane**. It is also critical to identify the peritoneal cavity and bowel just deep to the muscle layer.
6. **Inject local anesthetic subcutaneously for analgesia at the procedural site.**
7. **Insert the procedural needle with an in-plane approach from a lateral-to-medial direction.** Use a 22- or 25-gauge needle. Advance the needle through the external oblique and internal oblique muscles to the plane above the transverse abdominis muscle.
8. **Inject the medication between the internal oblique and transversus abdominis muscles.** Remove the needle and apply a dressing.

Tips and Safety Considerations

- Use doppler imaging to identify the satellite arteries to avoid inadvertent puncture and intravascular injection.
- Avoid a needle trajectory that is too steep, to prevent perforation of the peritoneal cavity.

Postprocedure Management

A lower extremity neurological examination to rule out an unintended femoral nerve blockade. Patients should also be made aware of the potential of an ineffective block. Additionally, patients should also be counseled on and monitored for potential complications such vascular injury leading to hematoma formation, local anesthetic toxicity (rare), infection, nerve injury, and peritoneal perforation causing small or large bowel perforation (especially in patients with thin abdominal walls).

References

1. Tsai HC, Yoshida T, Chuang TY, et al. Transversus abdominis plane block: an updated review of anatomy and techniques. Biomed Res Int. 2017;2017:8284363. doi:10.1155/2017/8284363
2. Rafi AN. Abdominal field block: a new approach via the lumbar triangle. Anaesthesia. 2001;56(10):1024–1026.
3. Soliz JM, Lipski I, Hancher-Hodges S, Speer BB, Popat K. Subcostal transverse abdominis plane block for acute pain management: a review. Anesth Pain Med. 2017;7(5):e12923. doi:10.5812/aapm.12923
4. Young MJ, Gorlin AW, Modest VE, Quraishi SA. Clinical implications of the transversus abdominis plane block in adults. Anesthesiol Res Pract. 2012;2012:731645. doi: 10.1155/2012/731645
5. Rozen WM, Tran TM, Ashton MW, Barrington MJ, Ivanusic JJ, Taylor GI. Refining the course of the thoracolumbar nerves: a new understanding of the innervation of the anterior abdominal wall. Clin Anat. 2008 May;21(4):325–33. doi:10.1002/ca.20621. PMID: 18428988.

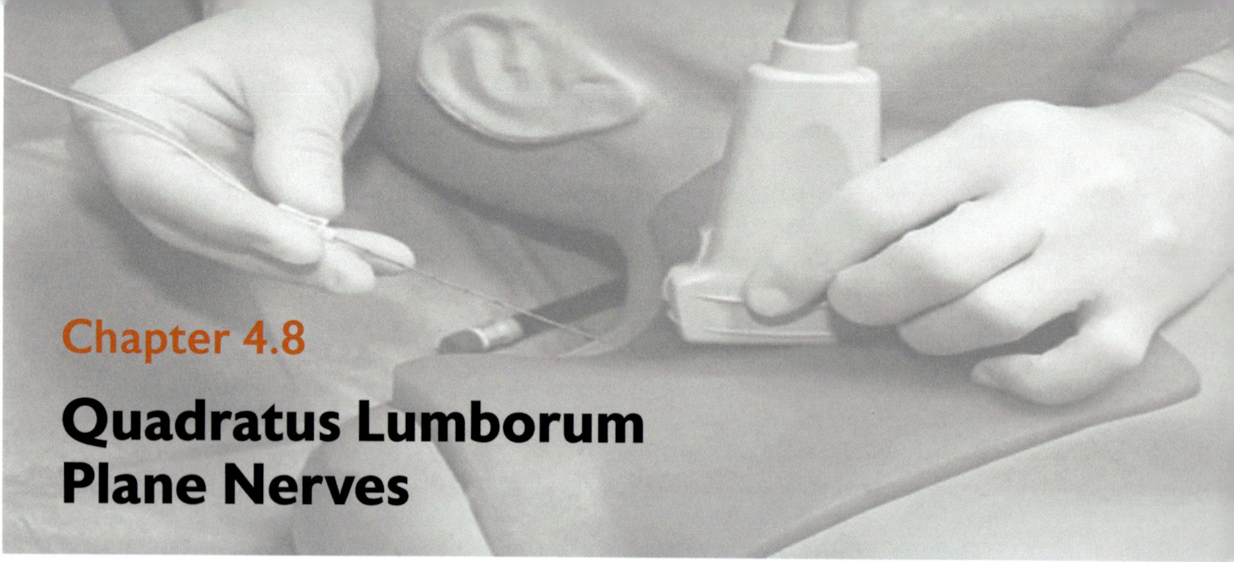

Chapter 4.8

Quadratus Lumborum Plane Nerves

Akshat Gargya

Contents

Introduction

The quadratus lumborum (QL) block is a fascial plane field block used for acute and chronic low thoracic and flank pain syndromes. Although the exact mechanism is unknown, the QL block is theorized to work by anesthetizing spinal nerves in a manner similar to a paravertebral block.[1–4]

Indications

Quadratus lumborum blocks can be used in cancer patients with chronic pain or undergoing lower abdominal surgeries like laparoscopic gynecological surgery, proctosigmoidectomy, and nephrectomy. The block can also be used for relieving pain for hip surgery and pathological fracture of the femoral neck.[2] In oncologic patients, common visceral referral patterns from renal masses can present with flank pain that can be relieved with this procedure. Other disease states that can improve after a QL block are T12 rib and lateral abdominal wall metastasis.

Critical Anatomy

Quadratus lumborum muscles form the posterior abdominal wall. They originate from the iliac crests and insert on the medial border of the 12th ribs and transverse processes of the first four lumbar vertebrae. Posteriorly, the QL muscle is surrounded by thoracolumbar fascia, separating it from the latissimus dorsi muscle laterally and the erector spinae muscles medially (Figures 4.8.1–2). Anteriorly, the quadratus lumborum muscle is separated from the psoas muscles by a thin fascial plane. Local anesthetic medications are injected anterior, lateral, or posterior to the QL muscle at the level of iliac crest (L4) and L2. Cadaveric models have shown that the medication spreads cranially to thoracic paravertebral space to block thoracic sympathetic trunk up to T9 level.[2] It is theorized that spread of medications to the thoracolumbar fascia often block sympathetic afferent fibers, contributing to its analgesic mechanism.[5]

Equipment and Patient Preparation

1. Monitors and Sterility

a. No specific monitors are needed for this procedure, but emergency resuscitation equipment should be available immediately. This includes ACLS drugs, supplemental oxygen, airway adjuncts, and suction.

b. Strict antiseptic technique should be observed including sterile probe cover, ultrasound gel, and sterile gloves. Chlorhexidine or other skin prep agent should be used to clean the skin prior to commencing the procedure.

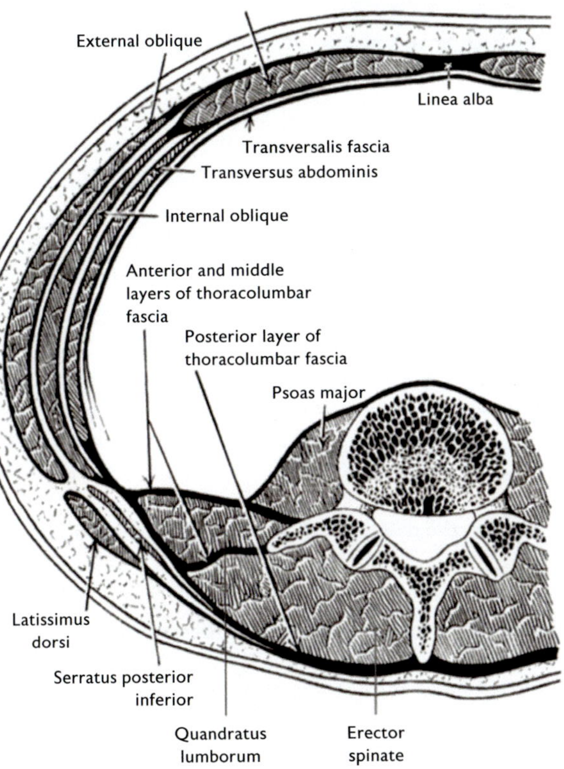

Figure 4.8.1 A horizontal section through the abdominal walls at the level of the second lumbar vertebra illustrating the locations of the erector spinae and quadratus lumborum muscles. (Reprinted with permission from Cunningham's Manual of Practical Anatomy: Thorax and Abdomen, 16th Edition)

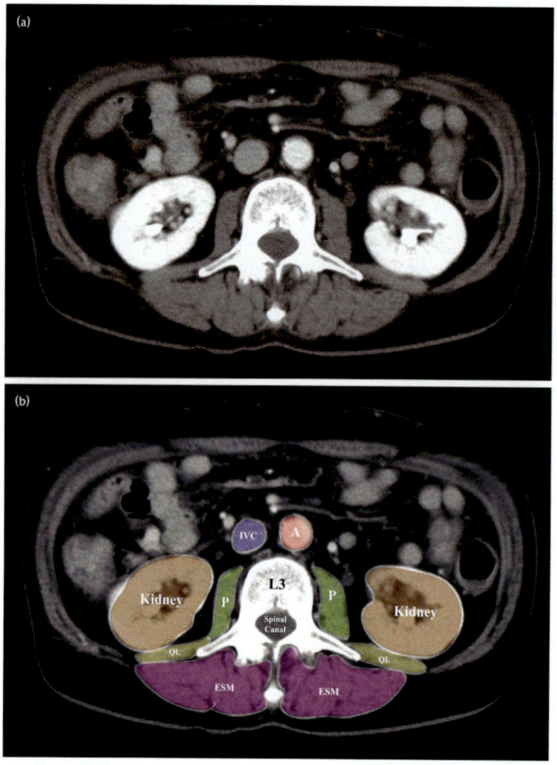

Figure 4.8.2 CT images of the quadratus lumborum muscle at the level of L3 transverse process (unlabeled - **a**, labeled - **b**). *IVC* inferior vena cava, *A* aorta, *P* psoas muscle, *QL* quadratus lumborum, *ESM* erector spinae muscle.

2. **Equipment**
   a. Probe: High-frequency linear array transducer (8–12 MHz) or low-frequency linear array transducer (2–5 MHz) depending on body habitus
   b. Needle type: 22- or 25-gauge, 2- to 3.5-inch needle
   c. Local anesthetic (2–4 mL): Lidocaine 1%–2%; ropivacaine 0.2%–0.5%; bupivacaine 0.25%–0.5%
   d. Adjuvant (1 mL): Nonparticulate or particulate steroid
3. **Position**
   a. Lateral decubitus (preferred) or supine

Step-by-Step Technique

QL Block (Figure 4.8.3)

1. **Prepare equipment and supplies, position the patient, and sterilize the procedural area with antiseptic solution.**
2. **Place the ultrasound probe in a transverse orientation just cephalad above the iliac crest.**
3. **Identify the posterior abdominal wall muscles and the transverse processes of L2, L3, and L4.** On ultrasound the "shamrock sign" is often visualized to identify the structures. The QL muscle forms the lateral leaf of the shamrock, the erector spinae muscles make up the posterior leaf, and the psoas major muscle makes the anterior leaf. The transverse processes of the L2–L4 vertebra represents the stem connecting the three leaves together.

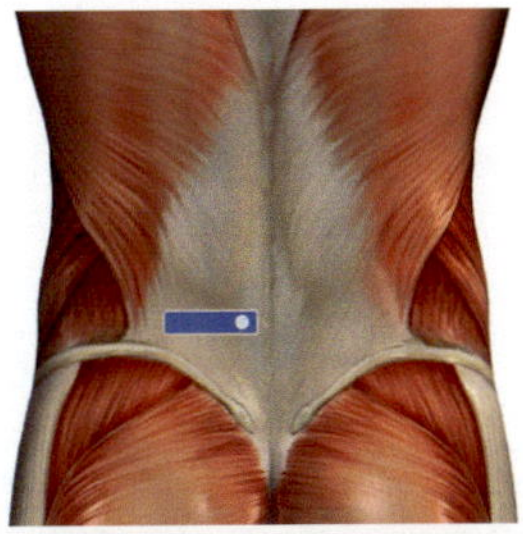

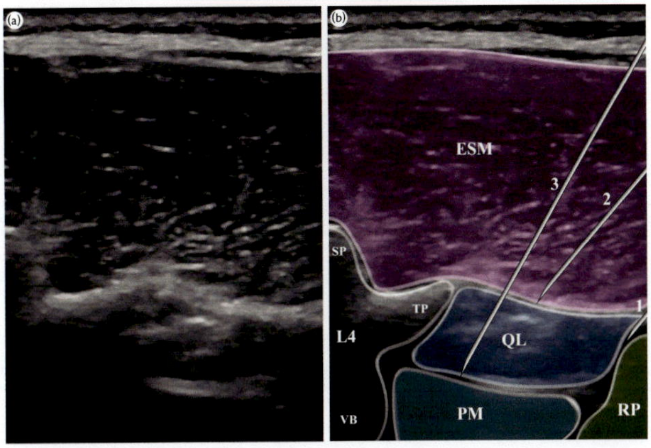

Figure 4.8.3 a, Ultrasound image of the posterior lumbar L4 region in an axial plane. **b,** Labeled ultrasound image of in-plane needle placement for a lateral/QL1 (needle #1), posterior/QL2 (needle #2), and anterior/transmuscular/QL3 (needle #3) quadratus lumborum plane block in short-axis. *ESM* erector spinae muscles, *QL* quadratus lumborum, *RP* retroperitoneal space, *PM* psoas major, *L4 SP* transverse process—*TP* transverse process—*VB* vertebral body.

4. **Identify the target fascial plane at the lateral QL muscle, which is also known as QL1.** (Figure 4.8.3—needle #1). For an anterior QL block (also known as the transmuscular QL, or QL3), the target is in the tissue plane between the QL and psoas muscles (Figure 4.8.3—needle #3) and in the plane between the quadratus lumborum and erector spinae muscles for posterior quadratus lumborum block (also known as the QL2, (Figure 4.8.3—needle #2).
5. **Inject local anesthetic subcutaneously for analgesia at the procedural site.**
6. **Insert the procedural needle with an in-plane approach from a posterior-to-anterior direction.** Use a 22- or 25-gauge needle. Consider using hydrodissection to verify correct needle placement in the desired fascial plane.
7. **Inject the medication around the QL muscle.** Remove the needle and apply a dressing.

Postprocedure Management

Patients should be counseled on and monitored for potential complications such vascular injury leading to hematoma formation (within the retroperitoneal space), local anesthetic toxicity (rare), infection, nerve injury, and peritoneal perforation. Additionally, patients should be made aware of the potential of an ineffective block.

References

1. Vidal E, Giménez H, Forero M, Fajardo M. Erector spinae plane block: a cadaver study to determine its mechanism of action. Revista Española de Anestesiología y Reanimación (English Edition). 2018;65(9):514–519.

2. Elsharkawy, H, El-Boghdadly, K, Kolli, S, Esa, WAS, DeGrande, S, Soliman, LM, Drake, RL. Injectate spread following anterior sub-costal and posterior approaches to the quadratus lumborum block: a comparative cadaveric study. Eur J Anaesthesiol. 2017;34:587–595.
3. Elsharkawy H, El-Boghdadly K, Barrington M. Quadratus lumborum block: anatomical concepts, mechanisms, and techniques. Anesthesiology. 2019;130(2):322–335. doi: 10.1097/ALN.0000000000002524.
4. Kot P, Rodriguez P, Granell M, et al. The erector spinae plane block: a narrative review. Korean J Anesthesiol. 2019;72(3):209–220. doi:10.4097/kja.d.19.00012
5. Benetazzo L, Bizzego A, De Caro R, Frigo G, Guidolin D, Stecco C. 3D reconstruction of the crural and thoracolumbar fasciae. Surg Radiol Anat. 2011;33:855–862.

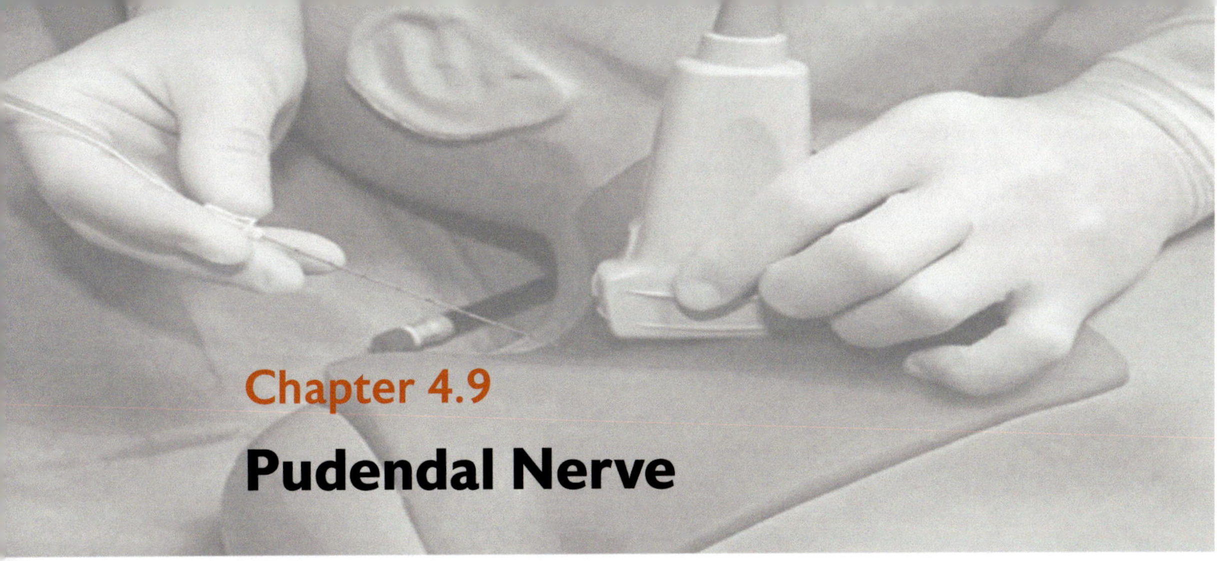

Chapter 4.9

Pudendal Nerve

Ajax Yang and Anthony Mazzola

Contents

Introduction

Pudendal neuralgia is a complex condition that significantly compromises the quality of life among men and women.[1–3] Pudendal neuropathy is a clinical diagnosis with symptoms classically reported as shooting or burning pain with sensory changes affecting the saddle region. Pain intensifies with sitting and decreases following a pudendal nerve block.[4] For the cancer patient, rectal or perineal tumors may result in somatic pain in the pudendal distribution. Neuralgias of this nerve can result from surgery or radiation in the perineal distribution.

On exam, there may be hyperalgesia, allodynia, and paresthesia. Symptoms are frequently unilateral; however, some patients present with bilateral pain. Regardless of symptom laterality, patients with pudendal neuralgia may benefit from a diagnostic block after exhausting the usual conservative medical management. In this chapter, the technical aspects of ultrasound-guided pudendal nerve interventions are discussed.

Indications and Technique

Compared to the conventional fluoroscopic landmark technique targeting directly adjacent to the tip of the ischial spine, ultrasound allows for the confirmation of injectate spread at the target between the sacrospinous and sacrotuberous ligaments at the ischial spine.[5] Evidence shows that fluoroscopic and ultrasound-guided block results are comparable in terms of reducing temperature and pinprick sensitivity.[6] A perioperative ultrasound-guided pudendal nerve block before transrectal ultrasound-guided prostate biopsy resulted in significantly less pain during both rectal probe insertion and prostate needle punctures.[7] Among oncological patients, pudendal nerve blocks have decreased radiation and chemotherapy-induced pudendal neuralgia.[8]

Diagnostic criteria have been proposed for pudendal neuralgia by pudendal nerve entrapment, which include five essential diagnostic criteria:[4] (1) Pain in the anatomical territory of the pudendal nerve; (2) The pain worsened by sitting; (3) The patient is not woken by the pain at night; (4) No objective sensory loss on clinical examination; (5) Positive anesthetic pudendal nerve block. Pudendal neuralgia often manifests as perineal, anal, or genital pain.

Critical Anatomy

The pudendal nerve is derived from the sacral plexus that is formed by the S2, S3, and S4 spinal nerves coalescing and coursing in an inferolateral trajectory anterior to the piriformis muscle (Figure 4.9.1). The pudendal artery, nerve, and vein form a bundle and travel in a space bordered by the sacrospinous ligament anteriorly and sacrotuberous ligament posteriorly next to the ischial spine. The pudendal nerve then wraps around the posterior portion of the sacrospinous ligament before entering the pudendal canal (Alcock's canal) formed by the obturator internus aponeurosis. The pudendal nerve is the most posterior structure within the canal. There are several locations where the pudendal nerve can be compressed including at the piriformis muscle, between the sacrospinous and sacrotuberous ligaments (most common), in the pudendal canal, and just below the inferior pubic ramus.[9,10] Although the pudendal nerve conducts both afferent sensory input and motor control of the pelvic floor musculature, external anal sphincter, and urethral sphincter; sensory dysfunction is observed more commonly in neuralgia of the nerve.[11] Because the pudendal nerve lies deeply in the pelvis, only the more proximal portion of the nerve is visible under ultrasound. Doppler ultrasound has been used to confirm the pudendal nerve location in relation to the pudendal artery and vein.[12,13] Optimal pudendal nerve injection was reported approximately 8 mm medial to the tip of the ischial spine and roughly 5 mm medial to the internal pudendal artery.[14] Distally, the pudendal nerve is further subdivided into three divisions: inferior anal nerve (also known as the rectal nerve), the perineal nerve, and the dorsal clitoral/penile nerve.[15]

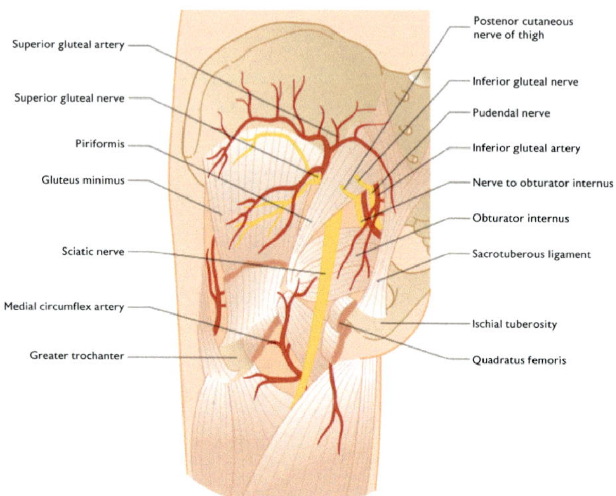

Figure 4.9.1 Dissection of the left gluteal region revealing the pudendal nerve. The gluteus maximus and gluteus medius have been removed and the quadratus femoris has been reflected. (Reprinted with permission from Cunningham's Manual of Practical Anatomy: Upper and Lower Limbs, 16th Edition)

Inferior Anal Nerve

The exact location of the inferior anal nerve is highly unpredictable. It can be found anywhere along the path of the pudendal canal and near the sacrospinous ligament. It traverses the ischioanal fossa to provide motor supply to the external sphincter and sensory innervation to the perianal skin, lower vagina, and the distal anal canal.

The Perineal Nerve

The perineal division courses in the inferior portion of the pudendal canal and provides both sensory and motor innervations as follows: sensation to labia/scrotum and muscular activation to levator ani, external anal sphincter, urethral sphincter, superficial transverse perineal muscle, bulbospongiosus muscle, ischiocavernosus muscle, and deep transverse perineal muscle.

Dorsal Clitoral or Penile Nerve

This branch of the pudendal nerve runs beneath the inferior ramus and pierces through the urogenital membrane. It then makes an acute cephalad turn to continue its course adjacent to the ischiocavernosus muscle and the inferior edge of the inferior pubic ramus. In females, the dorsal clitoral nerve innervates the clitoris. Similarly in males, the penile nerve innervates the corpus cavernosum and the skin of the penis. The motor branches supply the deep transverse perinei muscle and the urethral sphincter. The urethral branches supply the mucosa of the urethra.

Equipment and Patient Preparation

1. **Monitors and Sterility**
    a. No specific monitors are needed for this procedure, but emergency resuscitation equipment should be available immediately. This includes ACLS drugs, supplemental oxygen, airway adjuncts, and suction.
    b. Strict antiseptic technique should be observed including sterile probe cover, ultrasound gel, and sterile gloves. Chlorhexidine or other skin prep agent should be used to clean the skin prior to commencing the procedure.
2. **Equipment**
    a. Probe: Low-frequency linear array transducer (2–5 MHz) depending on body habitus
    b. Needle type: 22- or 25-gauge, 2- to 3.5-inch needle
    c. Local anesthetic (2–4 mL): Lidocaine 1%–2%; ropivacaine 0.2%–0.5%; bupivacaine 0.25%–0.5%
    d. Adjuvant (1 mL): Nonparticulate or particulate steroid
3. **Position**
    a. Prone

Step-by-Step Technique

1. **Prepare equipment and supplies, position the patient prone, and sterilize the procedural area with antiseptic solution.**
2. **Place the ultrasound probe in a transverse orientation to identify the posterior superior iliac spine**. By scanning caudally, the ilium appears as a hyperechoic line that traverses in a downward and outward direction (Figure 4.9.2).
3. **Continue to scan caudally to bring the greater sciatic notch and piriformis muscle in view.** At this level, the posterior portion of the ilium will appear as a curved structure (Figure 4.9.3).

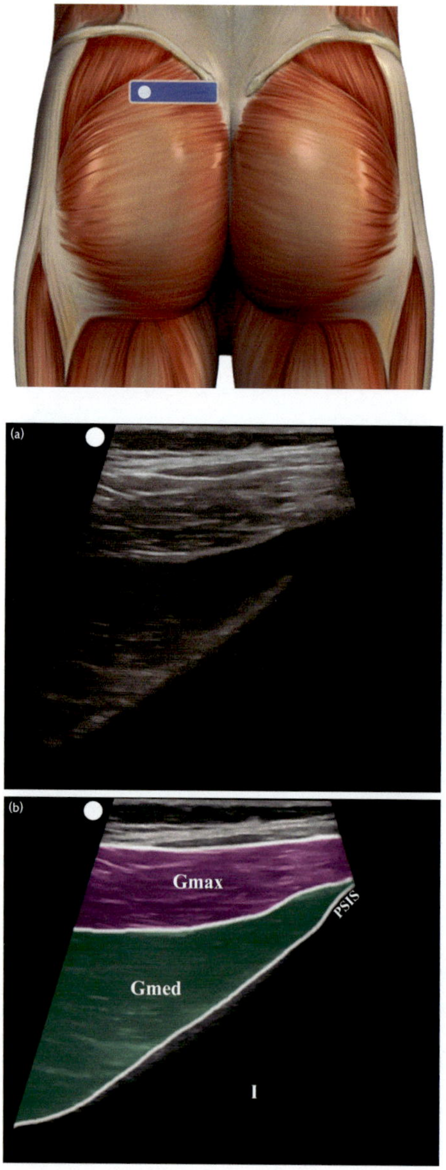

Figure 4.9.2 **a,** Ultrasound image of the posterior buttock in an axial plane. **b,** Labeled ultrasound image of the posterior gluteal muscles. *Gmax* gluteus maximus, *Gmed* gluteus medius, *PSIS* posterior superior iliac spine.

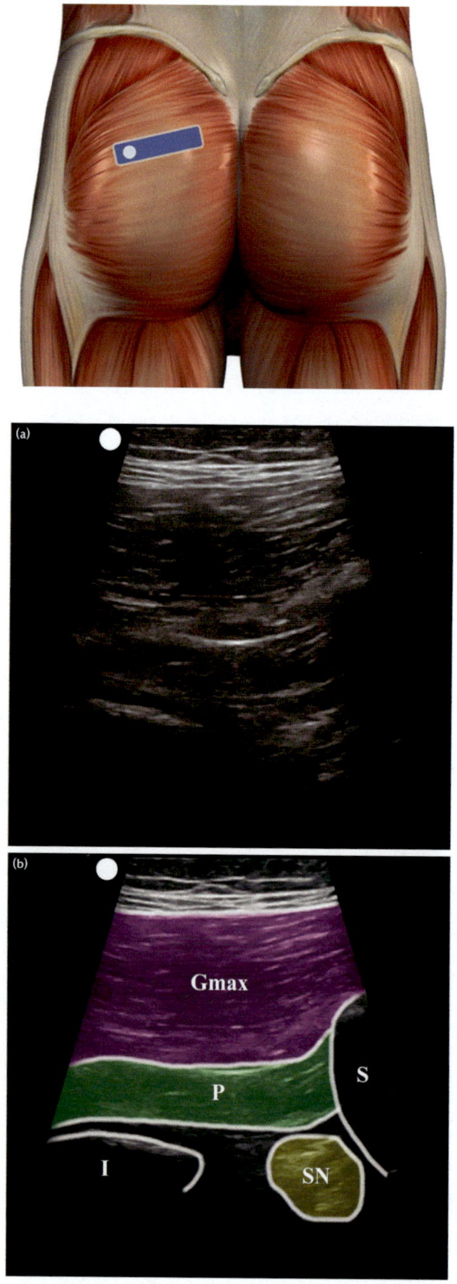

Figure 4.9.3 **a,** Ultrasound image of the posterior buttock in an axial oblique plane. **b,** Labeled ultrasound image of the piriformis muscle in long-axis and sciatic nerve in short-axis. *Gmax* gluteus maximus, *P* piriformis, *I* ilium, *SN* sciatic nerve (housed in the greater sciatic foramen), *S sacrum*.

4. **Identify the ischial spine.** By moving the probe further caudally, the curved hyperechoic line (the posterior rim of the ilium) will gradually transition into a straight line, which denotes the ischial spine (Figure 4.9.4).
5. **Identify the pudendal artery and the pudendal nerve medial to the ischial spine.**
6. **Inject local anesthetic subcutaneously for analgesia at the procedural site.**

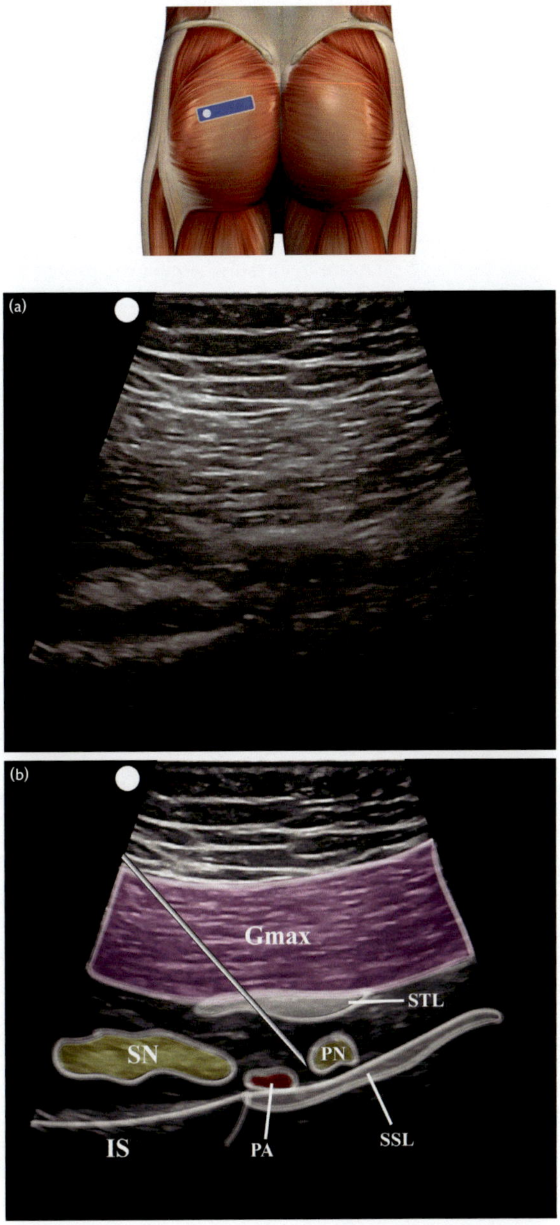

Figure 4.9.4 a, Ultrasound image of the posterior buttock in an axial oblique plane. **b,** Labeled ultrasound image of in-plane needle placement for a pudendal nerve block in short-axis. *Gmax* gluteus maximus, *STL* sacrotuberous ligament, *SN* sciatic nerve, *PA* pudendal artery, *PN* pudendal nerve, *IS* ischial spine, *SSL* sacrospinous ligament.

7. **Insert the procedural needle with an in-plane approach from a medial-to-lateral direction.** Once the needle tip pierces the sacrotuberous ligament, deposit the medication in the space formed by the sacrotuberous and sacrospinous ligaments (Figure 4.9.4).
8. **Inject the medication around the pudendal nerve.** Remove the needle and apply a dressing.

Tips

- Use doppler imaging to identify the pudendal artery, which is typically located lateral to the pudendal nerve, to avoid intravascular injection.

Safety Considerations

- Avoid a needle trajectory that is superficial and lateral to the ischial spine, where the sciatic nerve will typically be located.

Postprocedural Management

We recommend performing a lower extremity neurological exam before discharging the patient to assess strength, given the risk of inadvertent sciatic nerve block. Written instructions should be given to the patient to monitor any signs and symptoms of infection, hematoma, or neurological change. In situations where the pudendal nerve injection is performed for diagnostic purposes, patients should monitor the duration and degree of pain relief in relation to the type of local anesthetic used.

Further Reading

- Bellingham GA, Peng P. Pudendal and inferior cluneal nerve. In *Ultrasound for Interventional Pain Management*. Springer, Cham. 2020; pp. 109–119.
- Rofaeel A, Peng P, Louis I, et al. Feasibility of real-time ultrasound for pudendal nerve block in patients with chronic perineal pain. *Regional Anesthesia and Pain Medicine*. 2008;33:139–145.

References

1. Spinosa JP, Laurençon J, Kuhn G, Dubuisson JB, Riederer BM, et al. Sacral staged reflexes to localize the pudendal compression: an anatomical validation of the concept. *Rev Med Suisse*. 2006;2(84):2416–2418.
2. Amarenco G, Lanoe Y, Perrigot M, Goudal H. [A new canal syndrome: compression of the pudendal nerve in Alcock's canal or perineal paralysis of cyclists]. *Presse Med*. 1987;16(8):399.
3. Hibner M, Desai N, Robertson LJ, Nour M. Pudendal neuralgia. *J Minim Invasive Gynecol*. 2010;17(2):148–153.
4. Labat J-J, Riant T, Robert R, Amarenco G, Lefaucheur J-P, Rigaud J. Diagnostic criteria for pudendal neuralgia by pudendal nerve entrapment (Nantes criteria). *Neurourol Urodyn*. 2008;27(4):306–310.
5. Rofaeel A, Peng P, Louis I, et al. Feasibility of real-time ultrasound for pudendal nerve block in patients with chronic perineal pain. *Regional Anesthesia and Pain Medicine*. 2008;33:139–145.
6. Bellingham GA, Peng P. Pudendal and inferior cluneal nerve. In: Peng P, Finlaysen R, Lee SH, Bhatia A (eds), *Ultrasound for Interventional Pain Management*. Springer, Cham; 2020, pp. 109–119.
7. Adsan Ö, İnal G, Özdoğan L, Kaygısız O, Uğurlu Ö, Çetinkaya M. Unilateral pudendal nerve blockade for relief of all pain during transrectal ultrasound-guided biopsy of the prostate: a randomized, double-blind, placebo-controlled study. Urology. 2004;64(3):528–531.
8. Elahi F, Callahan D, Greenlee J, Dann TL. Pudendal entrapment neuropathy: a rare complication of pelvic radiation therapy. Pain Physician. 2013;16(6):E793–E797.
9. Robert R, Prat-Pradal D, Labat JJ, et al. Anatomic basis of chronic perineal pain: role of the pudendal nerve. *Surg Radiol Anat*. 1998;20(2):93–98.

10. Valovska A, Peccora CD, Philip CN, Kaye AD, Urman RD. Sacral neuromodulation as a treatment for pudendal neuralgia. *Pain Physician*. 2014;17(5):E645–E650.
11. Itza Santos F, Salinas J, Zarza D, Gómez Sancha F, Allona Almagro A. Update on pudendal nerve entrapment syndrome: an approach anatomic-surgical, diagnostic and therapeutic. *Actas Urológicas Españolas (English Edition)*. 2010;34(6):500–509.
12. Beco J, Mouchel J, Mouchel T, Spinosa J-P. Concerns about the use of colour doppler in the diagnosis of pudendal nerve entrapment. *Pain*. 2009;145(1–2):261; author reply 262.
13. Mollo M, Bautrant E, Rossi-Seignert A-K, Collet S, Boyer R, Thiers-Bautrant D. Evaluation of diagnostic accuracy of colour duplex scanning, compared to electroneuromyography, diagnostic score and surgical outcomes, in pudendal neuralgia by entrapment: a prospective study on 96 patients. *Pain*. 2009;142(1):159–163. doi:10.1016/j.pain.2009.01.019
14. Kovacs P, Gruber H, Piegger J, Bodner G. New, simple, ultrasound-guided infiltration of the pudendal nerve. *Diseases of the Colon and Rectum*. 2001;44(9):1381–1385.
15. Gray H, Williams PL, Bannister LH. *Gray's Anatomy: The Anatomical Basis of Medicine and Surgery*. Churchill Livingstone: Philadelphia; 1995.

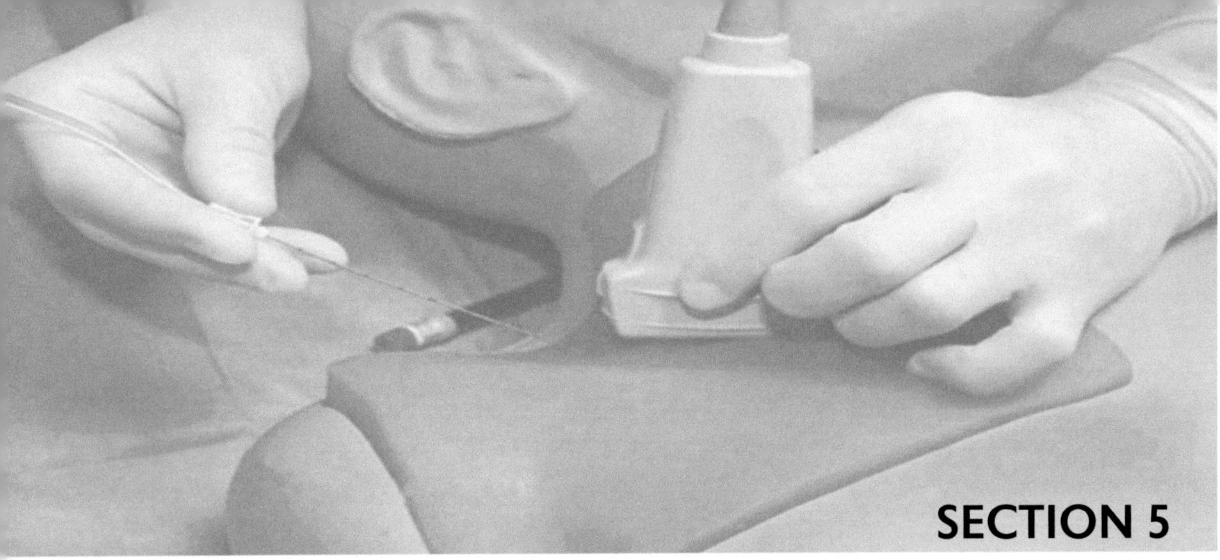

SECTION 5

NEUROAXIAL INTERVENTIONS

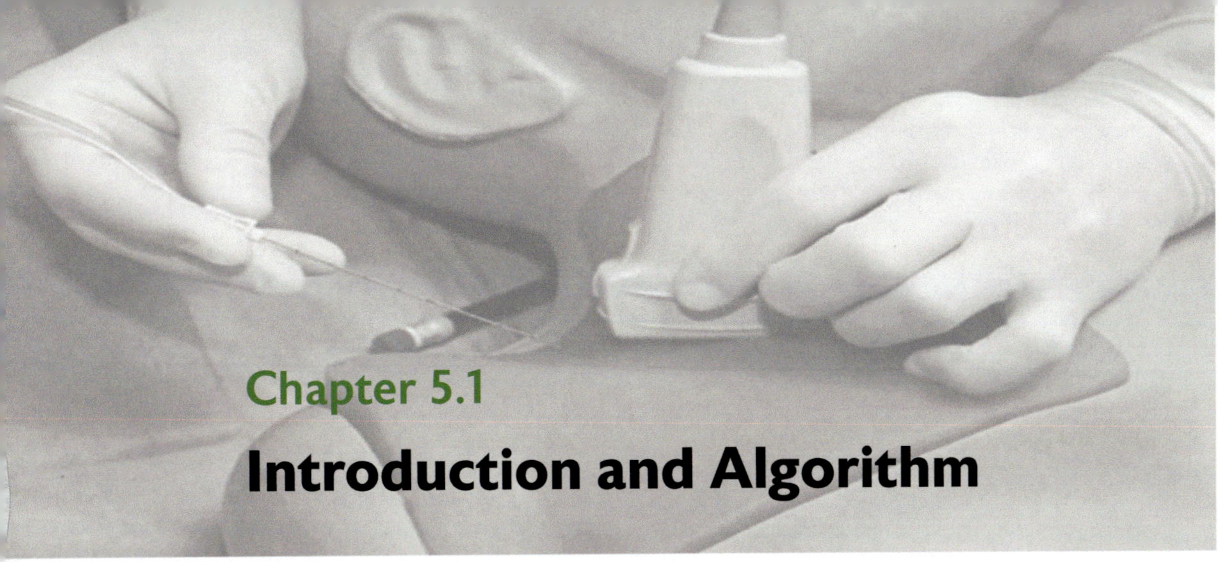

Chapter 5.1

Introduction and Algorithm

Amitabh Gulati

Contents

Introduction

The skeletal system is the third most common site of metastases in patients with systemic cancer, and the spine is the most frequently involved part of the skeleton.[1] Approximately 10% of all malignant tumor cases develop symptomatic spinal metastasis, with the most common primary tumors causing spinal metastasis being breast, prostate, lung, and thyroid cancer. The thoracic spine (70%) is the most common location of metastases, followed by lumbar spine (20%), and cervical spine (10%). Extradural lesions account for 90%–95% of spinal metastases.[2] The prognosis of patients with spinal metastases surviving beyond 2 years is about 10%–20%.

Clinical Presentation

The most common symptom that patients present with is back pain, usually preceding the onset of neurological symptoms. Pain can be either biological, radicular, or mechanical in nature at the time of presentation. Biological pain is due to proliferation of tumor cells in bone, usually the vertebral body, leading to damage of thick cortical bone and stretching of the periosteum. Radicular and spinal pain occur due to pressure on the spinal cord and nerve roots by disease, causing compression of neural structures. Finally, mechanical pain may occur due to processes like pathological fracture resulting in acute pain or spinal instability with or without compression of neural structures and articulating joints.

Historically, pain due to biological causes is predominantly nocturnal, usually reduces with activity, and responds to low-dose steroids. Mechanical pain due to structural instability usually increases with spinal mobility, while radicular pain occurs during weight bearing and tends to be relieved in recumbent position.[3] Neurological symptoms may present as motor or sensory deficits or both, and the clinical presentation can vary from paresthesias and numbness to paralysis with urinary and bowel incontinence. Often there is a need for urgent imaging and immediate treatment with radiation or surgery and intravenous steroids.

Investigations to elucidate the severity of metastatic spine disease include radiological and biochemical investigations. More specific serum studies, such as prostate-specific antigen (PSA) for prostate cancer, serum electrophoresis and beta-2-microglobulin for multiple myeloma, CA 19.9 for pancreatic cancer/gallbladder/bile duct tumors, CA 125 for ovarian cancer, and CA 15.3/CA 27.29 for breast cancer may point to specific pathology.[3,4]

MRI is the gold standard for evaluation of spinal metastasis and has the highest sensitivity (98.5%) and specificity (98.9%) in the detection and analysis of spinal metastases, with an accuracy of 98.7%.[2] PET imaging detects increased metabolic activity and can be used in clinical staging for metastatic disease. A nuclear bone scan can detect osseous metastatic lesions by identifying areas of increased osteoblastic activity in the skeleton. This study can be an excellent screening modality for diffuse bony involvement as well as individual lesions, since the entire skeletal system can be evaluated at once for the presence of osseous metastatic disease.[5] Histopathological confirmation through a core biopsy is mandatory in all patients with unknown primary lesions and, in patients with spinal cord compression, tissue analysis to evaluate tumor sensitivity to radiation therapy is also needed.

One of the most widely used decision paradigms for selecting appropriate management options for spinal metastatic disease based on patient presenting characteristics is referred to as the NOMS framework. This system considers neurologic, oncologic, mechanical, and systemic considerations to aid in determining optimal multidisciplinary therapy for patients suffering from metastatic spinal disease.[6] The neurologic assessment portion of the decision framework takes into consideration the degree of epidural spinal cord compression and myelopathy/radiculopathy through clinical and radiological evaluation. For the radiographic assessment, the Spine Oncology Study Group designed and validated a 6-point grading scale for the degree of epidural spinal cord compression.[7]

The oncologic assessment portion of the NOMS framework examines the responsiveness of tumors, depending on histology, to currently available treatment options. Tumors are categorized as radiosensitive or radioresistant based on their degree of response to conventional external beam radiation therapy. The mechanical assessment portion of the NOMS framework takes spinal stability into consideration. One of the most widely adopted systems is the Spine Instability Neoplastic Score (SINS) that is a spine instability scale specific to patients with cancer. According to this scale, a spine can be classified as stable (0–6), potentially unstable (7–12), or unstable (13–18).[8] The systemic assessment portion of the NOMS framework determines the ability of individual patients to tolerate different treatment modalities based on extent of metastatic disease, systemic illnesses/comorbidities, and tumor histology. Another well-known system is the Tokuhashi score, which has been validated as strongly predictive of patient prognosis across multiple cohorts.[9–10]

Management

The goals of treatment for patients with spine metastatic disease include palliation, analgesia, preservation of neurological function, and maintenance of spine stability with local tumor control.[11] Mainstays of therapy include medical management, surgical decompression, stabilization, and/or radiotherapy. Steroids can help reduce edema and improve neurologic symptoms, whereas bisphosphonates have been shown to reduce or delay skeletal events, such as pathologic fractures. Interventional options include peripheral nerve blocks, epidural/intrathecal infusions, and vertebral body augmentation, and a suggested algorithm for management is outlined in the next section.[12]

Surgery is considered when patients have instability. Before proceeding with surgical resections surgeons consider a patient's life expectancy, functional improvement, the degree of local control achievable by surgery, and the possible delay in adjuvant therapy due to surgical morbidity.[13] Minimally invasive spine procedures including vertebroplasty, kyphoplasty, and minimally invasive spine stabilization with percutaneous pedicle screws have been gaining acceptance. Vertebroplasty and kyphoplasty provide anterior column stability as well as pain relief, whereas minimally invasive spine stabilization provides both anterior and posterior column stability.[14] Additionally, spinal navigation systems for surgical resection have resulted in superior outcomes and less radiation for patients, revolutionizing surgery for spine metastases.[15]

Radiation plays an important role in the management of metastatic spinal cord disease. Three-dimensional conformal radiation therapy (3D- CRT) is the standard of practice to treat bone metastases. This approach is considered palliative due to the dose limitation required by the proximity of the spinal cord. Retreatment rates were 2.6 times higher for single-fraction radiotherapy and, therefore, multiple-fraction radiotherapy that produces a sustained response may be recommended for patients with oligometastatic disease or good prognosis.[16] Stereotactic body radiation therapy is a highly concentrated form of radiation that can irradiate target tissue at a high dose without affecting the surrounding normal tissue. Although there is a high risk of vertebral compression fractures, it involves minimal toxicity to the spinal cord and has a high local control rate of spinal metastases.[17]

Treatment Algorithm

The treatment algorithm is dependent on the anatomic structures involved, with radiologic imaging identifying potential pathology, which correlates with a patient's symptomatology. Interventional treatment options depend on the location of tumor, encroachment on specific neural structures, pain symptoms, and patient anatomic variability (Figures 5.1.1–3).

Spinal pain may arise from distinct anatomic locations including the vertebral body, posterior elements, neuroforaminal space, and lateral structures. Vertebral pain can be addressed with sympathetic chain blocks, epidural steroid injections, radiofrequency ablation of the tumor, vertebral augmentation, and basivertebral nerve ablation. Posterior element pain can be treated with medial branch blocks or radiofrequency ablation. Neuropathic pain arising from neuroforaminal involvement may be targeted with transforaminal or interlaminar epidural steroid injections. A recent review found that a transforaminal approach was better for pain relief than an interlaminar injection, but this is highly dependent on the tumor location.[18]

If there is multilevel involvement or the tumor location is lateral to the spine structures, fascial plane blocks such as erector spinae or quadratus lumborum blocks can be utilized. Pain that persists despite these interventions can be treated with more advanced pain management modalities including neuromodulation (spinal cord stimulation, peripheral nerve stimulation, or intrathecal drug delivery) and neurosurgical procedures such dorsal root entry zone (DREZ) lesioning.

Sacral pain may involve the sacroiliac joint space or the neural structures within the sacrum. If the joint space is involved, a lateral branch block followed by radiofrequency ablation would be the treatment of choice. However, if the joint space is not involved an intra-articular steroid injection would be ideal to address the pain symptoms. In both cases if the patient has minimal improvement, an intrathecal drug device implant may improve pain. Treatment of insufficiency fractures

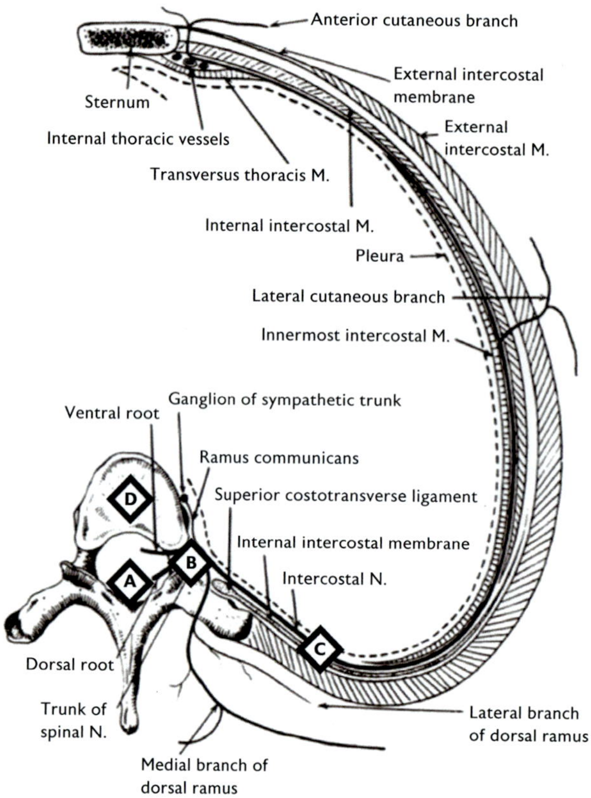

Figure 5.1.1 Interventional algorithm for lumbar spine pain based on location (A) intraspinal, (B) foraminal, (C) exiting nerve root and cutaneous branches, (D) vertebral.

may include ablations as discussed above and sacroplasty, especially for mechanical pain and instability. Involvement of neural elements can be treated initially with epidural steroid injections and consideration of a neuraxial intervention, including intrathecal drug delivery or spinal cord stimulation.

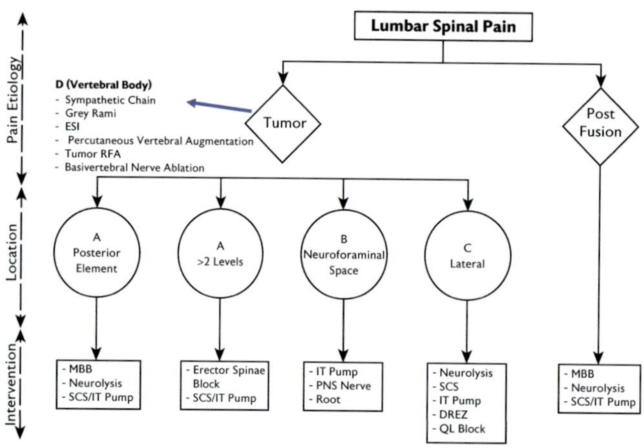

Figure 5.1.2 Interventional algorithm for lumbar spine pain based on location of the tumor represented by (A)–(D).

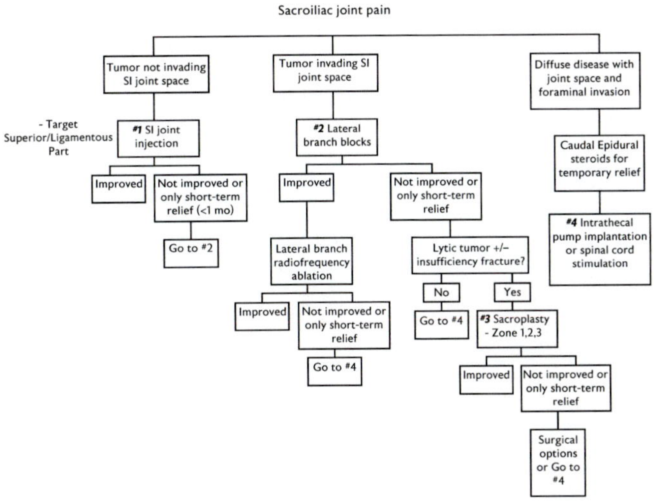

Figure 5.1.3 Interventional algorithm for sacroiliac joint based pain.

Contraindications

Absolute contraindications to sacroiliac joint injection and ablation are history of significant allergic reaction to the injected solutions, active infection over the site of injection, and patient refusal for the procedure.

Relative contraindications include patients on anticoagulants or with bleeding disorders, systemic infection, uncontrolled diabetes mellitus, anatomic abnormalities, and osteoporosis. Prior to proceeding with injection or ablation, patients should be able to provide informed consent and should be counseled on the expected results of the injections.

It is highly recommended that practitioners obtain clearance from the patient's primary care physician, cardiologist, neurologist, or oncologist prior to stopping anticoagulant and antiplatelet medications (Table 5.1.1).

Table 5.1.1 Contraindications to Neuraxial Procedures

Contraindications	Related Types
Absolute	• History of significant allergic reaction • Active infection over the site of injection • Patient refusal
Relative	• Use of anticoagulants • Coagulopathies • Systemic infection • Uncontrolled diabetes mellitus • Anatomic considerations

Conclusions

Management of patients with spine metastases requires a multidisciplinary approach and collaboration between various clinicians. These patients present with complex pain pathology, and delineating the cause of pain will guide which intervention is most appropriate. Pain physicians involved in management of these patients should utilize all modalities at their disposal, including interventional strategies, using an algorithmic approach.

References

1. Perrin RG, Laxton AW. Metastatic spine disease: epidemiology, pathophysiology, and evaluation of patients. Neurosurg Clin N Am. 2004;15:365–373.
2. Greenlee RT, Murray T, Bolden S, Wingo PA. Cancer statistics, 2000. CA: A Cancer Journal for Clinicians. 2000;50(1), 7–33.
3. Kurisunkal V, Gulia A, Gupta S. Principles of management of spine metastasis. Indian J Orthop. 2020;54(2):181–193.
4. Fridley JS, Syed S, Niu T, Leary OP, Gokaslan ZL. Presentation of spinal cord and column tumors. Neurooncol Pract. 2020;7(Suppl 1):i18–i24.
5. York JE, Walsh GL, Gokaslan ZL. Metastatic tumors. In: Benzel EC, Stillerman CB, eds. The Thoracic Spine. St Louis, MO: Quality Medical Publishing; 1999:392–411.
6. Laufer I, Rubin DG, Lis E, Cox BW, Stubblefield MD, Yamada Y, Bilsky MH. The NOMS framework: approach to the treatment of spinal metastatic tumors. Oncologist. 2013;18(6):744–751.
7. Bilsky MH, Laufer I, Fourney DR, Groff M, Schmidt MH, Varga PP, et al. Reliability analysis of the epidural spinal cord compression scale. J Neurosurg Spine. 2010;13:324–328.
8. Fourney DR, Frangou EM, Ryken TC, Dipaola CP, Shaffrey CI, Berven SH, et al. Spinal instability neoplastic score: an analysis of reliability and validity from the spine oncology study group. J Clin Oncol. 2011;29:3072–3077.
9. Yilmazlar S, Dogan S, Caner B, Turkkan A, Bekar A, Korfali E. Comparison of prognostic scores and surgical approaches to treat spinal metastatic tumors: a review of 57 cases. J Orthop Surg Res. 2008;3:37.
10. Leithner A, Radl R, Gruber G, et al. Predictive value of seven preoperative prognostic scoring systems for spinal metastases. Eur Spine J. 2008;17(11):1488–1495.
11. Kumar A, Weber MH, Gokaslan Z, Wolinsky JP, Schmidt M, Rhines L, et al. Metastatic spinal cord compression and steroid treatment. Clin Spin Surg. 2017;30(4):156–163.
12. Hortobagyi GN, Theriault RL, Lipton A, et al. Long-term prevention of skeletal complications of metastatic breast cancer with pamidronate: protocol 19 Aredia breast cancer study group. Journal of Clinical Oncology. 1998;16:2038–2044.
13. Klekamp J, Samii H. Surgical results for spinal metastases. Acta Neurochirurgica (Wien). 1998;140:957–967.
14. Ishida Y, Shigematsu H, Tsukamoto S, Morimoto Y, Iwata E, Okuda A, Kawasaki S, Tanaka M, Fujii H, Tanaka Y, et al. Impairment-driven cancer rehabilitation in patients with neoplastic spinal cord compression using minimally invasive spine stabilization. World J. Surg. Oncol. 2020;18:187.
15. Burström G, Persson O, Edström E, Elmi Terander A. Augmented reality navigation in spine surgery: a systematic review. Acta Neurochir. 2021;163:843–852.
16. Chow E, Zeng L, Salvo N, Dennis K, Tsao M, Lutz S. Update on the systematic review of palliative radiotherapy trials for bone metastases. Clin. Oncol. 2012;24:112–124.
17. Shiloh R, Krishnan M. Radiation for treatment of painful bone metastases. Hematol. Oncol. Clin. N. Am. 2018;32:459–468.
18. Oh DC, Rispoli L, Ghosh P, Gulati A. Epidural steroid injections for the management of spinal malignancy-related pain: a pragmatic review and retrospective study. Pain Pract. 2021;21(3):285–298.

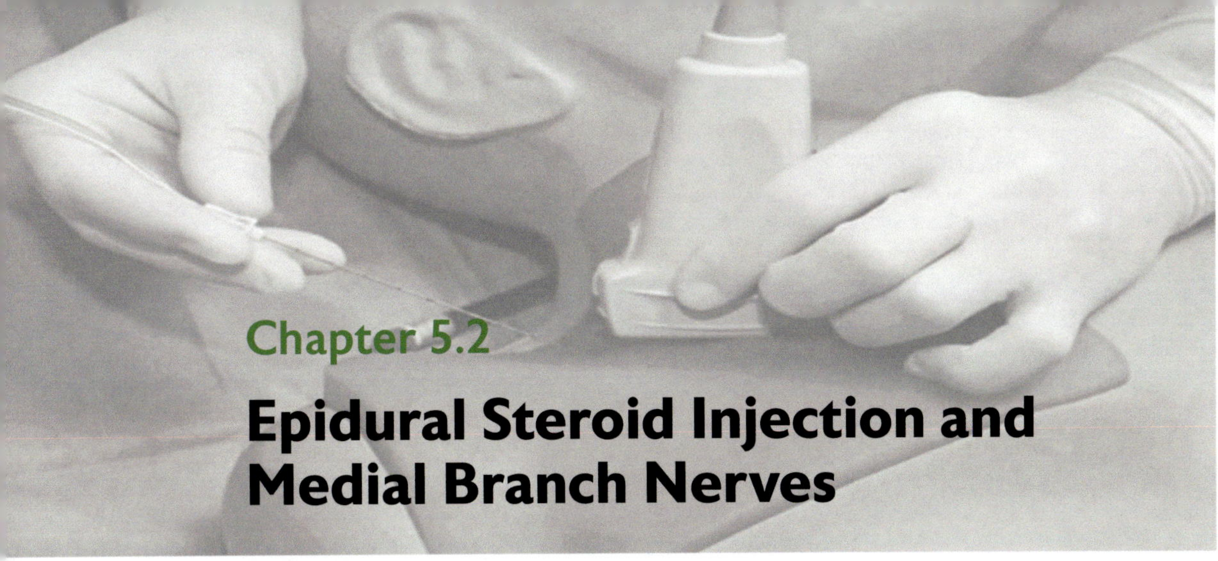

Chapter 5.2

Epidural Steroid Injection and Medial Branch Nerves

Ankur A. Patel

Contents

Introduction

Low back pain in the cancer population can stem from a number of causes. These include treatment-related sequelae like postsurgical pain and radiation changes, primary and metastatic tumor burden, pathologic fractures, and physical deconditioning. Frequently, muscular deconditioning will accelerate nononcologic painful processes such as degenerative disc disease, spondylosis, and spinal stenosis.[1] Management begins with conservative options like rehabilitation and pharmacological agents including nonsteroidal anti-inflammatory drugs, neuropathic agents, and opioid therapy. If pain is refractory to conservative measures, interventional spine procedures including epidural steroid injections (ESIs) and medial branch blocks (MBBs) can be performed. This chapter reviews the indications and techniques for these procedures in the oncologic population.

The ESI procedure consists of entering the epidural space by either the interlaminar, transforaminal, or caudal approach and injecting a combination of local anesthetic and steroid (particulate or nonparticulate). An MBB is a common extraspinal injection performed near the facet joint to treat joint degeneration causing axial low back pain. Fluoroscopic guidance is currently the gold standard for performing both ESIs and MBBs. However, ultrasound guidance is becoming more common in clinical practice with the advantages of avoiding radiation and being able to directly view musculature, ligaments, nerves, and vasculature. Additionally, ultrasounds are portable, allowing procedures to be performed at the bedside in the cancer population.

Critical Anatomy

The vertebral column is made of seven cervical, twelve thoracic, and five lumbar vertebrae; the sacrum; and the coccyx. Each vertebra is composed of six major components: the vertebral body, pedicles, laminae, spinous process, transverse processess, and articular processes. Adjacent vertebral bodies are separated by an intervertebral disc, with notable exceptions of C1/C2 and the fused sacrum. Together, the elements of the vertebra enclose and protect the spinal canal and the spinal cord within it. The spinal cord has three protective meninges known as the pia, arachnoid, and dura. The pia layer is the innermost layer and directly adheres with the spinal cord. After the pia mater is the subarachnoid space, which houses cerebral spinal fluid, and the arachnoid mater. The outermost and thickest layer is the dura mater. The dura is separated from the periosteum of the vertebral canal by the epidural space, which is the target of an ESI.

The epidural space is triangular in shape and contains spinal nerves, the vertebral plexus of veins, spinal arteries, lymphatics, areolar connective tissue, and epidural fat.[2,3] The posterior margin of the epidural space is formed primarily by the ligamentum flavum, facet joints, and laminae. The anterior margin consists of the posterior longitudinal ligament, posterior aspects of the vertebral bodies, and intervertebral discs. Laterally, the space is bounded by the pedicles and intervertebral foramen.[2]

When performing an ESI, three common approaches can be taken: interlaminar, transforaminal, or caudal. The interlaminar approach consists of introducing a needle within the interlaminar space and penetrating the skin, subcutaneous tissue, supraspinous ligament, interspinous ligament, and ligamentum flavum to reach the epidural space. Careful attention is needed when engaging the ligamentum flavum to ensure the needle is not advanced too far anteriorly resulting in dural puncture. A "loss of resistance technique" is utilized when engaging the ligamentum flavum to safely pass through and enter the posterior epidural space.

The ligamentum flava are paired, dense ligamentous structures connecting the lamina of two neighboring vertebrae that fuse into the ligamentum flavum. The ligamentum flavum is approximately 5 mm thick (anterior to posterior).[4] The ligament is thinnest in the cervical region, becoming thicker in the thoracic region and thickest in the lumbar region.[4] Throughout the ligamentum flavum, there are midline gaps due to an inconsistent fusion to allow for the exit of venous structures. This lack of fusion is increasingly present in the cervical and thoracic levels, which may pose a risk for dural puncture. A cadaveric study by Lirk et al. evaluated 52 vertebral column specimens to determine the incidence of midline gaps at various spinal levels.[5] The study revealed that the gaps in the ligamentum flavum are frequent in the cervical and high thoracic level, with highest incidence at C5–C6. This data suggests interventionalists cannot rely on the ligamentum flavum as the barrier to the epidural space, especially when performing cervical and high thoracic interlaminar ESI via a direct midline approach. An extradural space dorsal to the ligamentum flavum exists as the space of Okada. This retrodural space communicates with the extradural interspinous space and bilateral zygapophyseal joint.[6,7] This space can produce a false loss of resistance with contrast extravasation into the space of Okada and bilateral facet joints.

With the transforaminal approach, the exiting nerve root at the foramen is targeted with an oblique needle approach. This approach is complicated by neighboring vasculature that is vulnerable to injury. The artery of Adamkiewicz is of high concern in the low thoracic and high lumbar spine.

It typically passes through a neuroforamen between T9 and L2, although there is a high degree of anatomical variability.[8] It is the major vascular supply to the anterior thoracolumbar spinal cord and its injury can lead to paralysis, urinary incontinence, and bowel incontinence.[8] Additionally, the artery of Adamkiewicz is most commonly situated in the ventral superior or middle portion of the foramen, suggesting the more traditional supraneural or subpedicular ("safe triangle") approach may not be the safest approach.[9] In the cervical spine, the vertebral artery is the major vasculature of concern. It arises from the subclavian artery, enters the transverse foramen at the level of C6, and travels superiorly to the foramen magnum before entering the cranium. Normally, the vertebral artery is found anterior to the ventral ramus of the cervical nerve root and cervical zygapophyseal joint; however, anatomical anomalies have been reported.[10] Regardless of the approach, ESIs should use a multiplanar approach to ensure proper needle placement and trajectory.

Between the vertebral bodies lie intervertebral discs, which are formed from three major components: the annulus fibrosus, nucleus pulposus, and vertebral endplates. Compared to those of the cervical and thoracic spine, the vertebral bodies and intervertebral discs of the lumbar spine have a greater surface area for increased load-bearing and tension.[11] With increased stress, the intervertebral discs frequently suffer degenerative changes that can lead to herniation of the nucleus pulposus, resulting in nerve root irritation or compression.

Posteriorly, the articulation of the superior and inferior articular processes of two concurrent vertebral bodies forms a pair of facet joints, otherwise known as the zygapophyseal joint. The facet joint is a diarthrodial joint with opposing cartilage surfaces surrounded by a ligamentous capsule that facilitates load transfer and constrains motions within the spine.[12,13] The synovium and capsule of the facet joint have extensive nociceptive receptors, which transmit pain signals through the medial branches of the dorsal rami of the spinal nerves.[14] As the spinal nerves exit through the intervertebral foramina, they divide into four branches: the dorsal ramus, ventral ramus, meningeal branch, and rami communicantes. The dorsal ramus further divides into a medial and lateral branch. The medial branch continues posteriorly along the lateral border of the superior articular process of the lower vertebra and gives rise to small articular branches before entering the fibro-osseous canal, innervating the inferior and lateral aspects of the facet joint.[15] The fibro-osseous canal is bounded by the dorsal surface of the transverse process anteriorly, mamillary process medially, accessory process laterally, and the mammillary accessory ligament dorsally.[15,16] Upon exiting the fibro-osseous canal, the medial branch continues medially and caudally and gives rise to more small articular branches that innervate the medial and superior aspect of the subadjacent facet joint.[15]

Given the pathway of the medial branch and the rise to the articular branches, each facet joint in the thoracic and lumbar spine is innervated by two medial branches: one medial branch exiting at the level of the joint and the other branch one level above. Unlike the other dorsal rami, the dorsal ramus of L5 travels along the groove formed by the superior articular process of S1 and the sacral ala before branching into the lateral and medial branches.[15] Its medial branch continues toward the caudal aspect of the L5–S1 facet joint. Due to this, the dorsal ramus of L5 is the target for L5–S1 MBB or radiofrequency ablation (RFA). In contrast to those in the thoracic and lumbar spine, facet joints in the cervical spine below C4 are innervated by the medial branch above and below the joint level (e.g., the C4–C5 facet joint is innervated by the C4 and C5 medial branches).[17] The C2–C3 facet joint is innervated by the third occipital nerve, which is the superficial medial branch of the C3 dorsal ramus.[18]

Indications

ESIs have traditionally been used for diagnostic and therapeutic purposes in patients who have pain caused by irritation of a spinal nerve root. Degenerative changes from deconditioning, surgical treatment, pathological fractures, radiation treatment, and primary oncologic disease can all lead to neuropathic pain of spinal origin. Corticosteroids are commonly used to treat neuropathic pain from spinal nerve compression. The mechanism of action by which steroids improve cancer-related pain is believed to be through decreasing edema (possibly related to tumor burden), decreasing release of neuroinflammatory peptides, and tumoricidal effects.[19] Treatment with oral steroids may lead to undesired systemic side effects, such as immunosuppression, gastritis, osteoporosis, hyperglycemia, insomnia, gastritis, and more. These side effects are even more common in the oncologic population because steroids are frequently part of cancer treatments. Epidural steroid injections allow for a more targeted delivery of steroids, often resulting in lower total steroid doses with similar therapeutic outcomes. A retrospective review of 76 cancer patients by Oh et al. found level 3 evidence for epidural steroid injections for malignancy-related pain.[1] Specifically, thoracic epidural steroid injections provided at least moderate relief to all cancer patients and excellent pain relief to approximately 56% of patients. In this same study, lumbar epidural steroid injections provided moderate pain relief to 86% of cancer patients. Caudal epidural steroid injections provided the least relief, and the transforaminal approach resulted in the best pain relief in the oncological population.

Breast, prostate, and lung cancer commonly metastasize to bone. It is estimated that approximately 30% of cancer patients develop symptomatic spinal metastasis and up to 90% have metastatic spinal tumor burden at the time of death. Spinal tumor burden leads to pathologic compression fractures, spinal nerve and spinal cord compression and irritation, and invasion of facet joints. Moreover, cancer treatments can lead to radiation neuritis, postsurgical pain, and muscular deconditioning exacerbating degenerative changes. All of these changes can lead to low back pain.[20] Rispoli et al. presented a case presentation of thoracic lumbar MBB and cryoablation with excellent pain relief, which may also apply to MBBs in the cervical and lumbar spine.[21]

Cases

Case #1—Epidural Disease

A 61-year-old female with lung adenocarcinoma and metastatic lesions to the bone, liver, adrenal glands, and gastrointestinal tract had worsening neurologic symptoms from epidural disease at T9 and T10. She had a recent T9–T10 decompression with kyphoplasty and T8–T11 posterior fusion. The most recent MRI total spine revealed worsening epidural disease at T9 and unchanged L3 and S1 metastases causing mild epidural and neural foraminal impingement (Figure 5.2.1). The patient was admitted to the hospital with severe back pain and left posterolateral lower extremity radicular pain. Her pain prevented her from tolerating radiation to the spine. When interventional pain procedures were considered, additional imaging revealed epidural disease with central stenosis from L3 to L5. However, T12–L3 was free of epidural metastases and appropriate for intervention. The patient underwent an L2–L3 interlaminar ESI with the injectate directed caudally. On follow-up a week later, the patient noted a significant improvement in her overall pain. She still noted bouts of 10 out of 10 pain, but these exacerbations were significantly less frequent.

Case #2—Osseous Metastasis

A 64-year-old female with metastatic left-sided breast cancer to lymph nodes, bilateral knee joints, left ileum, sacrum, pelvis, and L5 presented to the clinic with left lower extremity radicular pain. The onset of pain was noted around the same time as the patient's radiation treatment. The most recent CT lumbar spine revealed unchanged left L5 vertebral body, pedicle, and posterior element metastasis with no significant epidural or foraminal disease, which was corroborated on the PET scan. An MRI total spine also revealed unchanged grade 1 anterolisthesis of L4–L5 with disc bulges

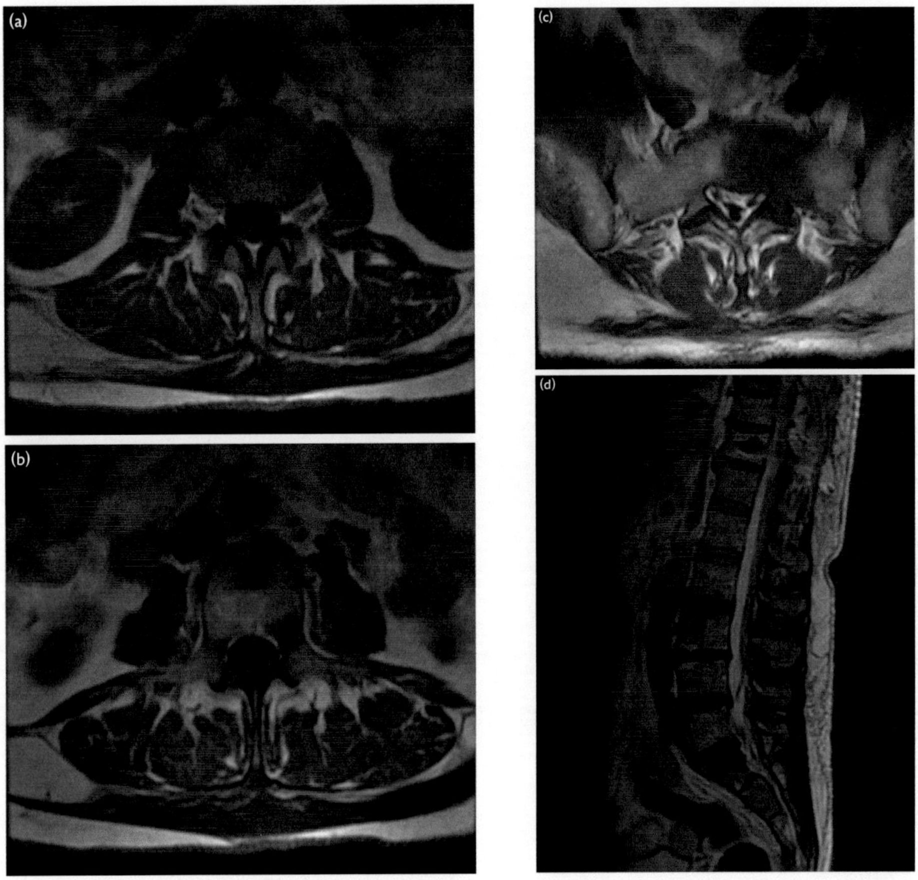

Figure 5.2.1 MRI thoracolumbar spine revealing L3, S1, and S1 metastases causing mild epidural and neural foraminal impingement. **a,** T2 axial image at L2/3 interspace. **b,** T2 axial image at L3. **c,** T2 axial image at L5/S1 interspace. **d,** T2 sagittal image.

at L2–L3 and L5–S1. Based on the patient's presentation and history of metastasis/radiation to the L5 region, it was deemed the pain was likely stemming from the L5 nerve root (Figure 5.2.2). An L5/S1 interlaminar ESI was performed approaching from the right side aimed toward the midline. This approach was chosen based on the safety of having no epidural disease and no osseous disease in the right portion of the posterior arch at L5. At the 1-month follow-up, the patient noted greater than 50% improvement in overall pain symptoms and an increased ability to participate in physical therapy.

Equipment and Patient Preparation

1. Monitors and Sterility

a. No specific monitoring is required during this procedure. It is highly advised that vital signs including blood pressure, heart rate, respiratory rate, and pulse oximetry are obtained prior to starting the procedure to ensure the patient is hemodynamically stable. A set of vitals is often taken post procedure as well.

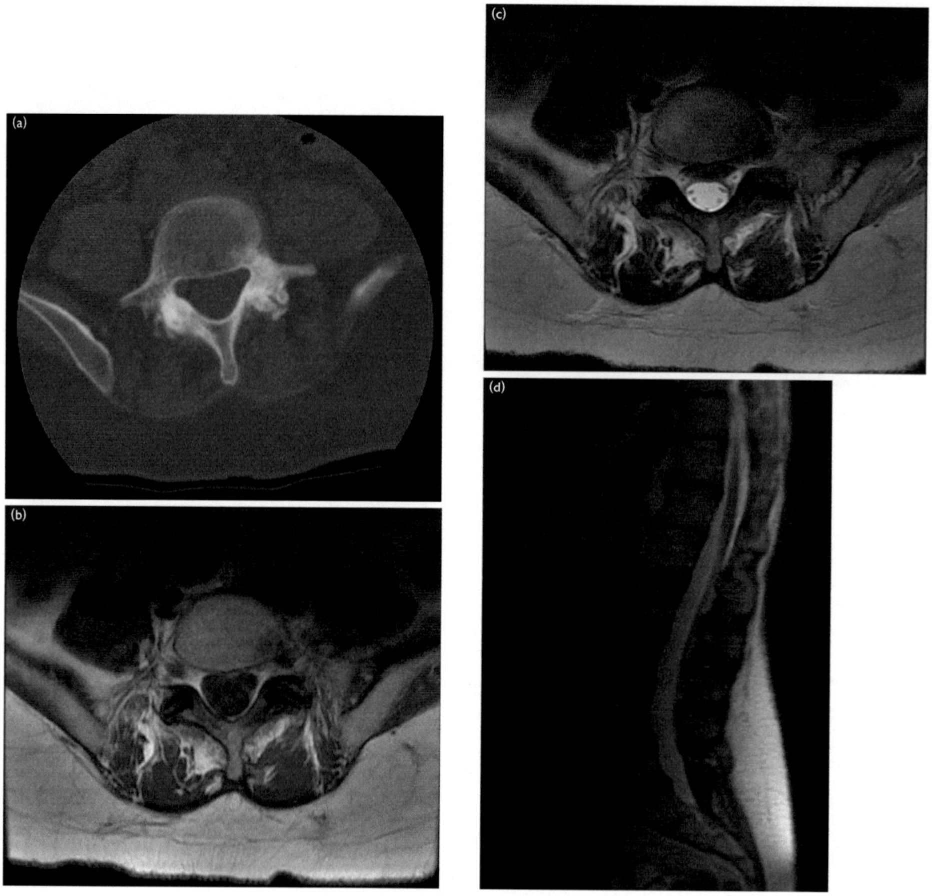

Figure 5.2.2 Imaging revealing grade 1 anterolisthesis of L4–5 with disc bulges at L2–3 and L5–S1in a patient with a history for metastasis/radiation to the L5 region. **a,** CT axial image at L5. **b,** MRI T1 axial image at L5/S1 interspace. **c,** MRI T2 axial image at L5/S1 interspace. **d,** MRI thoracolumbar T2 sagittal image.

b. Strict antiseptic technique should be observed including sterile draping, probe cover, ultrasound gel, gloves, and gauze. Chlorhexidine or another skin prep agent should be used to clean the skin prior to commencing the procedure.

2. **Imaging modalities:**
   a. Ultrasound
      i. Probe: linear probe (7–12 MHz) or curvilinear (2–5 MHz), which is used to achieve greater depth
   b. Fluoroscopy
3. **Needle type:**
   i. Local anesthetic: 27- or 30-gauge 1.5-inch needle
   ii. Epidural: 20-gauge 3.5-inch Tuohy needle with inner stylet for interlaminar approach and 22- or 25-gauge 3.5-inch spinal needle for transforaminal approach
   iii. Medial Branch Block: 22- or 25-gauge 3.5-inch needle spinal needle with inner stylet

4. **Patient position:** Prone
5. **Injectate:**
   a. Local anesthetic (0–2.0 mL): Lidocaine 1%–2%; Ropivacaine 0.2%–0.5%; Bupivacaine 0.25%–0.5%
   b. Adjuvant (0.5–1.0 mL): particulate or nonparticulate steroid
   c. Normal Saline (0–4 mL)

Step-by-Step Technique

Cervical Epidural Steroid Injection—Interlaminar Approach—Fluoroscopy

1. **Prepare equipment and supplies, position the patient prone, and sterilize the procedural area with antiseptic solution.** Consider placing a support beneath the chest to facilitate cervical flexion and patient comfort.
2. **Obtain an anteroposterior (AP) view to mark the C7–T1 level.** A caudal or cephalad tilt should be used to maximize the interlaminar space, and an oblique tilt should be used to ensure midline visualization of the space. Planned needle insertion should be midline or 1–1.5 cm lateral to the midline.
3. **Inject the skin and underlying tissues with local anesthetic**.
4. **Insert the Tuohy needle parallel to the image intensifier.** The needle should be engaged in firm tissue. Ensure the needle is not advanced too far ventrally until the contralateral oblique (CLO) or lateral safety views have been obtained.
5. **Once correct needle placement has been confirmed in the AP view, obtain either a CLO view or lateral safety view.** The CLO view visualizes the ventral interlaminar line (VILL) and the lateral view visualizes the spinolaminar line as the most dorsal needle placement while maintaining safety.
6. **Slowly advance the needle in 1 mm increments while checking for loss of resistance**. Loss of resistance may be performed with air or saline per the preference of the proceduralist.
7. **After loss of resistance, aspirate to rule out intravascular needle placement and inject contrast under fluoroscopy to confirm an epidural flow pattern.** Epidural contrast spread characteristically follows exiting nerve roots and is heterogeneous with epidural fat bubbles. Contrast should be confirmed to be epidural in more than one view.
8. **Inject the desired medications epidurally.**
9. **Flush and withdraw the Tuohy needle and apply a bandage.**
10. **Monitor vital signs for at least 30 minutes to ensure the patient is hemodynamically stable to be discharged.**

Tips

- A CLO view is obtained by obliquing the fluoroscope about 50°–60° opposite of the side of the needle. In this view, the ventral laminar margin and VILL should be identified. The VILL connects the ventral margins of two adjacent laminas.
- The lateral view is obtained by obliquing the fluoroscope to 90° to visualize the spinolaminar line.
- Preprocedural review of imaging studies is recommended to ensure adequate epidural space for needle placement at the targeted level.
- Multiview imaging of the AP, CLO, and/or lateral views should be used to ensure accurate needle placement and trajectory.

Safety Considerations

- Cervical interlaminar ESI is recommended to be performed at C7–T1, regardless of the level of pathology. The cervical epidural space is the largest in diameter between C7–T1, and the ligamentum flavum is reliably located between C7–T1.
- Ventral to the VILL or spinolaminar line is the posterior epidural space. Careful attention should be taken when LOR has been obtained to avoid puncturing the dura.

Thoracic Epidural Steroid Injection—Interlaminar Approach—Fluoroscopy

1. **Prepare equipment and supplies, position the patient prone, and sterilize the procedural area with antiseptic solution.** Consider placing a support beneath the chest to maximize thoracic flexion and patient comfort.
2. **Obtain an AP view and mark the desired level.** This level should be confirmed by counting the vertebral bodies from either T1 or T12. Once confirmed, tilt the fluoroscope in caudal or cephalad direction and oblique left or right to optimize the interlaminar space. Mark the needle insertion, which should be either midline or 1–1.5 cm ipsilateral to the midline of the interlaminar space.
3. **Inject the skin and underlying tissues with local anesthetic**.
4. **Insert the Tuohy needle parallel to the image intensifier.** The needle should be engaged in firm tissue. Ensure the needle is not advanced too far ventrally until the CLO or lateral safety views have been obtained.
5. **Once correct needle placement has been confirmed in the AP view, obtain either a CLO view or lateral safety view.** Ensure the needle is not unsafely ventral.
6. **Slowly advance the needle in 1 mm increments while checking for loss of resistance.** Loss of resistance may be performed with air or saline per the preference of the proceduralist.
7. **After loss of resistance, aspirate to rule out intravascular needle placement and inject contrast under fluoroscopy to confirm an epidural flow pattern.** Epidural contrast spread characteristically follows exiting nerve roots and is heterogeneous with epidural fat bubbles. Contrast should be confirmed to be epidural in more than one view.
8. **Inject the desired medications epidurally.**
9. **Flush and withdraw the Tuohy needle and apply a bandage.**
10. **Monitor vital signs for at least 30 minutes to ensure the patient is hemodynamically stable to be discharged.**

Tips

- A CLO view is obtained by obliquing the fluoroscope about 50°–60° opposite of the side of the needle. In this view, the ventral laminar margin and VILL should be identified. The VILL connects the ventral margins of two adjacent laminas.
- The lateral view is obtained by obliquing the fluoroscope to 90° to visualize the spinolaminar line.
- Preprocedural review of imaging studies is recommended to ensure adequate space for needle placement at the targeted level.
- Multiview imaging of the including AP, CLO, and/or lateral views should be used to ensure accurate needle placement and trajectory.

Safety Considerations

- Ventral to the VILL or spinolaminar line is the posterior epidural space. Careful attention should be taken when LOR has been obtained to avoid puncturing the dura.

Lumbar Epidural Steroid Injection—Interlaminar Approach—Fluoroscopy

1. **Prepare equipment and supplies, position the patient prone, and sterilize the procedural area with antiseptic solution.** Consider placing a support beneath the abdomen to reduce the lumbar lordotic curve.
2. **Obtain an AP view and mark the confirmed level.** A caudal or cephalad tilt and left or right oblique should be used to maximize the visualization of the interlaminar space. Planned needle insertion should be midline or 1–1.5 cm lateral to the midline.
3. **Inject the skin and underlying tissues with local anesthetic**.
4. **Insert the Tuohy needle parallel to the image intensifier.** The needle should be engaged in firm tissue. Ensure the needle is not advanced too far ventrally until the CLO or lateral safety views have been obtained.
5. **Once the needle tip has been confirmed in the AP view, obtain either a CLO view or lateral safety view.**
6. **Slowly advance needle in 1 mm increments while checking for loss of resistance**. Loss of resistance may be performed with air or saline per the preference of the proceduralist.
7. **After loss of resistance, aspirate to rule out intravascular needle placement and inject contrast under fluoroscopy to confirm an epidural flow pattern. Contrast is injected under continuous fluoroscopy guidance to confirm flow pattern.** Epidural contrast spread characteristically follows exiting nerve roots and is heterogeneous with epidural fat bubbles. Contrast should be confirmed to be epidural in more than one view.
8. **Inject the desired medications epidurally.**
9. **Flush and withdraw the Tuohy needle and apply a bandage.**
10. **Monitor vital signs for at least 30 minutes to ensure the patient is hemodynamically stable to be discharged.**

Tips

- A CLO view is obtained by obliquing the fluoroscope about 50°–60° opposite of the side of the needle. In this view, the ventral laminar margin and VILL should be identified. The VILL connects the ventral margins of two adjacent laminas.
- The lateral view is obtained by obliquing the fluoroscope to 90° to visualize the spinolaminar line.
- Preprocedural review of imaging studies is recommended to ensure adequate space for needle placement at the targeted level.
- Multiview imaging of the AP, CLO, and/or lateral views should be used to ensure accurate needle placement and trajectory.

Safety Considerations

- Ventral to the VILL or spinolaminar line is the posterior epidural space. Careful attention should be taken when LOR has been obtained to avoid puncturing the dura.

Lumbar Epidural Steroid Injection—Transforaminal Supraneural Approach—Fluoroscopy

1. **Prepare equipment and supplies, position the patient prone, and sterilize the procedural area with antiseptic solution.** Consider placing a support beneath the abdomen to reduce lordotic curvature and increase patient comfort.
2. **Obtain an AP view and mark the confirmed level.** Caudal or cephalad tilt should be used to align the superior endplate.

3. **Oblique the fluoroscope and identify the foramen.** The target will be inferior to the pedicle and lateral to the pars interarticularis.
4. **Inject the skin and underlying tissues with local anesthetic.**
5. **Insert a spinal needle parallel to the image intensifier.** The needle should be engaged in firm tissue. Ensure the needle is not advanced too far ventrally until the lateral safety view has been obtained.
6. **An AP view is obtained to ensure the needle has not advanced past the midpedicular line.** Advancing the needle medial to the midpedicular line can lead to damage of the spinal nerve.
7. **Obtain a lateral safety view to determine the depth of the needle placement.** Advance the needle until it is within the intervertebral foramen.
8. **Once the position is confirmed, aspirate and inject contrast.** Contrast injection should be performed under continuous fluoroscopy to rule out intravascular needle placement. Epidural flow is confirmed by its spread around the spinal nerve and beneath the pedicle into the midline epidural space.
9. **Inject the desired medications epidurally.**
10. **Flush and withdraw the needle.**
11. **Monitor vital signs for at least 30 minutes to ensure the patient is hemodynamically stable to be discharged.**

Tips

- Vascular injection can be difficult to visualize and can be more readily identified with the use of digital subtraction.

Safety Considerations

- The needle should be directed to the superior aspect of the foramen to avoid spinal nerve injury. The "safe triangle" or supraneural technique can be used to avoid spinal nerve injury; however, this technique does not avoid vascular injury.
- Needle placement medial to the midpedicular line may result in dural puncture.

Caudal Epidural Steroid Injection—Fluoroscopy

1. **Prepare equipment and supplies, position the patient prone, and sterilize the procedural area with antiseptic solution.** Consider placing a support beneath the chest to facilitate cervical flexion and patient comfort.
2. **Palpate the sacral cornu and mark the sacral hiatus between them.** AP fluoroscopy can be utilized to confirm the location.
3. **Inject the skin and underlying tissues with local anesthetic.**
4. **Insert a spinal needle at a 45° angle cephalad between the sacral cornu.** Advance the needle with progressive lessening of the angle. The needle should feel firmly engaged within the posterior sacrococcygeal ligaments.
5. **Obtain a lateral fluoroscopic view to ensure the needle is in the sacral hiatus.**
6. **Aspirate to rule out intravascular needle placement and inject contrast.** Flow is typically seen 1–2 levels cephalad. Epidural spread characteristically follows exiting nerve roots and is heterogenous with epidural fat bubbles.
7. **Inject the desired medications epidurally.**
8. **Flush and withdraw the needle and apply a bandage.**

Tips

- Avoid too steep of a needle angle to avoid penetrating sacrum and bowel.

Safety Considerations

- It is critical to not advance past S3 to avoid dural puncture.

Caudal Epidural Steroid Injection—Ultrasound

1. **Prepare equipment and supplies, position the patient prone, and sterilize the procedural area with antiseptic solution.** Consider placing a support beneath the chest to facilitate cervical flexion and patient comfort.
2. **Place the probe in an axial plane at the level of the gluteal folds in the middle of the buttock region.** The sacral hiatus should be visualized between two adjacent sacral cornua as shown in Figure 5.2.3.
3. **Center the probe between the sacral cornua and rotate the 90° over the sacral hiatus to visualize it in long-axis.**
4. **Inject the skin and underlying tissues with local anesthetic.**
5. **Insert a 22- or 25-gauge 2- to 3.5-inch needle with an ultrasound-guided in-plane approach.** As the needle is advanced, a palpable "pop" will be felt as it passes through the sacrococcygeal ligament into the sacral canal (Figure 5.2.4).
6. **Aspirate to rule out intravascular needle placement and inject the desired medications epidurally.** It is important to note that the needle cannot be visualized once in the sacral canal due to obstruction of the ultrasound waves by the sacrum.
7. **Flush and withdraw the needle and apply a bandage.**

Tips

- The injection can also be performed out-of-plane with the transducer in an axial plane, which may make it easier to ensure the needle is the center of the canal.

Safety Considerations

- Avoid too steep of a needle angle to avoid penetrating sacrum and bowel.
- Minimize pushing the needle past the palpable "pop" of the sacrococcygeal ligament to prevent dural puncture, which is possible cephalad to the S3 level.

Lumbar Medial Branch—Ultrasound

1. **Prepare equipment and supplies, position the patient prone, and sterilize the procedural area with antiseptic solution.** It is recommended to place a pillow underneath the abdomen to minimize lumbar lordosis.
2. **Identify and count the desired facet joints.** Palpate the posterior superior iliac spine (PSIS). Place the probe over the PSIS in the axial plane. At the level of the PSIS, the sacrum will be visualized as shown in Figure 5.2.5.
3. **While maintaining visualization of the sacrum, translate the probe cephalad and medial to visualize the L5–S1 facet joint (Figure 5.2.6).** Lateral to the L5–S1 facet joint will be the sacral ala, which is the target for the dorsal ramus of L5 (Figure 5.2.7). Note this is on or close to the tip of the PSIS.

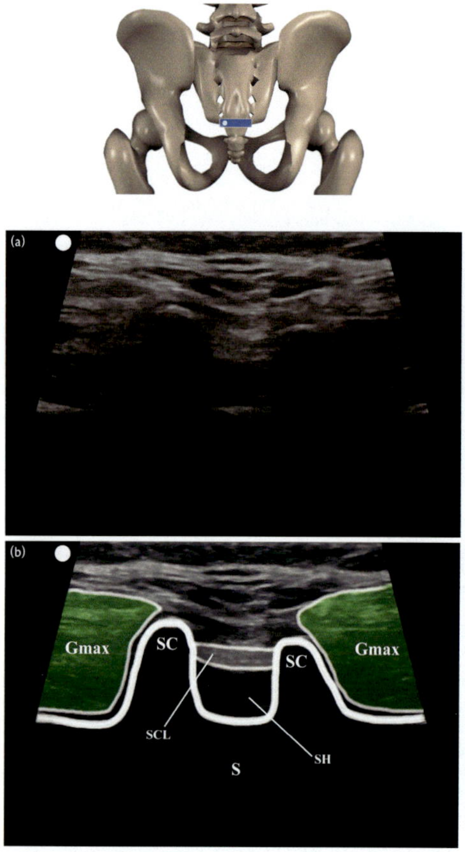

Figure 5.2.3 a, Ultrasound image of the sacral hiatus at the level of the cornua in an axial plane. **b,** Labeled transverse ultrasound image of sacral hiatus. *Gmax* gluteus maximus, *SC* sacral cornua, *SCL* sacrococcygeal ligament, *SH* sacral hiatus, *S* sacrum.

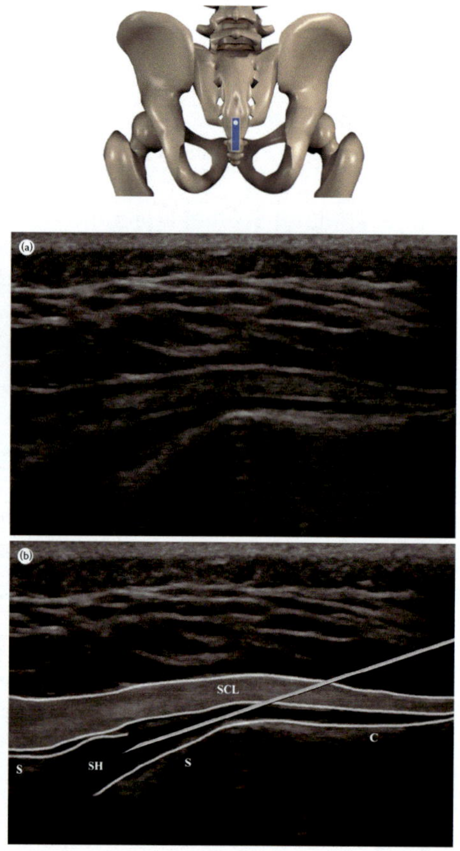

Figure 5.2.4 a, Ultrasound image of the sacral hiatus at the level of the cornua in a sagittal plane. **b,** Labeled longitudinal ultrasound image of in-plane needle placement for a caudal epidural. *SCL* sacrococcygeal ligament, *S* sacrum, *SH* sacral hiatus, *C* coccyx.

4. **Continue translating the probe cephalad to view the L4–L5 facet joint.** Once the L4–L5 facet joint is identified, the probe can be translated slightly caudad to identify the transverse process of L5, the superior articular process of L5, the facet joint capsule of the L4–L5, the inferior articular process of L4, and the spinous process of L4. The L4 medial branch can be targeted at the junction of the cephalad border of the transverse process of L5 and the lateral border of the superior articular process of L5 (Figure 5.2.8). The process can be continued as the probe is translated cephalad identifying the medial branches of L1–L3.
5. **Once the targeted medial branch is identified, inject the skin just lateral to the ultrasound probe and underlying tissues with local anesthetic.**
6. **For L1–L4 medial branches, insert a 22- or 25-gauge needle with an in-plane approach.** The spinal needle should be inserted at a 40°–45° angle at the lateral end of the transducer and advanced in the medial direction to the junction of the transverse process and the superior articular process. The transducer can then be rotated 90° to obtain the sagittal view to confirm the needle placement.

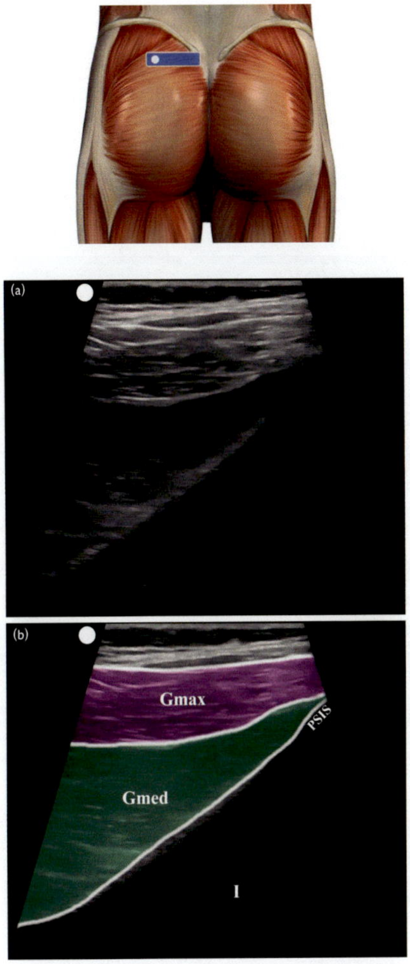

Figure 5.2.5 **a,** Ultrasound image of the posterior buttock in an axial plane. **b,** Labeled ultrasound image of the posterior gluteal muscles. *Gmax* gluteus maximus, *Gmed* gluteus medius, *PSIS* posterior superior iliac spine.

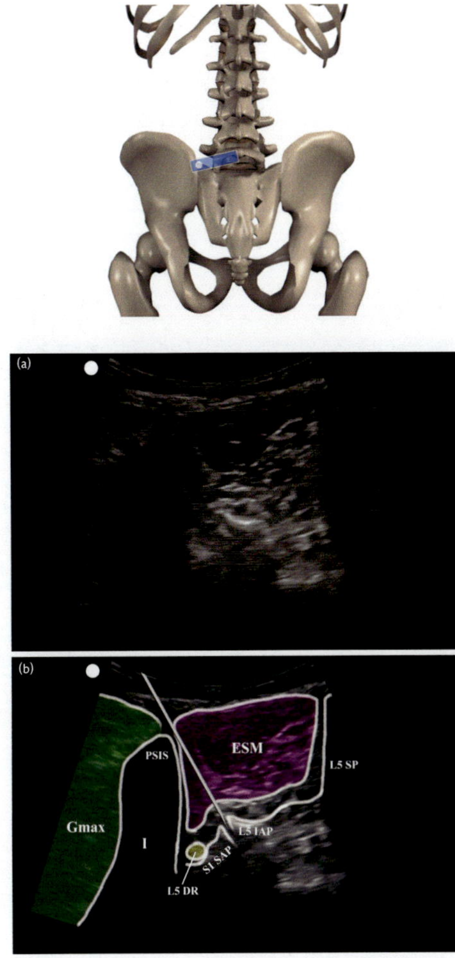

Figure 5.2.6 **a,** Ultrasound image of the lower back at the L5–S1 level in an axial oblique plane. **b,** Labeled ultrasound image of in-plane needle placement of the L5–S1 facet joint in short-axis. *Gmax* gluteus maximus, *ESM* erector spinae muscles, *PSIS* posterior superior iliac spine, *I* ileum, *L5 SP* L5 spinous process, *L5 IAP* L5 inferior articular process, *L5 DR* L5 dorsal ramus, *S1 SAP* S1 superior articular process.

7. **Aspirate to rule out intravascular needle placement and inject the desired medications.**
8. **Flush and withdraw the needle and apply a bandage.**

Tips

- For the L5 dorsal ramus block, the approach is similar to the L1–L4 MBB, except the target is the junction of the cephalad border of sacral ala and lateral border of the superior articular process. The approach is from medial to lateral due to the iliac crest.

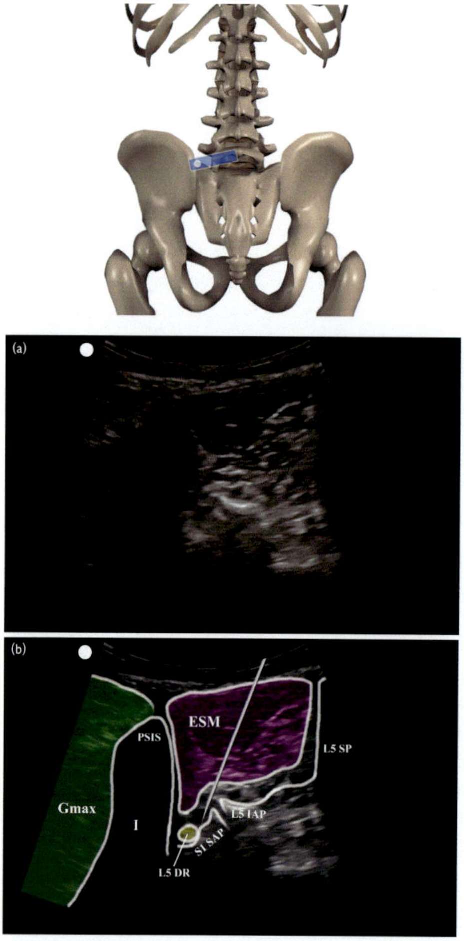

Figure 5.2.7 a, Ultrasound image of the lower back at the L5–S1 level in an axial oblique plane. **b,** Labeled ultrasound image of in-plane needle placement of the L5 dorsal ramus in short-axis. *Gmax* gluteus maximus, *ESM* erector spinae muscles, *PSIS* posterior superior iliac spine, *I* ileum, *L5 SP* L5 spinous process, *L5 IAP* L5 inferior articular process, *L5 DR* L5 dorsal ramus, *S1 SAP* S1 superior articular process.

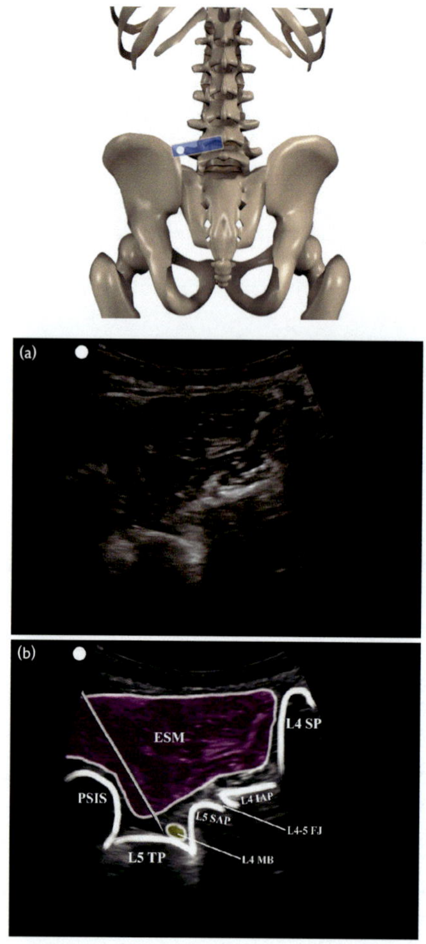

Figure 5.2.8 a, Ultrasound image of the lower back at the L4–5 level in an axial oblique plane. **b,** Labeled ultrasound image of in-plane needle placement for an L4 medial branch block in short-axis. *ESM* erector spinae muscles, *L4 SP* L4 spinous process, *L4 IAP* L4 inferior articular process, *L5 SAP* L5 superior articular process, *L4-5 FJ* L4-5 facet joint, *PSIS* posterior superior iliac spine, *L4 MB* - likely location of L4 medial branch nerve, *L5 TP* L5 transverse process.

Lumbar Selective nerve root (transforaminal)—Ultrasound Approach

1. **Prepare equipment and supplies, position the patient prone, and sterilize the procedural area with antiseptic solution.** Consider placing a support beneath the abdomen to reduce lordotic curvature and increase patient comfort.
2. **Identify and count the desired levels.** Palpate the PSIS. Place the probe over the PSIS in the axial plane. At the level of the PSIS, the sacrum will be visualized as shown in Figure 5.2.5.
3. **While maintaining visualization of the sacrum, translate the probe cephalad and medial to visualize the L5–S1 facet joint (Figure 5.2.6).** Lateral to the L5–S1 facet joint will be the sacral ala (Figure 5.2.7). Please note this is on or close to the tip of the PSIS.

4. **Continue translating the probe cephalad to view the L4–L5 facet joint.** Once the L4–L5 facet joint is identified, the probe can be translated slightly caudad to identify the transverse process of L5, superior articular process of L5, facet joint capsule of the L4–L5, inferior articular process of L4, and spinous process of L4 (Figure 5.2.8).
5. **Continued translating cephalad to the desired transforaminal level (**Figure 5.2.9**).** Count by identifying the cephalad and caudad facet joints of each level.
6. Once the desired level is identified, inject the skin just lateral to the ultrasound probe and underlying tissues with local anesthetic.

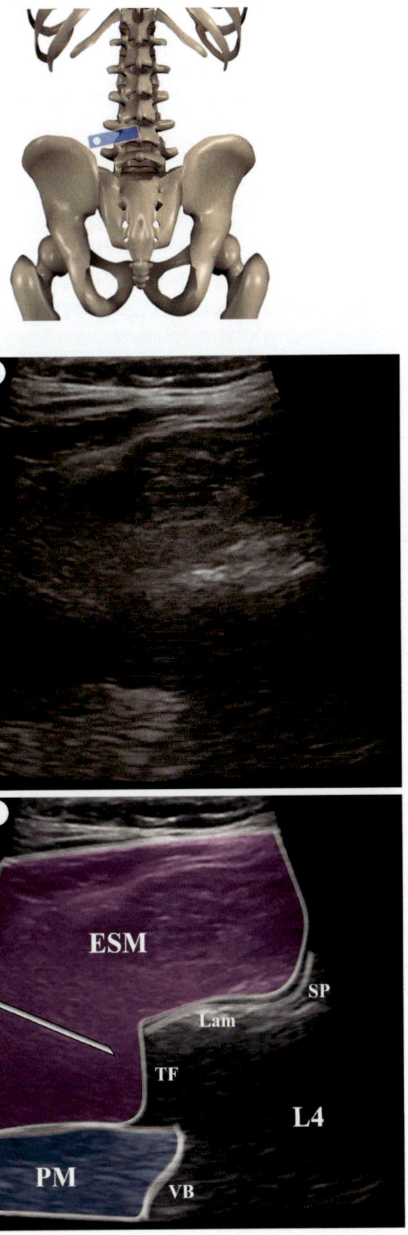

Figure 5.2.9 a, Ultrasound image of the lower back at the L4 level in an axial oblique plane. **b,** Labeled ultrasound image of in-plane needle placement for an L4 nerve root block. *ESM* erector spinae, *L4 SP-Lam-TF-VB* L4 spinous process—lamina—transforaminal space—vertebral body, *PM* psoas muscle.

7. **For L1–L5 nerve roots, insert a 22- or 25-gauge 3.5-inch spinal needle with an in-plane approach.** The spinal needle should be inserted at a 40°–45° angle at the lateral end of the transducer and advanced in the medial direction toward the inferolateral margin of the lamina (Figure 5.2.9).
8. **Aspirate to rule out intravascular needle placement and inject the desired medications.**
9. **Flush and withdraw the needle and apply a bandage.**

Safety Considerations

- Be sure to turn on doppler to identify any satellite arteries before proceeding with the procedure.

Postprocedure Management

Patients may experience increased pain postprocedurally, which is managed conservatively with rest, ice packs, and acetaminophen. Other serious side effects specifically after ESI include postural headache due to possible dural puncture from improper needle placement. If patients experience postural headaches, conservative measures such as rest and hydration are recommended for 24–48 hours. If symptoms persist longer than 48 hours, an epidural blood patch can be performed depending on the risk/benefits and chemotherapeutic agent the patient is receiving. In extremely rare cases, patients may experience nerve injury, epidural hematoma, infection of the procedural site, or allergy to injected medication.

Immediately after the procedure, patients may experience signs of orthostasis with sudden changes in position. Vital signs should be checked and observed for up to 30 minutes to ensure patients are hemodynamically stable and able to be discharged. Patients should be instructed to go to the emergency room if they develop fever, increased swelling, redness, drainage from the site of injection, bowel or bladder incontinence, or sudden weakness or numbness in the lower extremities.

Further Reading

- Furman MB, Berkwits L, Cohen I, Goodman B, Kirschner J, Lee T, Li P (2018) Atlas of Image-Guided Spinal Procedures. In: Torres L, Lin PS, Furman MB (eds), Lumbar Zygapophysial Joint Innervation—Anatomy Diagram and Lesion Zone Diagram. Philadelphia PA; 2018: 281–284.
- Patel V (2015) Transforaminal Epidural Steroid Injection. In Diwan S, Staats P (eds), Atlas of Pain Medicine Procedures. Philadelphia, PA: McGraw Hill; 2015: 200–210.
- Irwin D, Gofeld M (2011) Ultrasound-Guided Lumbar Facet Nerve Block and Intra-articular injection. Atlas of Ultrasound-Guided Procedures in Interventional Pain Management.
- Greher M (2019) Lumbar Medial Branches and L5 Dorsal Ramus. In: Peng P (ed) Ultrasound for Interventional Pain Management: An Illustrated Procedural Guide. Springer Nature, S.I. Cham: Switzerland, 169–185.

References

1. Oh DC, Rispoli L, Ghosh P, Gulati A. Epidural steroid injections for the management of spinal malignancy-related pain: a pragmatic review and retrospective study. *Pain Pract.* 21(3), 285–298 (2021).
2. Richardson J, Groen GJ. Applied epidural anatomy. *Contin. Educ. Anaesthesia, Crit. Care Pain.* 5(3), 98–100 (2005).
3. Ellis H. The anatomy of the epidural space. *Anaesth. Intensive Care Med.* 7(11), 402–404 (2009).
4. Cramer GD. Chapter 5—The cervical region [Internet]. In: *Clinical Anatomy of the Spine, Spinal Cord, and Ans (Third Edition)*. Cramer GD, Darby SA (Eds.), Mosby, Saint Louis, 135–209 (2014).
5. Lirk P, Kolbitsch C, Putz G, et al. Cervical and high thoracic ligamentum flavum frequently fails to fuse in the midline. *Anesthesiology.* 99(6), 1387–1390 (2003).

6. Stolzenberg DS, Greis AC. The space of Okada with bilateral facet joint arthrograms during a lumbar interlaminar epidural injection. *Pain Med. (United States)*. 19(3), 636–637 (2018).
7. Jiao J, Bailey IM, Beckworth WJ, Sandhu D, Nguyen P. The retrodural space of Okada and unusual contrast flow. *PM R*. 11(12), 1357–1359 (2019).
8. Goodman BS, Posecion LWF, Mallempati S, Bayazitoglu M. Complications and pitfalls of lumbar interlaminar and transforaminal epidural injections. *Curr. Rev. Musculoskelet. Med*. 1(3–4), 212–222 (2008).
9. Mandell JC, Czuczman GJ, Gaviola GC, Ghazikhanian V, Cho CH. The lumbar neural foramen and transforaminal epidural steroid injections: an anatomic review with key safety considerations in planning the percutaneous approach. *Am. J. Roentgenol.* 209(1), W26–W35 (2017). doi:10.2214/AJR.16.17471. Epub 2017 May 15. PMID: 28504548.
10. Gitkind AI, Olson TR, Downie SA. Vertebral artery anatomical variations as they relate to cervical transforaminal epidural steroid injections. *Pain Med. (United States)*. 15(7), 1109–1114 (2014).
11. Frost BA, Camarero-Espinosa S, Johan Foster E. Materials for the spine: Anatomy, problems, and solutions. *Materials (Basel)*. 12(2), 253 (2019). doi:10.3390/ma12020253. PMID: 30646556; PMCID: PMC6356370.
12. Gellhorn AC, Katz JN, Suri P. Osteoarthritis of the spine: the facet joints. *Nat. Rev. Rheumatol.* 9(4), 216–24 (2013). doi:10.1038/nrrheum.2012.199. Epub 2012 Nov 13. PMID: 23147891; PMCID: PMC4012322.
13. Jaumard N V., Welch WC, Winkelstein BA. Spinal facet joint biomechanics and mechanotransduction in normal, injury and degenerative conditions. *J. Biomech. Eng*. 133(7), 071010 (2011). doi:10.1115/1.4004493. PMID: 21823749; PMCID: PMC3705911.
14. Binder DS, Nampiaparampil DE. The provocative lumbar facet joint. *Curr. Rev. Musculoskelet. Med*. 2(1), 15–24 (2009). doi:10.1007/s12178-008-9039-y. Epub 2009 Mar 31.
15. Shuang F, Hou SX, Zhu JL, et al. Clinical anatomy and measurement of the medial branch of the spinal dorsal ramus. *Med. (United States)*. 94(52), e2367 (2015). doi:10.1097/MD.0000000000002367. PMID: 26717379; PMCID: PMC5291620.
16. Demondion X, Vidal C, Glaude E, Subocz L, Francke JP, Cotten A. The posterior lumbar ramus: CT-anatomic correlation and propositions of new sites of infiltration. *Am. J. Neuroradiol.* 26(4), 706–10 (2005).
17. Conly JR, Baez-Cabrera LD, Cohen I, White BF, Furman MB. Chapter 30H—Cervical Zygapophysial Joint Innervation: Anatomy, Dissections, and Lesion Zone Diagrams. In: Furman MB (ed), *Atlas of Image-Guided Spinal Procedures*, 2nd ed. Springer: Cham Switzerland (2018), 505–14.
18. Narouze S. Chapter 22—Cervicogenic headache. In: Benzon HT, Raja SN, Liu SS, Fishman SM, Cohen SP (eds), *Essentials of Pain Medicine*, 4th ed. Elsevier: Philadelphia, PA; 2018:177–82.
19. Watanabe S, Bruera E. Corticosteroids as adjuvant analgesics. *J. Pain Symptom Manage*. 9(7), 442–5 (1994). doi:10.1016/0885-3924(94)90200-3.
20. Cohen SP, Raja SN. Pathogenesis, diagnosis, and treatment of lumbar zygapophysial (facet) joint pain. *Anesthesiology* 106(3), 591–614 (2007). doi:10.1097/00000542-200703000-00024.
21. Rispoli L, Rakesh N, Shah R, Gulati A. Interventional pain treatments in the management of oncologic patients with thoracic spinal tumor–related pain: a case series. *Pain Pract*. 19(8), 866–74 (2019). doi:10.1111/papr.12813. Epub 2019 Sep 3.

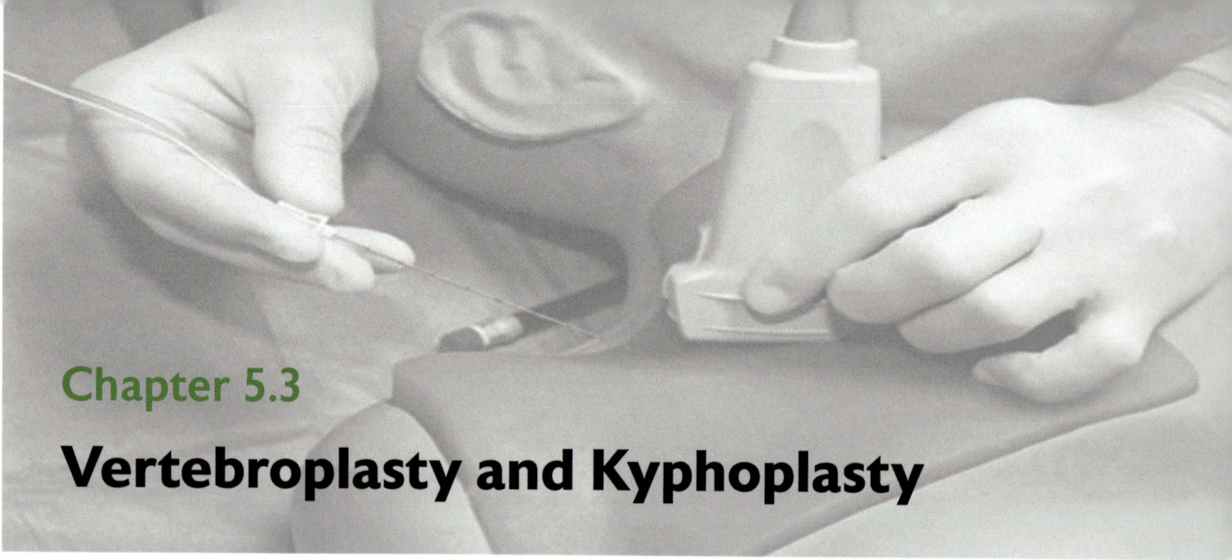

Chapter 5.3

Vertebroplasty and Kyphoplasty

Storm Horine and Priyanka Ghosh

Contents

Introduction

Percutaneous vertebroplasty was first performed in 1984 by Dr. Galibert for the treatment of severe radiculopathy related to a large vertebral hemangioma requiring structural reinforcement.[1] Since then, the procedure has undergone a variety of technical modifications and improvements. Vertebroplasty now involves percutaneous cement introduction, directly under pressure, to increase strength and stability of vertebral bodies with fractures. Kyphoplasty uses a percutaneous introducer to access the vertebral body, allowing various instruments to be used in the same space. This allows for tissue biopsy, ablation, balloon inflation, and cement deposition. Balloon inflation is particularly important as it creates a cavity by compressing cancellous bone, restores vertebral height, and permits more cement to be injected. Both vertebral augmentation techniques have been shown to be effective in improving pain and function with minimal side effects.[2]

There is also an emerging role for vertebral augmentation in cancer. Myeloma, breast, prostate, lung, and other malignancies may appear as osseous spine lesions and cause pathologic fracture. Vertebral compression fractures are found in 34-64% of patients at the onset of multiple myeloma and these fractures can lead to pain, disability, and decreased compliance with anticancer treatments.[3] Not only are pathologic lesions likely to worsen without intervention but also there is an exponential increase in risk of second vertebral fracture after suffering an initial fracture.[4,5] Conservative therapies are frequently inadequate, and vertebral augmentation has been shown to be safe and effective for treating pain for malignant spinal fractures.[2] For these reasons, vertebral augmentation is increasingly being recommended early in the course of cancer with spinal metastases.[6]

Indications

Many patients with vertebral fractures can heal well with conservative care, such as analgesics, physical therapy, and orthotic devices. However, a subset of patients fail conservative therapy and may benefit from vertebral augmentation. The ideal patient for these procedures has a symptomatic, painful vertebral fracture that is refractory to conservative management. Indications for kyphoplasty extend beyond symptom management because ablation may be considered as part of a treatment plan alongside surgery and radiation.[7]

Contraindications

Absolute contraindication to percutaneous vertebral augmentation include active systemic infection or sepsis, local infection at skin insertion site, uncorrectable coagulopathy, inability to hold anticoagulants, myelopathy, spinal instability, retropulsion of fracture fragments into the epidural space, severe allergy to cement or contrast, myelopathy, pregnancy, and patient refusal. Relative contraindications include more than 75% of vertebral body height loss, disruption of the posterior wall of the vertebral body, epidural extension of tumor, previous severe spinal stenosis, more than three compression fractures, inability to lie prone, and inability to tolerate anesthesia or sedation.

Critical Anatomy

Vertebral augmentation requires an in-depth understanding of relevant anatomy. The spinal column is composed of 33 vertebral bones that can be divided into five different regions based on structure: cervical, thoracic, lumbar, sacral, and coccygeal. The individual vertebrae can be further divided into an anterior vertebral body and a posterior vertebral arch. The posterior vertebral arch is composed of pedicles, inferior and superior articulating processes, lamina, and a midline spinous process.

The anterior vertebral body is the main weight-bearing component of the spinal column. The lumbar vertebrae bear the most weight and consequently have the largest vertebral bodies. Vertebral bodies are composed of spongy cancellous bone, which is covered by a thin layer of harder and denser cortical bone. The superior and inferior endplates of the vertebral bodies are composed of thick layers of cancellous bone that anchor to the intervertebral discs and allow exchange of solutes. The posterior vertebral body wall abuts the spinal canal. The anterior vertebral body wall is adjacent to the aorta or iliac arteries, depending on spinal level.

Radiologic diagnosis of vertebral compression fractures is complex but can be described using the AOSpine TL injury classification system.[8] This system categorizes fractures according to morphology of injury: Type A (compression), Type B (tension band disruption), and Type C (displacement/translation). Injuries are next graded on neurologic status of the patient and then finally given patient-specific modifiers. Type A compression injuries, the most relevant injury type for vertebral augmentation, are further divided into 5 subtypes. Subtype A0 refers to no fracture or clinically insignificant fractures. Subtype A1 is a wedge or impaction fracture of a single endplate without posterior vertebral body wall involvement. Subtype A2 is a fracture of both endplates but without posterior vertebral body wall involvement. Subtype A3 consists of a single endplate fracture with involvement of the posterior wall or spinal canal. Subtype A4 means fractures involve both endplates and the posterior wall.

Equipment and Patient Preparation

- Monitors:
  - Patients should be continuously monitored with pulse oximetry, electrocardiography, noninvasive blood pressure measurements, and capnography.
  - Patients should be given supplemental oxygen, and a peripheral intravenous line should be established.
  - Patients typically require moderate sedation or general anesthesia.
- Sterility:
  - Skin at the procedure site should be sterilized with a skin preparation agent such as chlorhexidine.
  - Antibiotic prophylaxis of cefazolin 2 grams or clindamycin 600 mg should be given intravenously prior to skin incision.
- Imaging: Fluoroscopy or computerized tomography scanning
- Needle: 11-gauge needle cannula for lumbar interventions, 13-gauge needle cannula for thoracic interventions, 22-gauge spinal needle
- Scalpel: #11 or #15 blade
- Miscellaneous: Orthopedic hammer
- Patient position: supine with head in contralateral rotation
- Local anesthetic (3 –4 mL):
  - Lidocaine 1%– 2% or bupivacaine 0.25% for local infiltration
- Adjuvant (0.5 –1 mL): non particulate steroid

Fluoroscopy and Procedural Equipment

Vertebral augmentation requires:

1. Fluoroscopy or computerized tomography scanning
2. Local anesthetic: lidocaine 1%– 2% or bupivacaine 0.25% for local infiltration
3. Contrast solution
4. Polymethylmethacrylate (PMMA) or other cement and cement-mixing system
5. Optional for kyphoplasty: introducer cannula instead of needle cannula, orthopedic balloon tamp with inflation syringe, hand-operated drill, biopsy needle, ablation electrode

Procedural Technique

Transpedicular Approach: The Most Common Technique

1. **Position the patient in prone position.** Place 1 –2 pillows beneath the abdomen to minimize lordotic curvature and ensure the patient is not rotated or laterally flexed.
2. **Obtain anterior-posterior fluoroscopic image of lumbar spine.** Visualize both the site of entry and target location of final catheter tip placement. Identify desired vertebral level and adjust cranio-caudal tilt to align the vertebral body endplates. Oblique the fluoroscope image to bring the pedicles to the middle of the vertebral body and to have the spinous process in the midline.
3. **Plan needle cannula or introducer trajectory.** The ideal skin entry point is at the superior lateral quadrant of the pedicle: at approximately 9 o'clock for the left pedicle and 3 o'clock for the right pedicle.
4. **Sterilize with skin preparation agent.**
5. **Anesthetize the entry site, planned trajectory, and periosteum with local anesthetic using the spinal needle.**

6. **Use #11 or #15 blade to make skin incision at needle introducer entry point.**
7. **Insert needle introducer and advance to the superior lateral quadrant of the pedicle.** Advance slowly and use both AP and lateral fluoroscopic imaging to guide needle placement.
8. **Advance needle introducer into bone using orthopedic hammer.** Check AP images for cranio-caudal and medial-lateral trajectory and check lateral images for depth assessment.
9. **Keep needle introducer lateral to the medial border of the pedicle and superior to the inferior border of the pedicle.** This trajectory ensures the safety of the spinal cord and spinal nerves by maintaining the needle introducer in the pedicle and away from the spinal canal and neuroforamen.
10. **With liberal AP and lateral fluoroscopic imaging, advance needle introducer through the pedicle and into the vertebral body.** Withdraw and correct needle trajectory as needed.
11. **Advance the needle introducer into the vertebral body.** For vertebroplasty, the optimal location of the needle for cement deposition is at the anterior one third of the vertebral body. For kyphoplasty, the optimal location for the introducer is at the posterior one-third of the vertebral body.
12. **For kyphoplasty, remove the needle from the introducer cannula, perform biopsy if desired, and insert a hand-operated drill.** Biopsies may be taken prior to drilling. Advance the drill with frequent imaging to the anterior one-quarter of the vertebral body. Do not advance into the anterior cortical surface.
13. **For kyphoplasty, remove the drill, perform ablation if desired, and insert orthopedic balloon tamp.** Ablation may be performed prior to balloon inflation. Balloon tamps are connected to locking syringes with digital manometers. Inflate the balloons slowly and under live or frequent fluoroscopic imaging. Inflate until reaching the edges of the vertebral body or until reaching a desired pressure. Do not exceed 400 PSI. Deflate and remove balloons.
    a. Note: Orthopedic balloons are filled with contrast for fluoroscopic visualization. The balloons may tear and expel the contrast. It is important to verify patients have no contrast allergies for this potential exposure.
14. **Mix cement based on manufacturer instructions and load into cement injector syringes.** Wait for desired cement consistency before injecting. Cement consistency hardens with time, which occurs faster at warmer temperatures.
15. **For vertebroplasty, inject contrast prior to cement and view with fluoroscopy.** Ensure the cement will not be injected into basivertebral veins, other vasculature, the intervertebral disc, or outside the boundaries of the vertebral body. Then, inject cement under lateral fluoroscopic visualization.
    a. Note: For safety, ensure there is no extravasation of cement into the epidural space and avoid deposition of cement in the posterior aspect of the vertebral body. This minimizes the risk of neurovascular compromise.
16. **For kyphoplasty, insert cement delivery syringes in the introducer cannulas and slowly inject cement under lateral fluoroscopic visualization.** Inject with frequent imaging to avoid injection into basivertebral veins, other vasculature, the intervertebral disc, or outside the boundaries of the vertebral body. Inject until cement delivery matches or slightly exceeds the volume of the cavity created by the orthopedic balloon tamp.
17. **Remove needle cannulas after re-inserting the stylet**. Avoid depositing a trail of cement by replacing the stylet into the needles and cannulas when removing them. Hold manual compression over access sites to prevent hematoma formation. Clean and cover with sterile dressing. Take final AP and lateral images to evaluate final cement deposition location.

Postoperative Management and Complications

Postoperatively, patients are typically given 2 hours of bedrest. Patients can receive intravenous nonsteroidal anti-inflammatory drugs, such as ketorolac, unless there is a patient-specific contraindication. Patients should have a thorough neurologic exam following vertebral augmentation to evaluate for nerve or spinal cord injury. Pain may improve immediately following surgery but more commonly improves within 24–72 hours. Patients should be counseled to report any sudden increase in back pain or new back pain, as it could indicate cement leakage or new fracture. Patients should be seen for follow-up in clinic within 3 weeks to assess the surgical site, pain, and mobility.

Complications shared with all surgical procedures include bleeding, infection, and injury to adjacent structures. One of the major complications is the extravasation of cement through vertebral body cortical defects. This can allow posterior spread to impinge on neural structures, anterior spread into vasculature, or superior/inferior spread into a disc space. Serious complication rate is approximately 2% and includes infection, hematoma, cement extension into the inferior vena cava or aorta, aortic puncture, cement pulmonary embolism, and neurologic injury to spinal cord or spinal nerves.[9]

References

1. Mathis JM, Belkoff SM, Deramond H. History and early development of percutaneous vertebroplasty. In: Mathis JM, Deramond H, Belkoff SM (eds), Percutaneous Vertebroplasty and Kyphoplasty. Springer, New York, NY; 2006: 3–8. https://doi.org/10.1007/0-387-36083-2_1
2. Sørensen ST, Kirkegaard AO, Carreon L, Rousing R, Andersen MØ. Vertebroplasty or kyphoplasty as palliative treatment for cancer-related vertebral compression fractures: a systematic review. Spine J. 2019;19(6):1067–1075. doi:10.1016/j.spinee.2019.02.012. Epub 2019 Feb 26. PMID: 30822527.
3. Anselmetti GC, Manca A, Montemurro F, et al. Percutaneous vertebroplasty in multiple myeloma: prospective long-term follow-up in 106 consecutive patients. Cardiovasc Intervent Radiol. 2012 Feb;35(1):139–145. doi:10.1007/s00270-011-0111-4. Epub 2011 Feb 9. PMID: 21305282.
4. Kyriakou C, Molloy S, Vrionis F, et al. The role of cement augmentation with percutaneous vertebroplasty and balloon kyphoplasty for the treatment of vertebral compression fractures in multiple myeloma: A consensus statement from the International Myeloma Working Group (IMWG). Blood Cancer J. 2019;9(3):27. Published 2019 Feb 26. doi:10.1038/s41408-019-0187-7
5. Lindsay R, et al. Risk of new vertebral fracture in the year following a fracture. JAMA. 2001;285:320–323.
6. Kam NM, Maingard J, Kok HK, Ranatunga D, Brooks D, Torreggiani WC, Munk PL, Lee MJ, Chandra RV, Asadi H. Combined vertebral augmentation and radiofrequency ablation in the management of spinal metastases: an update. Curr Treat Options Oncol. 2017;18(12):74. doi:10.1007/s11864-017-0516-7. PMID: 29143901
7. Masala S, Lunardi P, Fiori R, et al. Vertebroplasty and kyphoplasty in the treatment of malignant vertebral fractures. J Chemo. 2004;16:S30–3.
8. Vaccaro AR, Oner C, Kepler CK, Dvorak M, Schnake K, Bellabarba C, Reinhold M, Aarabi B, Kandziora F, Chapman J, Shanmuganathan R, Fehlings M, Vialle L; AOSpine Spinal Cord Injury & Trauma Knowledge Forum. AOSpine thoracolumbar spine injury classification system: fracture description, neurological status, and key modifiers. Spine (Phila Pa 1976). 2013;38(23):2028–2037. doi:10.1097/BRS.0b013e3182a8a381. PMID: 23970107.
9. Chew C, Craig L, Edwards R, Moss J, O'Dwyer PJ. Safety and efficacy of percutaneous vertebroplasty in malignancy: a systematic review. Clin Radiol. 2011;66(1):63–72.

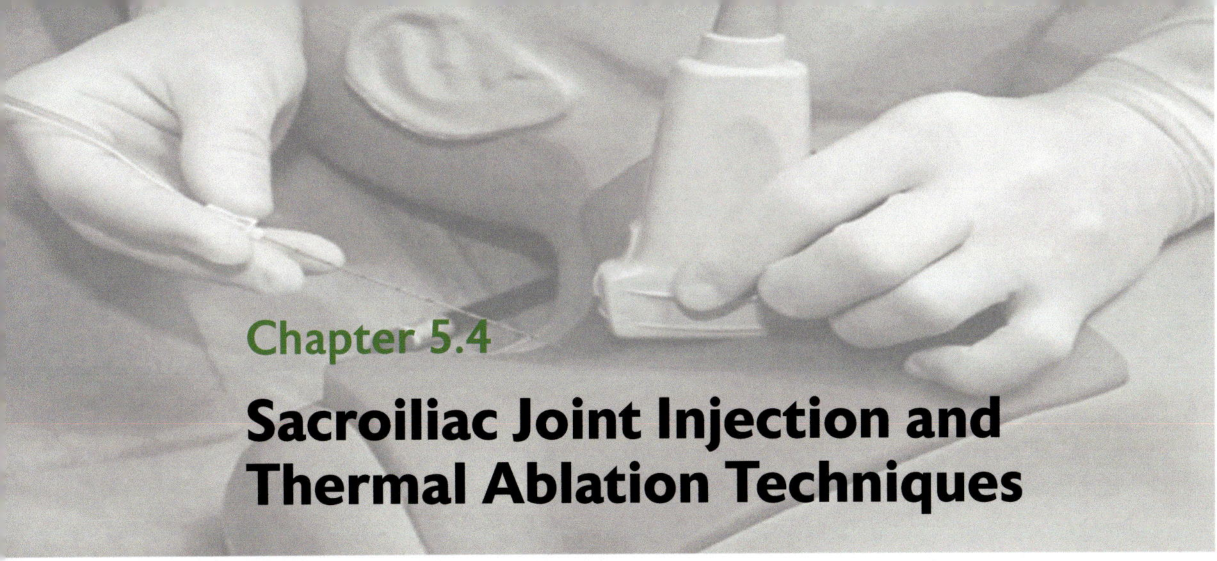

Chapter 5.4

Sacroiliac Joint Injection and Thermal Ablation Techniques

Ankur A. Patel

Contents

Introduction

The sacroiliac (SI) joint connects the bones of the sacrum and ilium, and is one of the largest axial joints in the body.[1] It is considered a diarthroidal joint, where the anterior third of the joint is a true synovial joint and the posterior two-thirds is composed of ligamentous structures.[1] It is a common source of lower back and buttock pain.[2–3] Sacroiliac joint dysfunction may be directly or indirectly related to tumor burden, metastatic lesions, sacral and pelvic fractures, nerve compression, or periosteal inflammation. Additionally, SI joint pain can be a result following oncological therapies such as surgical resection or radiation therapy.

SI joint interventions are safe and effective for SI joint induced axial low back pain when conservative therapy fails. This injection is commonly done with fluoroscopic guidance. However, recent studies have shown that ultrasound guidance may be a superior approach as it can target the ligaments connecting the joint and does not expose the patient to radiation.[4] In addition, ultrasound-guided interventions can be performed quickly at the bedside for patients with severe pain.

Critical Anatomy

The SI joint is a true diarthrodial synovial joint connecting the sacrum and ilium provides stability and load transfer between the spine and lower extremities. The joint consists of both fibrocartilage and hyaline cartilage surrounded by a fibrous capsule.[5] The overall stability of the SI joint is maintained by strong intrinsic and extrinsic ligaments.

The anterior SI ligament is an extension and thickening of the anterior joint capsule. Compared to the other ligaments of the joint, the anterior SI ligament is relatively weak and thin. It is often disrupted during injuries and serves as a common pain generator. The posterior SI ligament is thicker and stronger than the anterior SI ligament (Figures 5.4.1–2). As the posterior SI ligament extends from the sacrum, it forms a compact band known as the interosseous SI ligament in the superoposterior aspect of the joint.[6] This ligamentous network provides stability and limits motion within the SI joint. The SI joint also receives structural support from the piriformis, gluteus maximus, coccygeus, levator ani, paraspinals, and bicep femoris muscles. These muscles help stabilize the joint and transfer muscular forces from the upper to lower extremities. Since these muscles are functionally connected to the SI joint, their dysfunction or injury can greatly affect the stability and functionality of the SI joint. It is highly recommended that these muscles be evaluated for dysfunction and treated when managing patients SI joint pain.

The innervation of the SI joint has significant variability, leading to ambiguity in the medical literature. Some sources claim the anterior SI joint is innervated by L2–S2 ventral rami and the posterior SI joint is innervated by the lateral branches of the L4–S3 dorsal rami (1–2). However, a cadaveric study published in 2014 determined the posterior SI joint is innervated primarily by the S1–S3 lateral branches with occasional innervation by the L5 and S4 branches. These sacral nerves unite to form the posterior sacral network, a common target for SI joint RFA.[7–8]

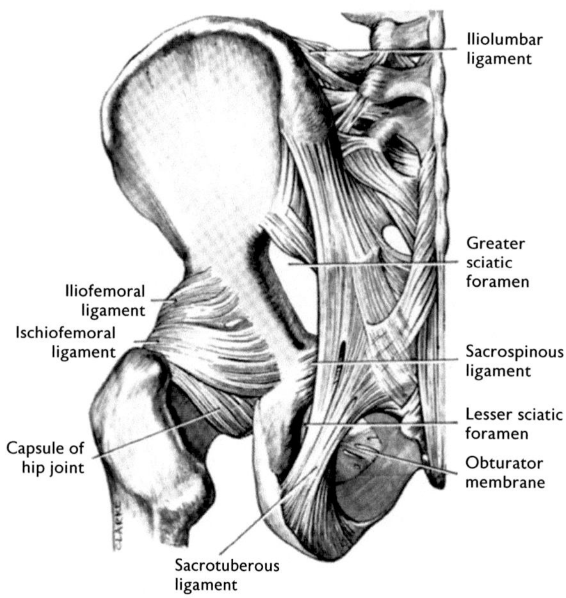

Figure 5.4.1 Dorsal view of the pelvic ligaments. (Reprinted with permission from Cunningham's Manual of Practical Anatomy: Upper and Lower Limbs, 16th Edition)

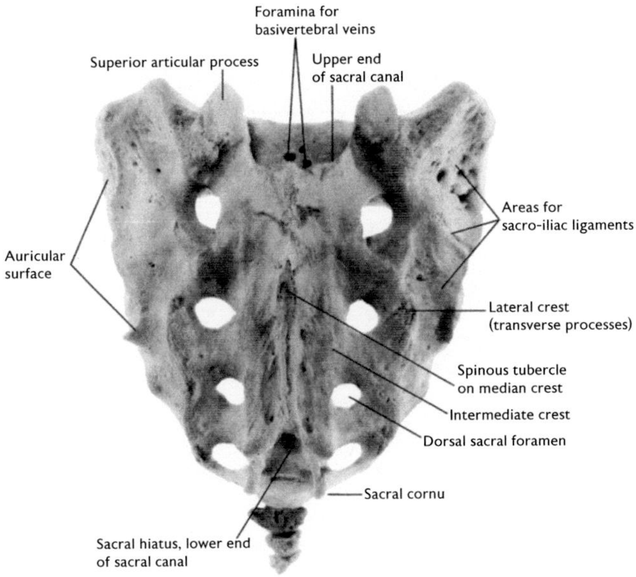

Figure 5.4.2 Dorsal surface of the sacrum and coccyx. (Reprinted with permission from Cunningham's Manual of Practical Anatomy: Thorax and Abdomen, 16th Edition)

Indications

SI joint injection is typically done for both diagnosis and treatment of SI joint pain in patients who have failed conservative modalities such as nonsteroid anti-inflammatory medications and physical therapy. We also recommend SI joint treatment for tumors and stable fractures causing pain in the sacrum and posterior ileum. Imaging can delineate the oncologic causes of SI joint pain. Physical examination maneuvers that evaluate SI joint dysfunction include SI compression, SI distraction, thigh thrust, flexion and abduction and external rotation (FABER), and Gaenslen's test. However, these provocative tests lack sensitivity and specificity to accurately diagnose SI joint dysfunction.[2–3] Given the overall low predictive power of these physical examination maneuvers, SI joint anesthetic blocks are considered the gold standard for diagnosing SI joint dysfunction.[5]

As discussed by Oh et al., there are two main approaches of ultrasound-guided SI joint injection: the superior and inferior approach.[9] The approach taken depends primarily on the location of tumor burden or fracture site (Table 5.4.1). Ligamentous pain and lesions in the superior portions of the sacrum, ilium, or SI joint are best targeted with a superior approach. Likewise, inferior lesions are best treated with an inferior approach. Additionally, tumors diffusely invading the SI joint are typically best treated with an inferior approach to allow medication to spread into the synovial portion of the joint. However, needles should not be driven through a tumor due to the risks of seeding the SI joint with cancer or causing bleeding.[10] Therefore, if a tumor overlies one portion of the joint, it is safest to only access the opposite portion of the joint.[9]

Equipment and Patient Preparation

1. Monitors and Sterility

a. No specific monitoring is required during this procedure. It is highly advised that vital signs, including blood pressure, heart rate, respiratory rate, and pulse oximetry be obtained prior to starting the procedure to ensure the patient is hemodynamically stable. A set of vital sign measurements is often taken post procedure as well.

Table 5.4.1 Indications for Sacroiliac Joint Injection and Ablation and Recommended Approach

Approach Recommended	Indications
Superior SI Joint Injection	• Superior bony disease of the sacrum or ilium • Fracture of superior sacrum or ilium • Ligamentous pain of SI joint • Tumor burden preventing accessing inferior SI joint over site of injection
Inferior SI Joint Injection	• Inferior bony disease of the sacrum or ilium • Fracture of inferior sacrum or ilium • Diffuse bony disease throughout superior and inferior SI joint • Tumor burden preventing accessing superior SI joint

b. Strict antiseptic technique should be observed including sterile draping, probe cover, ultrasound gel, gloves, and gauze. Chlorhexidine or another skin prep agent should be used to clean the skin prior to commencing the procedure.

2. **Equipment**
   a. Probe: High-frequency linear array transducer (8–12 MHz) or low-frequency linear array transducer (2–5 MHz)—depending on depth necessary
   b. Needle type
      i. Sacroiliac joint injection: 22- to 25-gauge 2- or 3.5-inch spinal needle
      ii. Sacroiliac radiofrequency ablation: 50 or 100 mm needle with 5 or 10 mm active tip
   c. Local anesthetic (2–4 mL): Lidocaine 1%–2%; ropivacaine 0.2%–0.5%; bupivacaine 0.25%–0.5%
   d. Adjuvant (1 mL): Particulate or non-particulate steroid
3. **Position**
   a. Prone

Step-by-Step Technique

Sacroiliac Joint Injection—Ultrasound-Guided Inferior Approach

1. **Prepare equipment and supplies, position the patient in the prone position, and clean the skin around the area of the block with antiseptic solution** It is recommended to place a pillow underneath the abdomen to minimize the natural lumbar lordosis.
2. **Place the probe midline in the transverse position just above the gluteal cleft. Move the transducer cephalad to visualize the sacral hiatus**. The sacral cornua should also be identified in this view as shown in Figure 5.4.3.
3. **Translate laterally toward the side of interest to visualize the lateral edge of the sacrum**. Tilting the probe cephalad may improve visualization of the ilium.
4. **Identify the cleft between the lateral sacrum and medial ilium, representing the posteroinferior aspect of the SI joint.** This is located at or slightly caudad to the S2 or S3 (based on anatomic variability) foramen (Figure 5.4.4).
5. **Inject local anesthetic subcutaneously for analgesia at the procedural site.**
6. **Insert the procedural needle with an in-plane approach from medial to lateral.** The needle is inserted at a 40°–45° angle and advanced until the needle is seen entering the joint space.

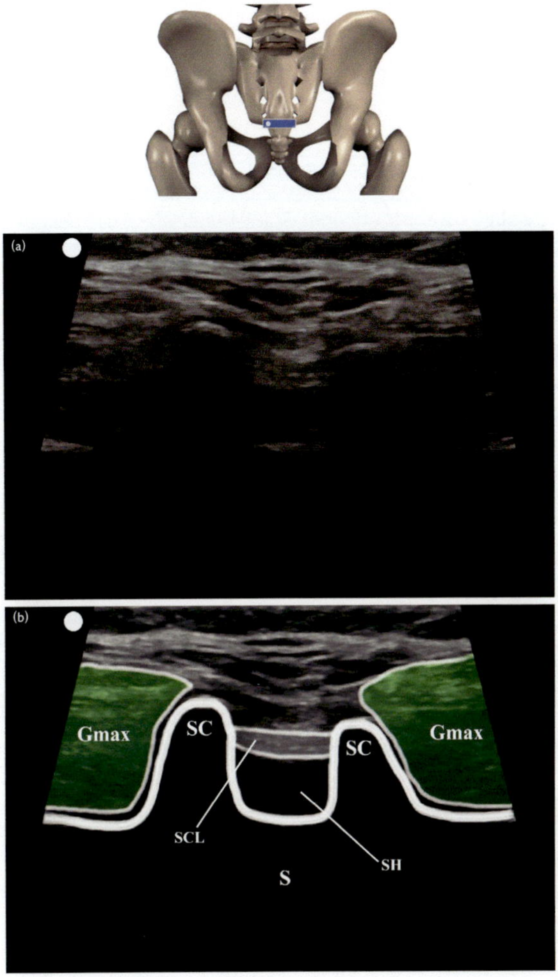

Figure 5.4.3 **a,** Ultrasound image of the sacral hiatus at the level of the cornua in an axial plane. **b,** Labeled transverse ultrasound image of sacral hiatus. *Gmax* gluteus maximus, *SC* sacral cornua, *SCL* sacrococcygeal ligament, *SH* sacral hiatus, *S* sacrum.

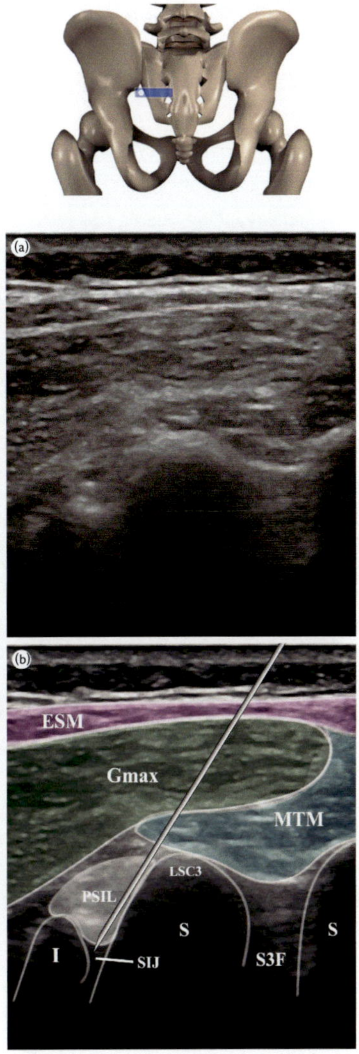

Figure 5.4.4 **a,** Ultrasound image of the inferior portion of the sacroiliac joint in an axial plane. **b,** Labeled ultrasound image of in-plane needle placement for an inferior approach sacroiliac joint injection. *ESM* erector spinae muscles, *Gmax* gluteus maximus, *MTM* multifidus, *I* ileum, *PSIL* posterior sacroiliac ligament, *SIJ* sacroiliac joint, *S* sacrum, *LSC3* lateral sacral crest at S3, *S3F* S3 foramen.

7. **Inject the medication in the SI joint.** Color doppler can be used to further visualize the spread of the injectate in the joint space.
8. **Remove the needle and apply a bandage.**

Tips and Safety Considerations

- Avoid inadvertent injection into the S2 or S3 foramen.
- Avoid advancing needle too ventral or through osteoporotic/metastatic bone, which can result in organ injury.

Sacroiliac Joint Injection—Ultrasound-Guided Superior Approach

1. **Prepare equipment and supplies, position the patient in the prone position, and clean the skin around the area of the block with antiseptic solution.** It is recommended to place a pillow underneath the abdomen to minimize the natural lumbar lordosis.
2. **Place the probe over the posterior superior iliac spine and translate the probe medially in longitudinal view.** In this view, the PSIS and spinous process of the sacrum should be visualized (Figure 5.4.5).
3. **Translate the probe medially and caudad to find the openings of the sacrum, representing the S1 sacral foramen (**Figure 5.4.6**).**
4. **Translate the probe further caudad to reveal the ligamentous or superior portion of the SI joint (Figure 5.4.7**). Moving further inferiorly will reveal the S2 foramen (Figure 5.4.8). Thus, the superior portion of the SI joint is located between the S1 and S2 foramen levels.
5. **Inject local anesthetic subcutaneously for analgesia at the procedural site.**
6. **Insert the procedural needle with an in-plane approach from medial to lateral.** The needle is inserted at a 45° angle at the medial end of the transducer and advanced laterally, under direction visualization, until the needle is seen entering the joint space.
7. **Inject the medicine into the SI joint.** Color duplex doppler can be used to further visualize the spread of the injectate in the joint space.
8. **Remove the needle and apply a bandage.**

Tips and Safety Considerations

- Avoid inadvertent injection into the S1 or S2 foramen.
- Avoid advancing needle too ventral or through osteoporotic/metastatic bone, which can result in visceral organ injury.

Sacroiliac Joint Radiofrequency Ablation

1. **Prepare equipment and supplies, position the patient in the prone position, and clean the skin around the area of the block with antiseptic solution.** It is recommended to place a pillow underneath the abdomen to minimize the natural lumbar lordosis.
2. **Place the probe midline in the transverse position just above the gluteal cleft and move the transducer cephalad to visualize the sacral hiatus (Figure 5.4.3).** The sacral cornua should also be identified in this view.
3. **Move the probe laterally to view the posterior sacral foramen of S4.** The fourth transverse sacral tubercle may be visualized.
4. **Move the prove cephalad to view the posterior sacral foramen of S3 and the third sacral lateral crest (LSC3) (Figure 5.4.9**). Mark the location of LSC3 on the patient's skin.

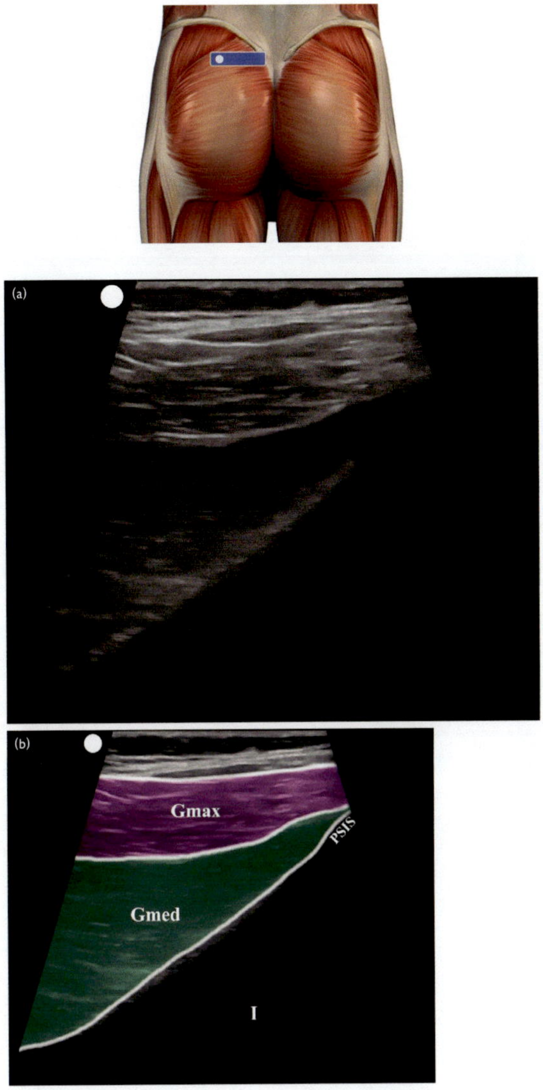

Figure 5.4.5 **a,** Ultrasound image of the posterior buttock in an axial plane. **b,** Labeled ultrasound image of the posterior gluteal muscles. *Gmax* gluteus maximus, *Gmed* gluteus medius, *PSIS* posterior superior iliac spine.

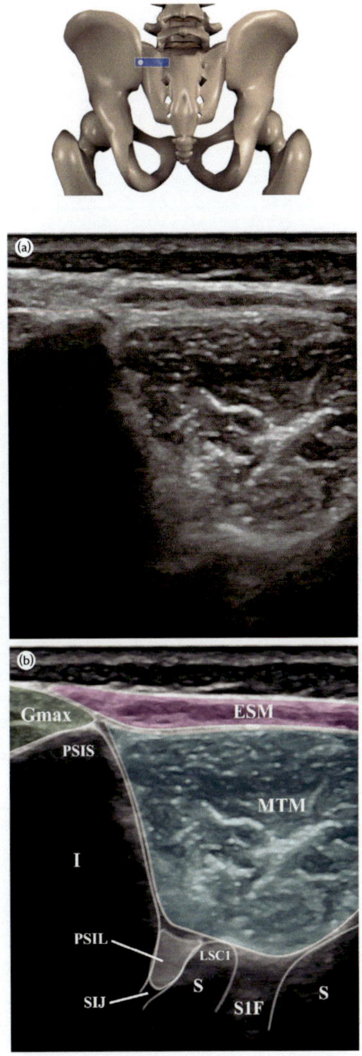

Figure 5.4.6 **a,** Ultrasound image of the sacroiliac joint at the S1 foramen level in an axial plane. **b,** Labeled ultrasound image of the S1 foramen. *Gmax* gluteus maximus, *ESM* erector spinae muscles, *MTM* multifidus, *PSIS* posterior superior iliac spine, *I* ileum, *PSIL* posterior sacroiliac ligament, *SIJ* sacroiliac joint, *S* sacrum, *LSC1* lateral sacral crest at S1, *S1F* S1 foramen.

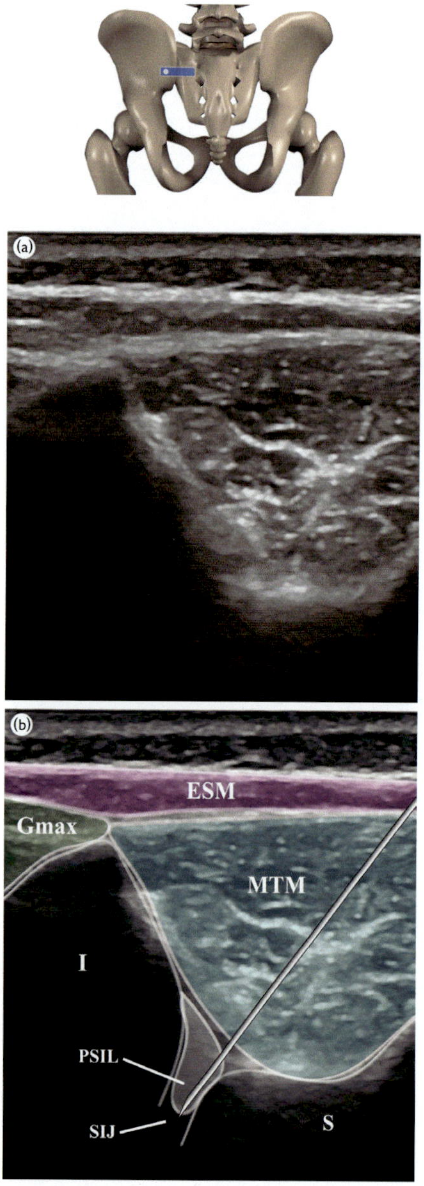

Figure 5.4.7 **a,** Ultrasound image of the superior portion of the sacroiliac joint in an axial plane between S1 and S2 foramina. **b,** Labeled ultrasound image of in-plane needle placement for a superior approach sacroiliac joint injection. *ESM* erector spinae muscles, *Gmax* gluteus maximus, *MTM* multifidus, *I* ileum, *PSIL* posterior sacroiliac ligament, *SIJ* sacroiliac joint, *S* sacrum.

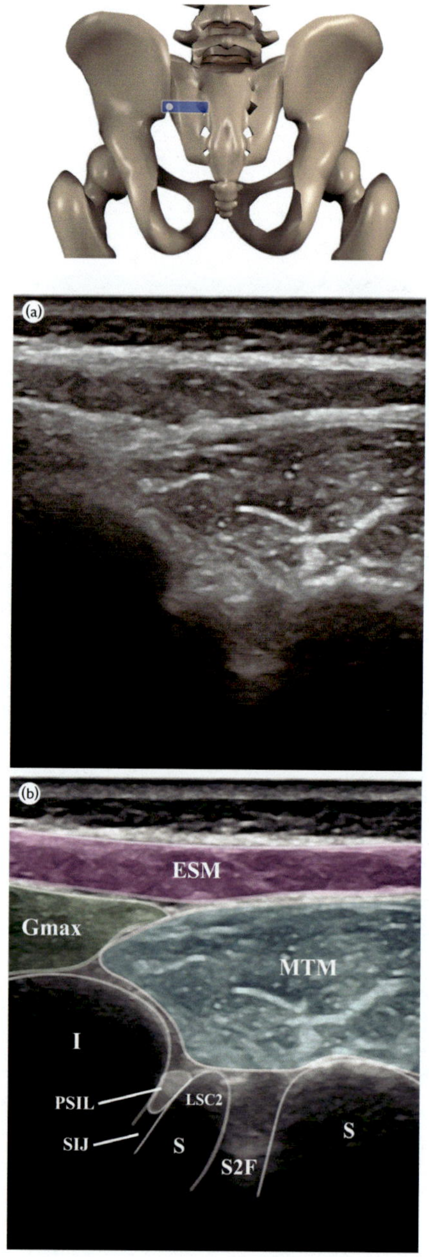

Figure 5.4.8 **a,** Ultrasound image of the sacroiliac joint at the S2 foramen level in an axial plane. **b,** Labeled ultrasound image of the S2 foramen. *ESM* erector spinae muscles, *Gmax* gluteus maximus, MTD multifidus, *I* ileum, *PSIL* posterior sacroiliac ligament, *SIJ* sacroiliac joint, *S* sacrum, *LSC2* lateral sacral crest at S2, *S2 LB* lateral branch of S2 nerve, *S2F* S2 foramen.

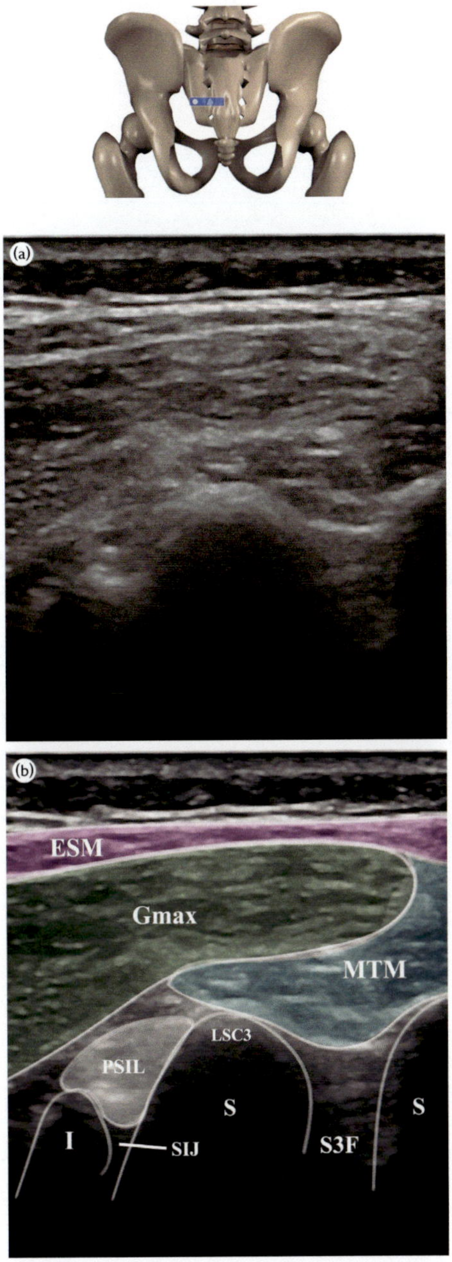

Figure 5.4.9 **a,** Ultrasound image of the sacroiliac joint at the S3 foramen level in an axial plane. **b,** Labeled ultrasound image of the S3 foramen. *ESM* erector spinae muscles, *Gmax* gluteus maximus, *MTM* multifidus, *I* ischium, *PSIL* posterior sacroiliac ligament, *SIJ* sacroiliac joint, *S* sacrum, *LSC3* lateral sacral crest at S3, *S3F* S3 foramen.

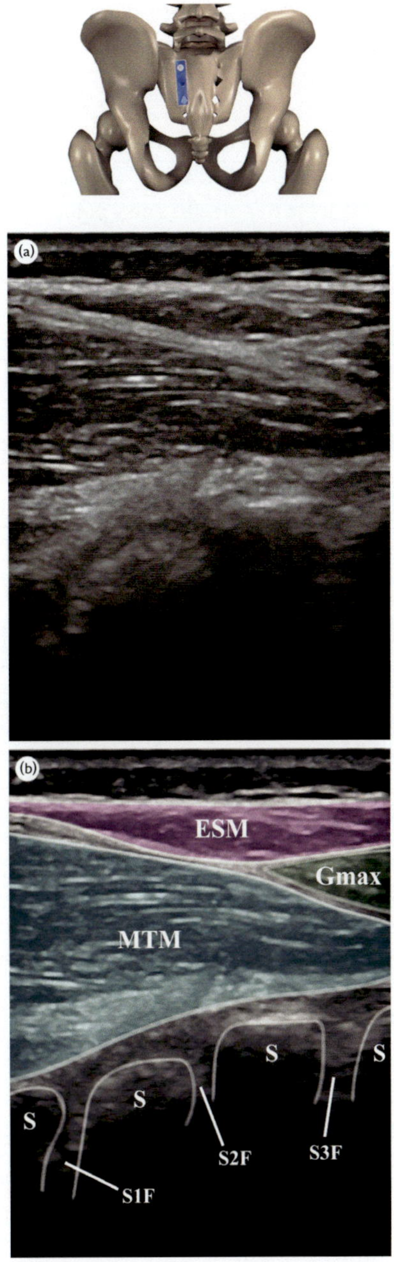

Figure 5.4.10 **a,** Ultrasound image of the sacral foramen in a sagittal plane. **b,** Labeled ultrasound image of the sacral foramen. *ESM* erector spinae muscles, *Gmax* gluteus maximus, *MTM* multifidus, *S* sacrum, *S1F* S1 foramen, *S2F* S2 foramen, *S3F* S3 foramen.

5. **Move the probe further cephalad to visualize the posterior sacral foramen of S2 and the second sacral lateral crest (LSC2) as shown in Figure 5.4.8**. Mark the skin at this site.
6. Move the probe further cephalad to view the posterior sacral foramen of S1 and the first sacral lateral crest (LSC1) (Figure 5.4.6). Again, mark the skin at this site.
7. **Create a line connecting the markings of LSC1, LSC2, and LSC3**. This is the target for the RFA of the lateral branches.
8. **Mark the RFA needle entry points along this line.** For standard ablation, the distance between each cannula should be approximately 8–10 mm. For bipolar ablation, it should be 15 mm.
9. **Place the probe in transverse orientation over the marked region.** The LSCs at the **targeted** level should be visualized immediately beneath the probe.
10. **Inject local anesthetic subcutaneously for analgesia at the procedural site.**
11. **Insert the procedural RFA needle using an out-of-plane approach to contact the desired LSC.**
12. **Once the cannula placement is confirmed under ultrasound, begin the ablation process.**
13. **Remove the needles and apply a dressing.**

Tips and Safety Considerations

- Avoid inadvertent needle placement into the S1–S3 foramen.
- The procedure can also be done in a sagittal plane by visualizing the sacral foramen (S1–S3) as shown in Figure 5.4.10. The transducer is then moved laterally to visualize bone, which is the lateral sacral crest of each respective foraminal level. The cannulas can then be placed in an in-plane approach starting from S1 down to S3.

Postprocedure Management

Patients may experience increased pain postprocedurally, which is managed conservatively with rest, ice packs, and over-the-counter acetaminophen. Patients may rarely experience excessive bleeding from the site of injection or allergy to anesthetic. Immediately after the procedure, patients may experience signs of orthostasis due to a sudden change in position. Patient's vital signs should be checked and observed for up to 30 minutes to ensure the patient is hemodynamically stable to be discharged. Patients should be instructed to go to the emergency room if they develop fever, signs of infection at the site of injection, or sudden weakness in the lower extremity.

Further Reading

- Loh E, Burnham R (2019) Sacroiliac Radiofrequency Ablation. In: Peng P (ed) ULTRASOUND FOR INTERVENTIONAL PAIN MANAGEMENT: an illustrated procedural guide. SPRINGER NATURE, S.l., pp 191–197.
- Finlayson R, Francisca M, Le-Beuffe, E (2019) Sacroiliac Joint and Sacral Lateral Branch Blocks. In: Peng P (ed) ULTRASOUND FOR INTERVENTIONAL PAIN MANAGEMENT: an illustrated procedural guide. SPRINGER NATURE, S.l., pp 185–190.

References

1. Cohen SP (2005) Sacroiliac Joint Pain: A Comprehensive Review of Anatomy, Diagnosis, and Treatment. Anesthesia and Analgesia 101:1440–1453.
2. Hamidi-Ravari B, Tafazoli S, Chen H, Perret D (2014) Diagnosis and Current Treatments for Sacroiliac Joint Dysfunction: A Review. Current Physical Medicine and Rehabilitation Reports 2:48–54.
3. Barros G, McGrath L, Gelfenbeyn M (2019) Sacroiliac Joint Dysfunction in Patients With Low Back Pain. Fed Pract. 36(8):370–375. PMID: 31456628; PMCID: PMC6707638.

4. Perry JM, Colberg RE, Dault SL, Beason DP, Tresgallo RA (2016) A Cadaveric Study Assessing the Accuracy of Ultrasound-Guided Sacroiliac Joint Injections. Physical Medicine and Rehabilitation 8:1168–1172.
5. Schneider BJ, Ehsanian R, Rosati R, Huynh L, Levin J, Kennedy DJ (2019) Validity of Physical Exam Maneuvers in the Diagnosis of Sacroiliac Joint Pathology. Pain Medicine. 21(2):255–260. doi:10.1093/pm/pnz183.
6. Frost S, Fortin J, Wheeler M (2006) The Sacroiliac Joint: Anatomy, Physiology and Clinical Significance. Pain Physician 9(1):61–67. PMID: 16700283.
7. Roberts SL, Burnham RS, Ravichandiran K, Agur AM, Loh EY (2014) Cadaveric Study of Sacroiliac Joint Innervation. Regional Anesthesia and Pain Medicine 39:456–464.
8. Robinson TJG, Roberts SL, Burnham RS, Loh E, Agur AM (2016) Sacro-Iliac Joint Sensory Block and Radiofrequency Ablation: Assessment of Bony Landmarks Relevant for Image-Guided Procedures. BioMed Research International 2016:1–7.
9. Oh DC, First L, Rakesh N, Oh H, Gulati A. (2020) Inferior and Intra-/Peri-Articular Superior Sacroiliac Joint Injection Approaches Under Ultrasound Guidance to Treat Metastasis-Related Posterior Pelvic Bone Pain. Pain Practice: The Official Journal of World Institute of Pain 20(7):769–776.
10. Narouze ST, Benzon HD, Provenzano DA, Buvanendran A, Andres J, Deer T, Rauck R, Huntoon M (2018) Interventional Spine and Pain Procedures in Patients on Antiplatelet and Anticoagulant Medications (Second Edition). Regional Anesthesia and Pain Medicine 43(3):225–262. doi:10.1097/AAP.0000000000000700. PMID: 29278603.

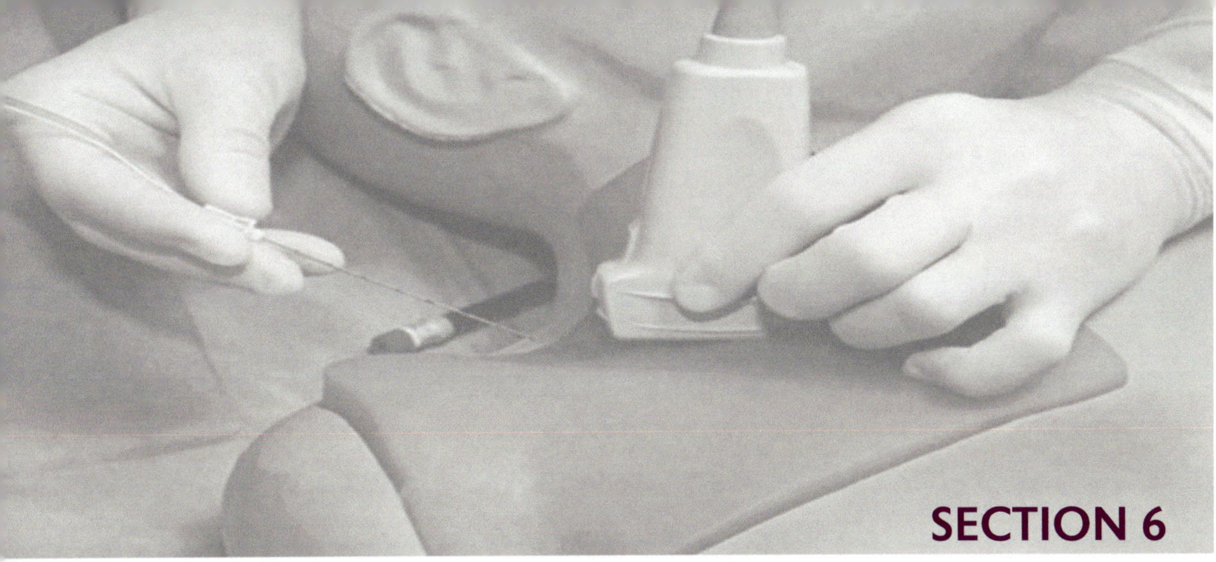

SECTION 6

EXTRA-AXIAL SECTION

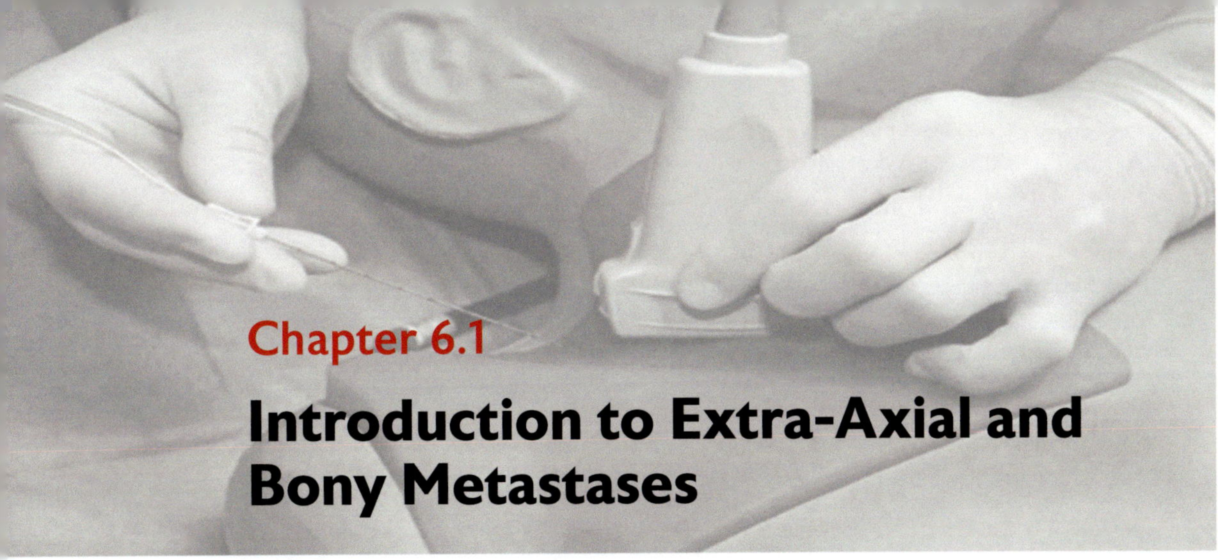

Chapter 6.1

Introduction to Extra-Axial and Bony Metastases

Manuel Cifrian Perez and Madeline Scanlon

Contents

Bone metastases are the most common malignant lesions involving the extra-axial skeleton, and their incidence is expected to increase in the future due to improved survival of cancer patients. Skeletal tumor morbidity includes pain, hypercalcemia, and pathological fracture.

Three types of fractures can occur in cancer patients: pathologic fractures, insufficiency fractures, and impending fractures. Pathologic fractures are a direct consequence of bone weakness due to the presence of bone metastases, which are usually lytic and located in weight-bearing bones. Fractures related to bone insufficiency result from bone reabsorption due to medical therapies or cytokines produced by the tumor. Lastly, impending fractures are painful bone metastases in weight-bearing areas, often requiring preventative treatment to avoid pathologic fracture.

Current modalities to treat oncologic bone pain and prevent fractures include RT, medical treatment, and surgery. Bone-targeting agents interfering with tumor-mediated osteolysis can reduce, but not completely remove, the risk of skeletal related events. Although radiotherapy is considered the best noninterventional treatment for bone metastases–related pain and has the most supporting evidence, it has several limitations. Pain relief typically occurs 1–2 weeks after completing radiotherapy, and some lesions are termed "radio-resistant," meaning they do not respond to RT. Even after completing RT, pain relief only occurs in less than 60% of treated patients. Newer techniques such as stereotactic body RT yield higher rates of local tumor control and pain management compared with standard external beam radiotherapy but present an increased risk of secondary fracture. Surgery can be the definitive solution in oligometastatic patients with slowly evolving disease and long life expectancy. However, surgical interventions carry a significant risk of infection, bleeding, and long recovery times, which may delay systemic therapies.

Management of bone tumors has been made easier by the development of numerous percutaneous techniques, consolidation, tumor ablation, and tumor decompression. Interventional procedures play an important role in managing bone metastases. These percutaneous techniques can be performed prior to radiation therapy, complementing their action due to similar but delayed effects on pain. They can also be used if radiation therapy has failed to relieve pain or in local recurrences.

The innervation of the bones of the appendicular skeleton is listed in Table 6.1.1.[1] This information is useful in determining which nerves should be targeted for blockade, stimulation, or ablation for specific painful bony lesions (Table 6.1.2). As an example, it is helpful to consider two bones that are highly susceptible to metastasis: the clavicle and the pubic symphysis. Although the innervation of the clavicle varies slightly based on the patient, it receives contributions from the subclavian nerve, lateral pectoral nerve, and supraclavicular nerves.[2] In our experience, the distal sensory branches of these nerves lie closest to the periosteum near the metastasis and can be targeted directly adjacent to the periosteum for optimized pain relief. Similarly, while the pubic symphysis is innervated variably by the iliohypogastric, ilioinguinal, genitofemoral, and pudendal nerves,[3] targeting the genitofemoral nerve near the pubic tubercle lateral to the pubic symphysis (fluoroscopic target) has been associated with a reduction of pain due to metastases at this location.

Percutaneous image-guided consolidation techniques play a major role for the management of bone metastases. Cementoplasty aims to stabilize bone and control pain by injecting acrylic cement into a weakened bone. This minimally invasive technique has proven its efficacy for bones like the acetabular roof and femoral condyles, which are submitted to compression forces. However, long cementoplasties of bone diaphyses, which are subject to torsion, should be treated with caution because cement cannot tolerate torsional and compressive forces. Osteolytic tumors of the acetabulum or condyles that are causing disability or a risk of fracture are excellent indications for the technique. For lesions of long bones, such as in the femoral diaphysis, surgical consolidation should be considered to avoid a pathological fracture. Radiation therapy does not provide consolidation nor pain relief and the therapeutic response is generally delayed. In contrast, cementoplasty allows fast consolidation and pain relief. When a bone tumor is associated with painful periosseous soft tissue invasion, cementoplasty can be combined with thermal ablation techniques of the peripheral nerves for optimal pain outcomes.

The main role of image-guided musculoskeletal tumor ablation is palliation of painful metastases secondary to advanced cancer disease. It can be considered potentially curative for benign tumors, such as osteoid osteomas, and for single metastases in poor surgical candidates. Alternatively, neurolysis may be achieved with percutaneous ethanol injection in selected cases to ablate osteolytic bone tumors and improve pain.

Radiofrequency ablation is achieved by altering the electric current at the tip of the electrode, causing local ionic agitation and subsequent frictional heat. Its use in bone tumors is mainly palliative but, in some cases, can be curative. For palliative treatment of painful bone metastases refractory to conventional therapies, the principal aim of radiofrequency ablation is to ablate the bone tumor interface where the source of pain is located. For painful bone metastases, significant pain relief is rapidly achieved in most cases. However, radiofrequency ablation should only be considered for patients with focal pain and a limited number of metastases. For lesions near neurological structures or other vulnerable organs, thermal insulation and temperature monitoring techniques are recommended. Carbon dioxide insufflation, hydrodissection, or balloon interposition can displace vulnerable organs away from the ablation zone and insulate them. Radiofrequency ablation can be combined with cementoplasty in weight-bearing areas such as the acetabulum, femoral condyles, distal tibia, talus, and calcaneus.

Microwave ablation uses electromagnetic waves to agitate ionic molecules and create frictional heat, resulting in tissue coagulative necrosis. Microwaves can propagate through many tissue types, even those with high impedance such as bone, with less susceptibility to heat-sink effects near vessels. Microwave ablation can achieve higher intratumor temperatures and larger ablation zones in less time than radiofrequency ablation.

Table 6.1.1 Bony Innervation and Peripheral Nerve Interventional Targets (Adapted from *NYSORA—Functional Regional Anesthesia Anatomy*)[1]

Bone	Innervation	Common Interventional Target
Scapula Anterior Posterior	Subscapular Nerve Suprascapular Nerve	Suprascapular Nerve
Clavicle Anterior Posterior	Supraclavicular Nerve Subclavian Nerve, Lateral Pectoral Nerve	Superficial Cervical Plexus Lateral Pectoral Nerve
Humerus Anterior Posterior	Axillary Nerve, Radial Nerve, Musculocutaneous Nerve Radial Nerve	As per innervation and location of lesion/tumor
Ulna Anterior Posterior	Anterior Interosseous Nerve (Median Nerve) Posterior Interosseous Nerve (Radial Nerve)	As per innervation and location of lesion/tumor
Radius Anterior Posterior	Anterior Interosseous Nerve (Median Nerve) Posterior Interosseous Nerve (Radial Nerve)	As per innervation and location of lesion/tumor
Carpal Bones Anterior Posterior	Ulnar Nerve Radial Nerve	As per innervation and location of lesion/tumor
Metacarpals Anterior Posterior	1st–4th: Median Nerve 5th: Ulnar Nerve 1st–3rd: Radial Nerve 4th–5th: Ulnar Nerve	As per innervation and location of lesion/tumor
Phalanges Anterior Posterior	1st–3rd Proximal, Middle, and Distal: Median Nerve 4th–5th Proximal, Middle, and Distal: Ulnar Nerve 1st Proximal, Middle, and Distal: Radial Nerve 2nd–3rd Proximal and Middle: Radial Nerve 2nd–3rd Distal: Median Nerve 4th–5th Proximal, Middle, and Distal: Ulnar Nerve	As per innervation and location of lesion/tumor
Pelvis Ilium Ischium Pubis	Ilioinguinal and Iliohypogastric Nerves, Sciatic Nerve Sciatic Nerve Iliohypogastric, Ilioinguinal, Genitofemoral, and Pudendal nerves	Ilioinguinal and Iliohypogastric Nerves, Lateral Sacral Branches, Genitofemoral Nerve
Femur Anterior Posterior	Femoral Nerve, Saphenous Nerve Obturator Nerve, Sciatic Nerve	As per innervation and location of lesion/tumor
Tibia	Saphenous Nerve, Common Peroneal Nerve, Tibial Nerve	As per innervation and location of lesion/tumor
Fibula	Tibial Nerve	Tibial Nerve
Tarsal, Metatarsals, Phalanges Dorsal Plantar	Superficial and Deep Peroneal Nerve Tibial Nerve, Sural Nerve	As per innervation and location of lesion/tumor

Table 6.1.2 Extra-Axial Cancer-Related Pain Treatment Options Based on Oncologic Status

Survivorship Pain	Active Cancer	Treatment-Related
• Corticosteroids • Viscosupplementation • Peripheral nerve stimulation • Nerve ablation • Regenerative medicine (for remission cases) • Neuraxial stimulation (spinal cord stimulation, dorsal root ganglion stimulation)	• Corticosteroids • Viscosupplementation • Nerve ablation (if musculoskeletal tumor invasion) • Peripheral nerve stimulation • Neuraxial stimulation (spinal cord stimulation, dorsal root ganglion stimulation) • Intrathecal pump • Surgical (Dorsal root exit zone lesioning, cordotomy)	• Corticosteroids • Viscosupplementation • Peripheral nerve stimulation • Nerve ablation • Regenerative medicine (if in remission) • Neuraxial stimulation

Cryoablation is the application of extreme cold to destroy cells by causing cellular and vascular injury. It can be used percutaneously under CT or MRI guidance. The major advantage of cryoablation over radiofrequency ablation is the precise visualization of the ice ball on both CT and MR imaging. Image guidance can be used to monitor the extension of the ice ball, check the proper covering of the tumor, and control the safety margin with adjacent vulnerable structures. Another major benefit is reduction of the postprocedural pain. Cryoablation is effective in sclerotic bone lesions, although the visualization of the ice ball is poor in these cases. In contrast to radiofrequency ablation, cryoablation is not contraindicated if metallic surgical hardware is contacting the targeted tumor.

Thorough familiarity with the different techniques and their indications in the oncologic population is essential for pain physicians. Thermal protection is crucial to prevent complications, particularly when performing thermal ablation procedures close to neural structures. Careful patient selection helps to determine whether the therapeutic intent is curative or palliative, and which technique is most suitable.

References

1. Carrera A, Lopez A, Sala-Blanch X, Kapur E, Hasanbegovic I, and Hadzic A. Functional regional anesthesia anatomy. Accessed January 1, 2022. https://www.nysora.com/foundations-of-regional-anesthesia/anatomy/functional-regional-anesthesia-anatomy/
2. Leurcharusmee P, Maikong N, Kantakam P, Navic P, Mahakkanukrauh P, Tran DQ. Innervation of the clavicle: a cadaveric investigation. *Reg Anesth Pain Med.* 2021;46(12):1076–1079.
3. Becker I, Woodley SJ, Stringer MD. The adult human pubic symphysis: a systematic review. *J Anat.* 2010;217(5):475–487.

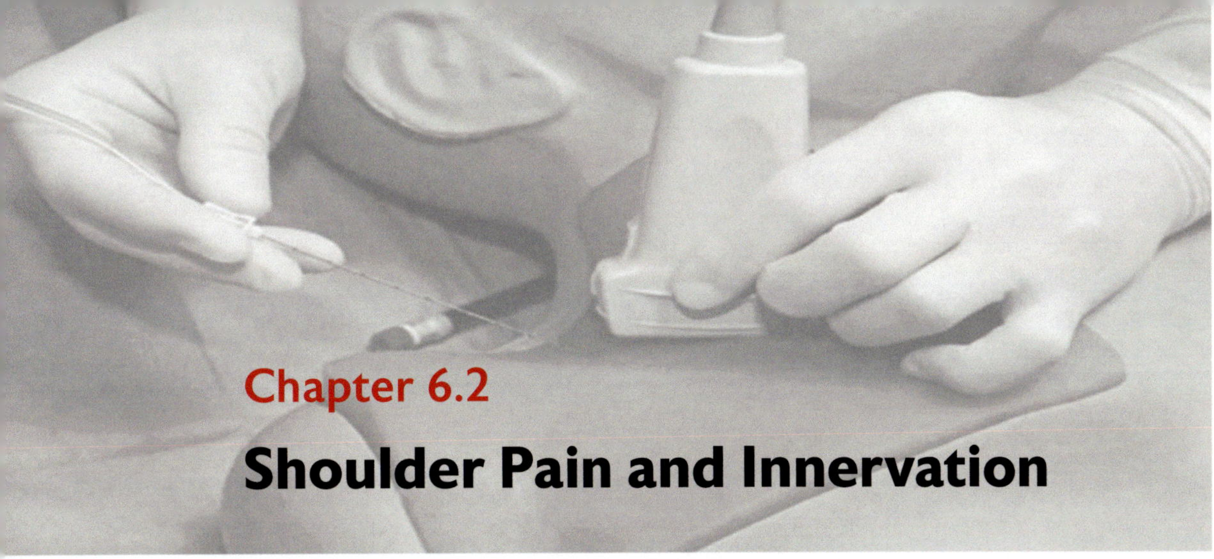

Chapter 6.2

Shoulder Pain and Innervation

Cory Ullger and Olga Komargodski

Contents

Introduction

The shoulder is a complex major joint with a high degree of mobility, needing many contributing muscles and innervating nerves. Chronic shoulder pain for a duration of more than one month was reported in 6.7% of the population[1] and it is estimated that 20% of the general population will suffer from shoulder pain throughout their lives.[2] Shoulder pain is the third most common musculoskeletal complaint after back and knee pain.[3]

Cancer pain related to the shoulder may result from direct tumor invasion, malignant infiltration of nerves, pathological fractures, and sequelae of cancer treatment including radiation-induced nerve injury, chemotherapy or postsurgical pain. Novel advancements in neuromodulation via intrathecal drug delivery and neurostimulation have augmented the ability to treat refractory shoulder pain. Ablative techniques for the management of cancer pain remain important in a select group of patients whose pain has proven intractable to these therapies, or in whom the implantation of a medical device is not feasible.[4].

Indications

Shoulder pain in the cancer patient may be divided into three distinct categories:

- Tumor-related pain
- Treatment-related pain
- Debility or pain unrelated to cancer

Common musculoskeletal causes of shoulder pain in the oncological patient include: osteogenic pain due to tumor burden, myofascial pain syndrome/trigger points, rotator cuff tendinitis, shoulder impingement syndrome, adhesive capsulitis, scapulothoracic bursitis, radiation-induced fibrosis, postsurgical pain (mastectomy, lymph node dissection surgery for head/neck/breast cancers, etc.), and hormonal therapy–induced arthralgias.[5]

Neuropathic shoulder pain may develop in the cancer patient due to mononeuropathies involving the axillary or suprascapular nerve, brachial plexopathy, or upper cervical radiculopathies—typically deriving from local tumor burden, radiation, or surgery.[6] Complex regional pain syndrome may also develop as a result of cancer- and treatment-related tissue trauma (Type I) or as a result of damage to a specific nerve (Type II).

The shoulder is the third most common site for primary bone tumors.[7] The most common area for a primary bone malignancy in the shoulder is the proximal humerus, followed by the scapula and clavicle.[8] In a review of 194 primary neoplasms of the shoulder 72% were benign and 28% were malignant.[9] Three indicators of potential malignancy were identified: older age, tenderness on palpation, and lesions of the scapula.[10] The shoulder can also be a site of metastatic lesions from lung cancer, breast cancer, renal cancer, hematologic malignancies, and others.[10] Referred pain from a lesion in the apical part of the lung, Pancoast tumor, may manifest in the shoulder.[11] Referred pain is important because a shoulder treatment may not alleviate the pain.

Cancer treatments such as surgery, radiation, and hormonal therapy, are common causes for shoulder pain in the cancer oncological population.[12–14] Up to 80% of patients report shoulder pain post lymph node dissection surgery for head and neck cancers,[15] the rates of pain are higher after radical lymph node dissection versus modified radical.[16] In patients with node negative breast cancer, up to 80% of patients report arm related pain symptoms; with a higher prevalence in those patients who have undergone breast surgery, axillary dissection, and radiation.[17]

Brachial plexopathy can be due to tumor invasion, radiation changes, chemotherapy, or trauma (18). Metastatic tumors leading to brachial plexopathy are extremely rare and generally arise from breast or lung cancers. Pain tends to be a pervasive issue as patients typically present in advanced stages. These tumors and the resulting pain are often difficult to treat.

Critical Anatomy

Based on Hilton's Law, at least 15 peripheral nerves or ventral rami may contribute to the innervation of the shoulder. The nerves supplying the shoulder mostly arise from the brachial plexus. Sensory innervation of the glenohumeral joint (GHJ), acromioclavicular joint (ACJ), and rotator cuff is carried by the articular branches of five nerves, which are the suprascapular nerve (SN), axillary nerve (AN), lateral pectoral nerve (LPN), musculocutaneous nerve, and subscapular nerve as shown in Figures 6.2.1–6.2.4.

The suprascapular nerve (SN) arises from the C5–C6 nerve roots and has afferent, efferent, and sympathetic fibers. It provides sensory fibers to 70% of the shoulder joint, including the posterior and superior regions of the GHJ, capsule, ACJ, the scapula and, variably, the overlying skin.[4] It also provides motor innervation for the supraspinatus and infraspinatus muscles.

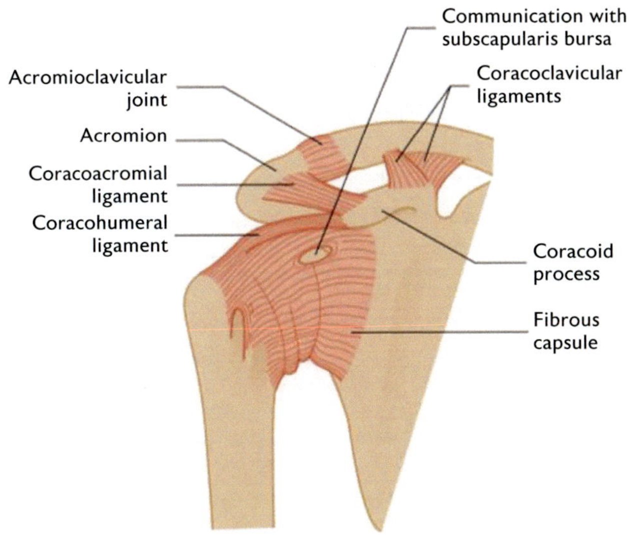

Figure 6.2.1 Diagram of the anterior aspect of the right shoulder joint capsule with surrounding ligaments. (Reprinted with permission from Cunningham's Manual of Practical Anatomy: Upper and Lower Limbs, 16th Edition)

The remainder of the innervation to the shoulder is from the axillary nerve, which provides sensory innervation to the anterior and inferior zones of the glenohumeral joint, with a relatively small contribution from the lateral pectoral, musculocutaneous, and subscapular nerves (5). The LPN branches course in a superior-lateral direction adjacent to thoracoacromial vessels across the superior aspect of the coracoid process and then descends into the anterior-superior GHJ.

A recent cadaveric dissection of the shoulder joint revealed proposed locations of the terminal branches of the SN, AN, and LPN (6). These studies identified anatomic safe zones to perform

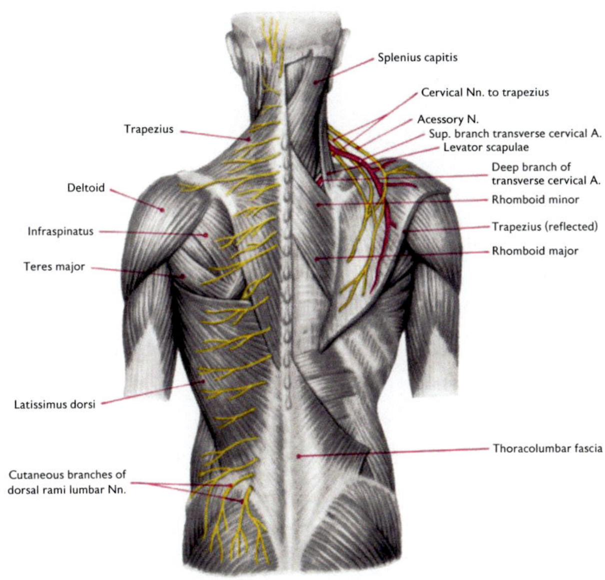

Figure 6.2.2 Dissection of the muscles and nerves of the back and shoulder. (Reprinted with permission from Cunningham's Manual of Practical Anatomy: Upper and Lower Limbs, 16th Edition)

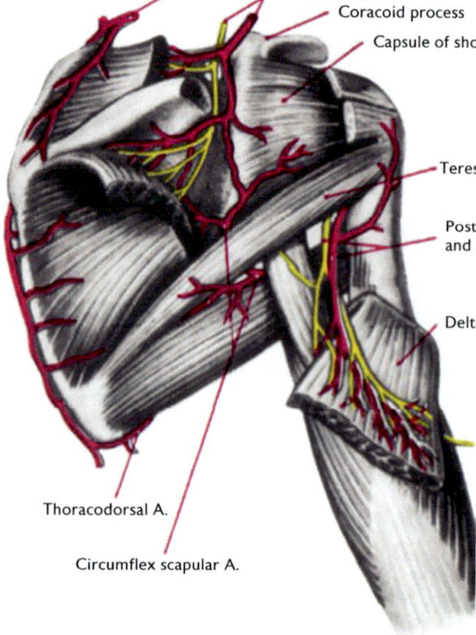

Figure 6.2.3 Neurovascular anatomy of the posterior shoulder with acromion removed. (Reprinted with permission from Cunningham's Manual of Practical Anatomy: Upper and Lower Limbs, 16th Edition)

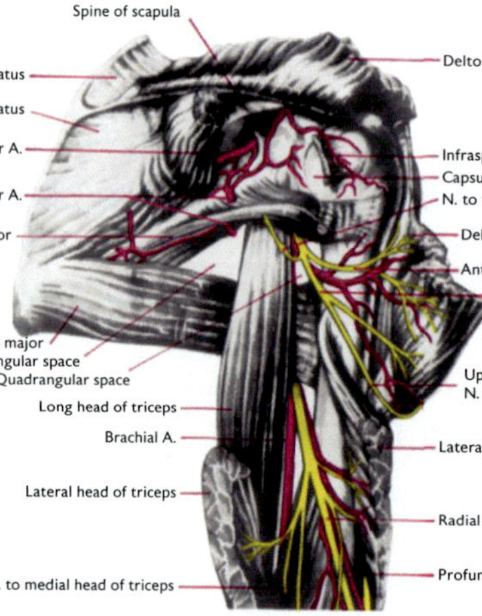

Figure 6.2.4 Dissection of the scapular region and back of arm revealing the neurovascular structures in the quadrangular and triangular spaces. The lateral head of the triceps has been divided to expose the spiral groove of the humerus. (Reprinted with permission from Cunningham's Manual of Practical Anatomy: Upper and Lower Limbs, 16th Edition)

anesthetic blocks and radiofrequency ablation. The sensory articular branches of the axillary nerve are found at the posterio-lateral aspect of the humerus overlying the teres minor. Blocking terminal branches in these safe zones is hypothesized to treat joint capsule pain while preserving the surrounding motor function.

Interventional Treatments

Conservative treatment options for shoulder pain include a course of physical therapy, ice/heat, anti-inflammatory medications, and rest. Interventional therapy should be planned as part of a comprehensive multimodal approach in cancer pain management that incorporates pharmacological, psychological, and behavioral therapy.

Indications

The most common interventional procedure for cancer related shoulder pain is likely a glenohumeral intra-articular injection. Local tumor burden may require modification to injection approach at the shoulder and thus being familiar with different approaches to the intra-articular space is paramount. Glenohumeral arthrosis is characterized by progressive and irreversible articular destruction and frequent involvement of the surrounding soft tissues.

When considering interventional treatments for shoulder pain due to active cancer or its treatments, a careful review of imaging and assessment of the cause of the pain syndrome is needed before choosing the best treatment (Tables 6.2.1, 6.2.2). In any case, collaboration with physical therapy and rehabilitation will be helpful in maximizing care for the oncologic patient.

Contraindications

The absolute contraindications to shoulder injections are patient refusal for the procedure, localized or systemic infection, and severe coagulopathy. Relative contraindications may include thrombocytopenia, anticoagulation, immunocompromised patients, distorted anatomy, prior nerve injury or damage, allergy to anesthetics, implanted pacemaker, allodynia, and inability to consent to the procedure. Table 6.2.3 outlines the contraindications and recommended treatment intervention to mitigate overall risk to the patient.

Equipment and Patient Preparation

1. **Monitors and Sterility**
    a. No specific monitoring is required during this procedure. It is highly advised that vital signs, including blood pressure, heart rate, respiratory rate, and pulse oximetry, be obtained prior to starting the procedure to ensure the patient is hemodynamically stable. A set of vitals is often taken post procedure as well.
    b. Strict antiseptic technique should be observed including sterile draping, probe cover, ultrasound gel, sterile gloves, and sterile gauze. Chlorhexidine or other skin prep agent should be used to clean the skin prior to commencing the procedure.
2. **Imaging modalities:**
    a. Ultrasound
        i. Probe: high-frequency linear array or low-frequency curvilinear array
3. **Needle type:**
    i. Local anesthetic: 27- or 30-gauge 1.5-inch needle
    ii. Nerve and joint injections: 22- to 25-gauge 2- to 3.5-inch spinal needle
4. **Patient position:** Seated, lateral decubitus or prone

Table 6.2.1 Shoulder Cancer–Related Pain Etiologies

Musculoskeletal	Neurologic	Vascular	Bone	Other
• Osteoarthritis (glenohumeral, acromioclavicular) • Shoulder impingement • Myofascial pain • Scapular dyskinesia • Bursitis (subdeltoid, scapulothoracic, subacromial) • Tendinopathy • Rotator cuff pathology • Contractures • Muscular tumor invasion • Postsurgical pain • Ligamentous damage and glenohumeral instability • Adhesive capsulitis • Labral damage	• Upper cervical radiculopathy • Polyneuropathy (CIPN) • Radiation-induced brachial plexopathy • Chemo/ immunotherapy-induced neuropathy • Leptomeningeal disease • Tumor invasion causing compression • Thoracic outlet syndrome • Mononeuropathy/ mononeuritis multiplex • Paraneoplastic neuropathy • Complex regional pain syndrome • Central pain syndrome	• Avascular necrosis • Hematoma	• Primary bone tumors • Metastasis • Osteoporosis • Insufficiency fracture • Pathological fracture	• Fibromyalgia • Graft-versus-host disease • Radiation dermatitis • Radiation-induced fibrosis • Lymphedema • Infection • Anxiety • Depression

Table 6.2.2 Shoulder Cancer–Related Pain Treatment Algorithm

Survivorship Pain	Active Cancer	Treatment-Related
• Corticosteroids • Viscosupplementation • Peripheral nerve stimulation • Total joint denervation • Regenerative medicine (for remission cases) • Prolotherapy (for tendinopathy) • Neuroaxial options (spinal cord stimulation, dorsal root ganglion stimulation)	• Corticosteroids • Viscosupplementation • Total joint denervation (if musculoskeletal tumor invasion) • Temporary peripheral nerve stimulation • Neuroaxial options (spinal cord stimulation, dorsal root ganglion stimulation) • Surgical (Dorsal root exit zone lesioning, cordotomy)	• Corticosteroids, viscosupplementation (musculoskeletal injury) • Neuromodulation before joint denervation (for nerve injury) • Follow survivorship (for remission cases) • Injection steroids vs viscosupplementation (if MSK injury)

Table 6.2.3 Contraindications to Shoulder Injections

Contraindications	**Related Types** *(recommended intervention)*
Absolute	Refusal for the procedure Localized or systemic infection Severe coagulopathy
Relative	Thromboctyopenia *(smaller needle gauge size)* Anticoagulation *(smaller needle gauge size)* Immunocompromised patients *(viscosupplementation instead of corticosteroids)* Distorted anatomy *(modified injection approach, consider neuromodulation)* Prior nerve injury or damage *(neuromodulation)* Allergy to anesthetics *(saline with injection)* Implanted pacemaker *(intrathecal drug delivery)* Allodynia *(neuromodulation)* Inability to consent to the procedure *(healthcare proxy)*

5. **Injectate:**
   a. Local anesthetic: Lidocaine 1%–2%; Ropivacaine 0.2%–0.5%; Bupivacaine 0.25%–0.5%
   b. Adjuvant: particulate or nonparticulate steroid

Procedure Techniques

A. Suprascapular Nerve Approach (Figure 6.2.5)

1. **With the patient in seated position and arm by the side, a low-frequency, linear ultrasound probe is placed in the axial oblique plane** in line over the lateral portion of the scapular spine.
2. **Translate the probe cranial and tilt the probe caudally to end in a coronal oblique plane on the superior posterior portion of the shoulder as shown in** Figure 6.2.6.
3. **Follow the scapular line medial to lateral until the suprascapular notch appears**. Then identify the suprascapular never and artery in the floor of suprascapular notch. The deep groove is the suprascapular notch. Below the transverse scapular ligament is the nerve. The suprascapular artery can often be visualized with doppler and is commonly seen above the ligamentous structure.
4. After anesthetizing the skin and needle track, the injectate **needle is advanced in-plane under direct ultrasound guidance through the supraspinatus muscle toward the suprascapular notch**, in a medial to lateral or lateral to medial direction, at an angle of 30°–45° to the vertical. Using doppler/PDI, take care to avoid the suprascapular artery. You may appreciate a tactile engagement as the needle pierces the transverse scapular ligament to target the SSN.
5. After aspiration is negative for heme and air, local anesthetic and adjuvant steroid mixture are injected slowly under visualization into the area.

Tips

- Special considerations: While anatomically guided suprascapular nerve blocks typically call for higher local anesthetic volumes for redundancy, with ultrasound guidance we recommend lower

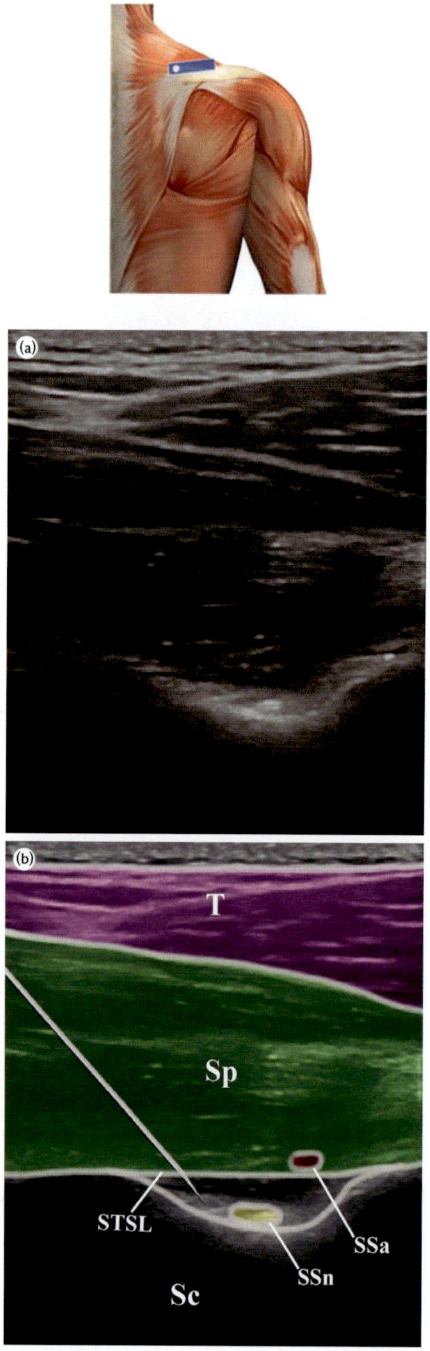

Figure 6.2.5 **a,** Ultrasound image of the posterior shoulder in a coronal oblique plane with a caudal tilt. **b,** Labeled ultrasound image of in-plane needle placement for a suprascapular nerve block in short-axis at the suprascapular notch. *T* trapezius, *Sp* supraspinatus, *STSL* superior transverse scapular ligament, *SSn* suprascapular nerve, *Sc* scapula.

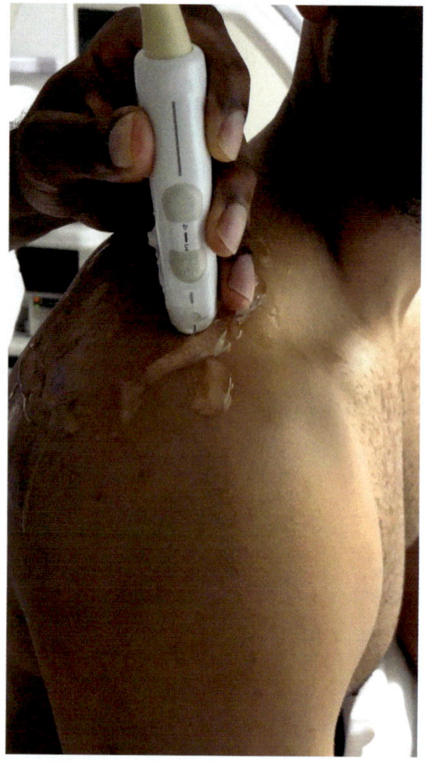

Figure 6.2.6 Ultrasound probe placement in a coronal oblique plane with tilt facing caudally to view the suprascapular notch.

local anesthetic volumes (less than 3 cc) to prevent local anesthetic overflow to the brachial plexus. Additionally, avoid angulating the needle too anterior to avoid pneumothorax, particularly if going out of plane posterior to anterior.

- Be sure to use doppler to search for and identify suprascapular artery near the target area to avoid during procedures.

Glenohumeral Joint Injection (Figure 6.2.7)

This technique may be performed posterior or anterior. Posterior technique will be described.

1. **The patient is seated with the ipsilateral arm crossing the chest or hanging at the side.** A linear or curvilinear (based on body habitus) probe is placed in a parallel position over the spinoglenoid notch caudal to the spine of the scapula.
2. **At this location, translate laterally to visualize the infraspinatus tendon deep to the deltoid**. The posterior part of the humeral head, glenoid, and labrum (triangular shaped) are visualized.
3. **After anesthesizing the skin, guide the needle toward the target intra-articular joint space. Final needle position will be deep the infraspinatus, just lateral to the glenoid labrum,** at the humeral head. Approach can be medial to lateral or lateral to medial. Note: the humeral head is covered with articular cartilage, and care should be taken not to advance the too far into the cartilage, as this would lead to possible resistance and possible tissue damage.
4. **Local anesthetic (typically 3–5 cc) with adjuvant steroid is used as the injectate.** The injectate will displace the posterior joint capsule and lift the infraspinatus superiorly. Color doppler can be used to observe flow caudad into the glenohumeral joint. If resistance is encountered on injection, the needle can be withdrawn for a small distance or the bevel of the needle can be rotated.

Tips

- Be sure to use doppler to search for and identify satellite vessels near the target area to avoid during procedures.

Safety Considerations

- Avoid piercing through the glenoid labrum, which will lead to worsening shoulder pain.

Axillary Nerve Approach (Figure 6.2.8)

1. **The probe is placed in a sagittal plane parallel to shaft of the humerus** and approximately 2 cm below the posterolateral part of the acromion on the dorsal side of the arm.
2. **Identify the surgical neck and the shaft of the humerus and the cross section of the posterior circumflex humeral artery (PCHA)**, using ultrasound doppler. Either inferior or superior to the posterior circumflex artery is the axillary nerve.
3. **The axillary nerve is located in close relation to the PCHA in the quadrangular space** between the teres minor muscle cranially, the deltoid muscle posteriorly, the long head of the triceps muscle caudally, and the shaft of the humerus anteriorly.
4. With the transducer parallel to the longitudinal axis of the humerus, the needle is advanced in-plane, caudad to cephalad, toward the axillary nerve.
5. After aspiration is negative, to ensure needle is not in the PCHA, local anesthetic is used to hydrodissect the nerve. Next, injectate containing local anesthetic only or local anesthetic with steroid is slowly injected. Note: keep volumes of local anesthetic low, 1–3 cc, as larger volumes may inadvertently result in motor block.

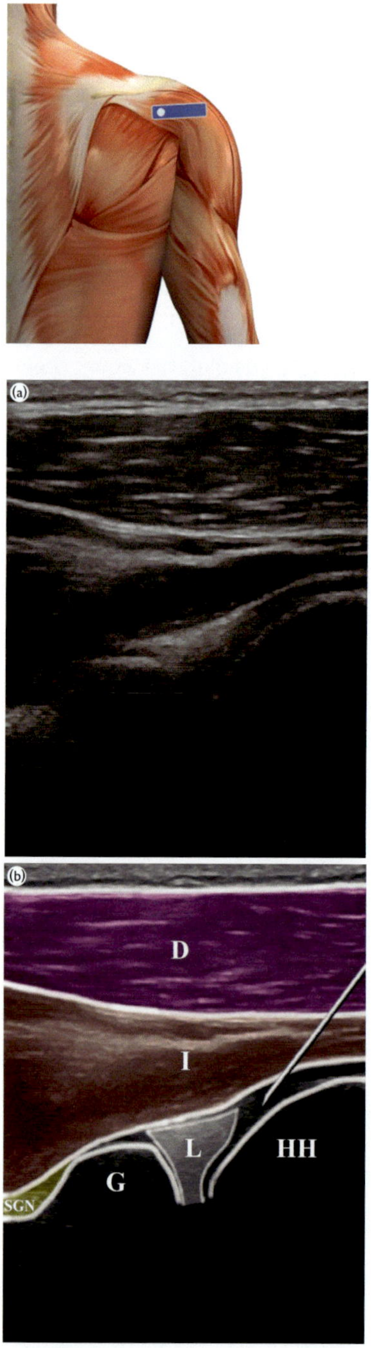

Figure 6.2.7 a, Ultrasound image of the posterior shoulder joint in an axial oblique plane. **b,** Labeled ultrasound image of in-plane needle placement for a posterior glenohumeral joint injection. *D* deltoid, *I* infraspinatus, *SGN* spinoglenonotch, *G* glenoid, *L* posterior labrum, *HH* humeral head.

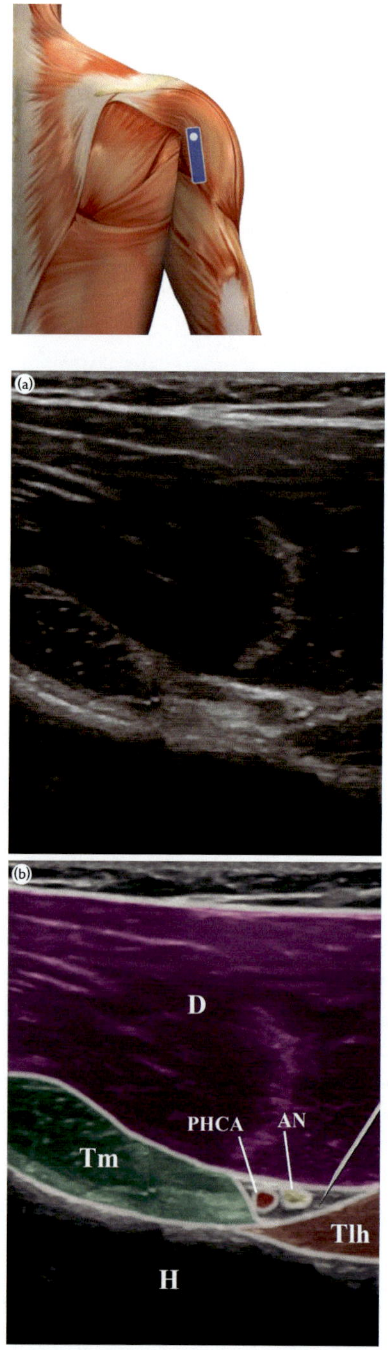

Figure 6.2.8 a, Ultrasound image of the posterior proximal arm in a sagittal plane. **b,** Labeled ultrasound image of in-plane needle placement for an axillary nerve block in short-axis. *D* deltoid, *Tm* teres minor, *PHCA* posterior humeral circumflex artery, *AN* axillary nerve, *Tlh* long head of triceps, *H* humerus.

Tips

- Be sure to use doppler to search for and identify posterior humeral circumflex vessels near the target area to avoid during procedures.

Acromioclavicular Joint (ACJ) Injection (Figure 6.2.9)

1. **Cross-arm/scarf test confirms anterior shoulder pain at the** acromioclavicular joint (ACJ).
2. **With the patient in supine or seated position, the ultrasound probe is placed in the coronal plane** in line over the ACJ.
3. **Center the ACJ and capsule in the middle of the screen;** it will appear as a hypoechoic space in-between the acromion and the distal clavicle. An effusion of the ACJ will appear as a "geyser sign" or "T."
4. **Under ultrasound guidance, the needle is directed from anterior to posterior in an out-of-plane approach.**
5. **Advance the needle until a change of resistance is encountered,** signaling the needle has entered the joint, and a hyperechoic dot signifying the needle is visualized under ultrasound. After identification, local anesthetic and adjuvant steroid mixture are injected slowly under visualization into the area.
6. **Special considerations:** Reduced volume (0.5–2 mL) of injectate recommended given the small joint space and concern for capsular distension/rupture with higher volumes. When performing out-of-plane technique, make sure to stop advancement of the needle once the needle tip is seen, to avoid inadvertent pneumothorax or placement of medication extracapsular. No local anesthetic may be necessary given the how superficial the structure is located.

Lateral Pectoral Nerve Approach (Figure 6.2.10)

1. **With the patient in supine position and arm abducted to 90 degrees, the ultrasound probe is placed in the sagittal plane** transverse to the clavicle. The probe is then translated caudally.
2. **Identify the pectoral musculature**, which will be visible at this level with the pectoralis major closest to the skin. The pectoralis minor is closest to the rib.
3. **Identify the medial pectoral and lateral pectoral arteries with doppler.** The nerves course along with the vasculature. Thus, they may be used as landmarks for the nerves. Of note, in this view, the lateral pectoral nerve will be located medial to the medial pectoral nerve. Use doppler to avoid the medial and lateral pectoral arteries as well as the pectoral branch of the thoracoacromial artery.
4. **To confirm correct placement of the needle tip hydrodissection can be utilized.** This is recommended due to precision required to deposit medication in close proximity to the nerve and to avoid the complication of pneumothorax by placing the needle too deep. Placement is confirmed when the injectate is seen to separate the pectoralis major and minor. A 22- or 25-gauge 1.5- to 3.5-inch needle in an in-plane approach is used to deposit injectate.
5. **Of note, injectate may spread to the medial pectoral,** which is also contained within the plane of the pectoralis major and minor. For ablative and neuromodulation procedures, the lateral pectoral nerve is located medially to the medial pectoral nerve as shown in Figure 6.2.10.

Tips

- Be sure to use doppler to search for and identify pectoral vessels near the target area to avoid during procedures.

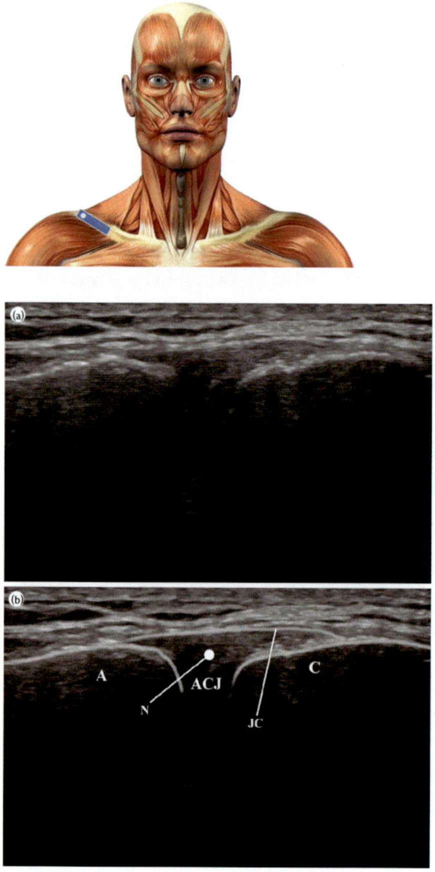

Figure 6.2.9 **a,** Ultrasound image of the acromioclavicular joint in a coronal plane. **b,** Labeled ultrasound image of an out-of-plane needle placement for an acromioclavicular joint injection. *A* acromion, *ACJ* acromioclavicular joint, *C* clavicle, *N* needle tip, *JC* acromioclavicular joint capsule.

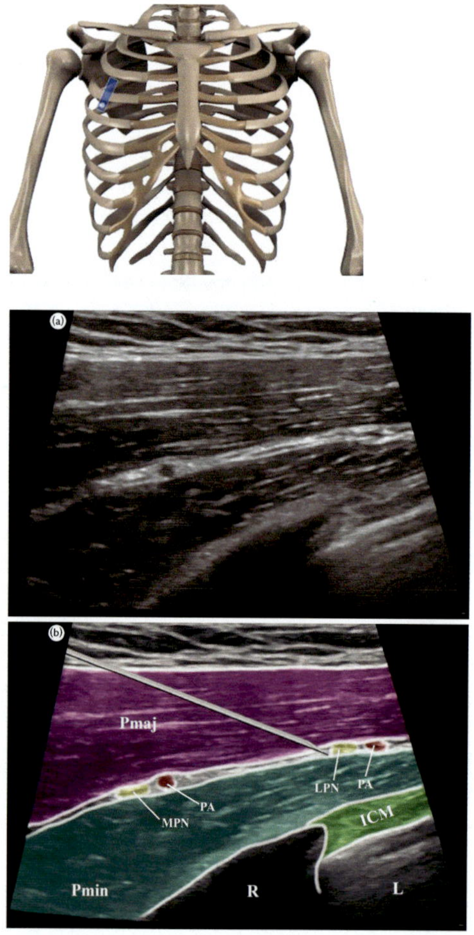

Figure 6.2.10 **a,** Ultrasound image of the anterior thorax at the level of the 3rd rib in a sagittal oblique plane. **b,** Labeled ultrasound image of an in-plane needle placement for a lateral pectoral nerve block in short-axis. *Pmaj* pectoralis major, *MPN* medial pectoral nerve, *LPN* lateral pectoral nerve, *PA* pectoral branch of the thoracoacromial artery, *Pmin* pectoralis minor, *ICM* intercostal muscles, *R* rib, *L* lung.

Neurotomy of the Suprascapular Nerve

Pulsed radiofrequency ablation or cryoablation may be performed at the suprascapular nerve. Conventional radiofrequency is typically avoided at the suprascapular nerve due to the contribution to motor function at the shoulder. However, if there is lack of access to pulsed radiofrequency or cryoablation, and in cases where there is already minimal functional use of the affected upper extremity due to significant disease burden in the oncological patient, use of the limb is not expected to improve, and decreased motor function would not impart significant change in debility, conventional radiofrequency ablation may be considered. While approach to the suprascapular nerve can be performed perpendicular to the suprascapular notch at the suprascapular fossa, the preferred approach is parallel via spinoglenoid notch:

Nerve Block Technique

1. The patient is seated in a chair with a low back or beach chair. Widely prep the posterior and superior shoulder.
2. Palpate the posterior shoulder, identify the subacromial space, and place the transducer just inferior to the spine of the scapula.
3. Orient the ultrasound transducer in the oblique axial plane, angled slightly superiorly toward the humeral head, parallel and inferior to the spine of the scapula. Translate the probe medially until the spinoglenoid notch is centered in the screen.
4. Anesthetize the overlying skin by making a skin wheal. Take care not anesthetize deep, as this will interfere with sensory and motor testing.
5. A. Out-of-plane technique: Advance pulsed/cryoablation needle out-of-plane utilizing the "walk-down technique." Insert the needle superficially until the tip is seen, withdraw and approach deeper—again stopping once needle tip is visualized, repeating until needle tip is visualized at the target spinoglenoid notch.

   B. In-plane technique: Keeping the spinoglenoid notch in the center of the screen, rotated the probe slowly 90 degrees. The spinoglenoid notch is seen as a hypoechoic region. If the osseous border of the scapula is seen, translate probe slightly medial or lateral until the foramen becomes visible. Next, advance pulsed/cryoablation needle in-plane from caudad to cephalad toward the opening at the spinoglenoid notch. Note: while a linear probe may be adequate for those with less tissue, in patients with a larger habitus, a curvilinear probe may be prudent to allow constant needle visualization deep. At this point the transducer is rotated back 90 degrees in transverse view and the hyperechoic needle tip is seen at the entrance of the spinoglenoid notch.
6. Holding the needle steady, at this point the ultrasound transducer is translated cephalad past the spine of the scapula, positioned over the scapular fossa, and tilted posterior until the suprascapular notch is clearly visualized.
7. The needle is then advanced slowly, out of plane, until a hyperechoic needle tip is visualized within the suprascapular notch deep to the transverse scapular ligament. Take care to advance the needle in small increments so as not to miss the hyperechoic flash as the needle tip comes under the transducer and to avoid advancing the needle too far anterior, which could result in unintentional pneumothorax. The needle may be spun clockwise and counterclockwise if you are having difficulty visualizing the needle tip.
8. At this point, remove inner cannula of the needle, attach an empty syringe and aspirate to ensure placement outside of the suprascapular artery, which runs parallel to the suprascapular nerve.
9. Sensory testing is performed at 50–100 Hz with 0.1–1.0 V resulting in paresthesias at the posterior and lateral shoulder. Motor testing, at 2 Hz with 1–1.5 V, is performed resulting in muscle contractions of the supraspinatus/infraspinatus. Reposition needles as necessary. If there is motor stimulation of brachial plexus with paresthesias/contraction of the distal upper extremity, needle may have been advanced too far anterior and the needle should be slightly withdrawn and then retested. After satisfactory response, infiltrate the needle with 1 mL of 2% lidocaine, and allow adequate time for anesthesia to take effect.
10. Ablation techniques:
    a. Pulse radiofrequency ablation: Settings: 42°C Duration: 120 seconds Cycles: 3
    b Cryoablation: temperature at or below (-)40°C, 60 to 90 second freeze, then 30–60 thaw cycle and repeat minimum 3 times.

Neurotomy of the Axillary Nerve

Pulsed radiofrequency ablation or cryoablation may be performed at the axillary nerve. Again, conventional radiofrequency is typically avoided at the axillary nerve given the significant contribution to motor function at the shoulder. Approach to the axillary nerve can be performed perpendicular as described above, or parallel, as described below. Conceptually, parallel placement should result in superior lesion or increased stimulation, however there is currently no evidence to confirm this:

Nerve Block Technique

1. The patient is seated (in a chair with a low back or beach chair) or placed in the prone position with the shoulder slightly abducted to obtain access to the medial aspect of the arm. Widely prep the posterior shoulder.
2. Palpate the posterior shoulder, identify the subacromial space, and place the transducer just inferior to the spine of the scapula.
3. Parallel Approach:
   a. In-plane technique: Center the axillary nerve in the center of the screen. Slowly rotate the transducer 90 degrees until the axillary nerve is seen in-plane. Advance pulsed/cryoablation needle in-plane from medial to lateral, just above the axillary nerve.
   b. Out-of-plane technique: Center the axillary nerve in the center of the screen. Advance pulsed/cryoablation needle out-of-plane utilizing the "walk-down technique." Insert the needle superficially until the tip is seen, withdraw and approach deeper—again stopping once needle tip is visualized, repeating until needle tip is visualized just superficial to the target axillary nerve.
4. At this point, remove inner cannula of the needle, attach an empty syringe and aspirate to ensure placement outside of the posterior circumflex humeral artery, which runs parallel to the axillary nerve.
5. Sensory testing is performed at 50–100 Hz with 0.1–1.0 V resulting in paresthesias at the anterolateral shoulder. Motor testing, at 2 Hz with 1–1.5 V, is performed resulting in muscle contractions of the deltoid. Reposition needles as necessary. After satisfactory response, infiltrate the needle with 1 mL of 2% lidocaine, and allow adequate time for anesthesia to take effect.
6. Ablation techniques:
   a. Pulse radiofrequency ablation: Settings: 42°C Duration: 120 seconds Cycles: 3
   b. Cryoablation: maximum temperature (-)40 C, 60 to 90 second freeze, then 30–60 thaw cycle and repeat minimum 3 times

C5–C7 Selective Nerve Root Block

Pre-existing cervical degenerative changes, metastases, and neurotoxic chemotherapy commonly damage the upper cervical brachial plexus, C5 and C6 nerve roots. The nerve roots may be targeted with blockade using local anesthetic and/or corticosteroid. Ablative techniques may be used rarely for uncontrollable malignant pain or consider neuromodulation techniques.

Chemical and Electrical Spinal Neuromodulation

In-depth discussion of these advanced techniques is outside the scope of this chapter. If patient fails to respond to injections and peripheral nerve stimulation, consider for dual lead spinal cord stimulation with leads to the top of C2, dorsal root ganglion stimulation at C5 or C6 (off-label, recommended for advanced practitioners only with 100 + DRG lead placements, and possibly in conjunction with neurosurgery), or chemical neuromodulation with intrathecal drug therapies (with catheter tip to C5–C7 or in the upper thoracic spine but with medication/flow reaching the lower cervical roots).

When to Refer Out

Discuss with radiation oncology for local tumor burden control. Consider referral to interventional radiology for cementoplasty for impending pathological fractures of the humerus, etc. For refractory cases, consider referral to neurosurgery for cordotomy.

Algorithms

Anterior shoulder pain—target the axillary nerve (anterior-lateral) and lateral pectoral nerve (anterior-superior)

Posterior shoulder pain—target the suprascapular nerve (posterior lateral)

References

1. Cunningham LS, Kelsey JL. Epidemiology of musculoskeletal impairments and associated disability. Amer J of Publ Hlth 1984;74:574–579.
2. Urwin M, Symmons D, Allison T, et al. Estimating the burden of musculoskeletal disorders in the community: the comparative prevalence of symptoms at different anatomical sites, and the relation to social deprivation. Ann Rheum Dis 1998;57:649–655.
3. van der Windt DA, Koes BW, de Jong BA, Bouter LM. Shoulder disorders in general practice: incidence, patient characteristics, and management. Ann Rheum Dis 1995;54:959–964.
4. Brown DE. Pain relief by suprascapular nerve block in glenohumeral arthritis. Scand J Rheumatol 1988;17:411–415.
5. Halata Z, Bauman K. Mechanoreceptors of the shoulder joint: structure and function. In: DiGiacomo G, Pouliart N, Costantini A, Vita A, et al., eds., Atlas of Functional Shoulder Anatomy. Milan, Italy: Springer; 2008: 206–208.
6. Eckmann MS, Bickelhaupt B, Fehl J, Benfield JA, Curley J, Rahimi O, Nagpal AS. Cadaveric study of the articular branches of the shoulder joint. Reg Anesth Pain Med 2017;42(5):564–570.
7. Öztürk R, Arıkan ŞM, Toğral G, Güngör BŞ. Malignant tumors of the shoulder girdle: Surgical and functional outcomes. J Orthopaedic Surgery 2019;27(2). doi:10.1177/2309499019838355
8. Barlow IW, Newman RJ. Primary bone tumors of the shoulder: an audit of the Leeds Regional Bone Tumor Registry. J R Coll Surg Edinb 1994;39:51–54.
9. Cleeman E, Auerbach JD, Springfield DS. Tumors of the shoulder girdle: a review of 194 cases. J of Should and Elb Surg 2005;14(5):460–465. doi:10.1016/j.jse.2005.02.003
10. Soker G, Soker E, Gulek B, Acikalin A, Asut E, Kaya O, Dilek O, Yilmaz C. Rotator cuff metastases: a report of two cases with literature review. N Am J Med Sci 2014;6(12):653–656.
11. Ronan L, D'Souza S. Pancoast's tumour presenting as shoulder pain in an orthopaedic clinic. BMJ Case Rep 2013;2013:bcr2012008131. Published 2013 Feb 5. doi:10.1136/bcr-2012-008131
12. Gheita TA, Ezzat Y, Sayed S, El-Mardenly G, Hammam W. Musculoskeletal manifestations in patients with malignant disease. Clin Rheumatol 2010;29(2):181–188.
13. Sano H, Hatori M, Mineta M, Hosaka M, Itoi E. Tumors masked as frozen shoulders: a retrospective analysis. J Shoulder Elbow Surg 2010;19(2): 262–266.
14. Robinson D, Halperin N, Agar G, Alk D, Rami K. Shoulder girdle neoplasms mimicking frozen shoulder syndrome. J Shoulder Elbow Surg 2003;12(5):451–455.
15. Lauchlan DT, McCaul JA, McCarron T. Neck dissection and the clinical appearance of post-operative shoulder disability: the post-operative role of physiotherapy. Eur J Canc Care 2008;17(6):542–548.
16. Gane EM, Michaleff ZA, et al. Prevalence, incidence, and risk factors for shoulder and neck dysfunction after neck dissection: a systematic review. Eur J Surg Oncol 2017;43(7):1199–1218. doi: 10.1016/j.ejso.2016.10.026. Epub 2016 Nov 17. Review.
17. Yap KP, McCready DR, Narod S, Manchul LA, Trudeau M, Fyles A. Factors influencing arm and axillary symptoms after treatment for node negative breast carcinoma. Cancer 2003;97(6):1369–1375.
18. Jaeckle KA. Neurologic manifestations of neoplastic and radiation induced plexopathies. Semin Neurol 2010;30:254–262.

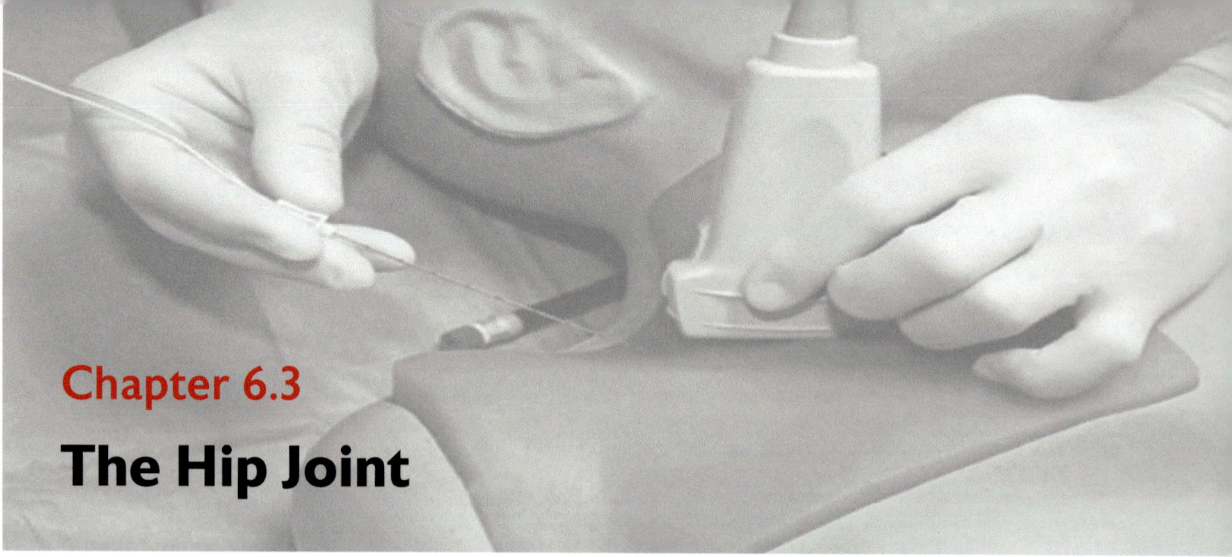

Chapter 6.3
The Hip Joint

Frank V. Schirripa

Contents

Introduction

When the hip joint and its supportive dynamic and static surrounding structures are inflamed or damaged, both active cancer patients and survivor patients may complain of pain in the joint, which may refer to the groin, buttocks, or thigh. Commonly, intra-articular corticosteroid injections are performed under image guidance using anatomic landmarks, but this usually requires an intact hip joint capsule with normal anatomy for consistent success.[1] While regenerative medicine techniques have the capacity to improve arthritic and musculoskeletal injuries for hip pain patients, performing these treatments in active cancer patients may be contraindicated. Oncologic patients may have hip pain from deconditioning and weakening of the joint from direct invasion of the bone or surrounding tendons, ligaments, or muscles from primary or metastatic disease. If surgery and radiation treatments do not alleviate the pain, there should be consideration for ablation of the obturator and femoral nerve branches innervating the joint.[2–6]

Indication

Proximal femur tumors are benign 68% of the time in comparison to pelvic tumors, which are malignant 62% of the time. Metastatic disease to both anatomical locations most commonly occurs after age 40. Proximal femur tumors are typically more superficial in nature and present earlier than pelvic tumors, which are usually deeper anatomically.[7] Malignant osseous tumors can present with pain and impaired range of motion if near a joint.[8] Intra-articular soft tissue tumors present similarly to other pathologies causing joint destruction, including restricted range of motion and pain.[7] Either as a result of malignancy, or a consequence of treatment/recovery, oncologic patients may present with hip pain. This pain is often multifactorial and requires thorough evaluation and diagnosis Tables 6.3.1 and 6.3.2. It is important to note that cancer patients have the potential to develop early arthropathies secondary to radiation and chemotherapy.[9–10]

Additionally, primary tumor invasion of supporting musculature such as the iliopsoas and gluteus can lead to direct somatic pain. Surgical excision of the tumor burden can cause muscle and ligamentous weakness, which will alter the patient's overall gait biomechanics and kinetic chain. This can lead to pain from muscle contractures, worsening osteoarthritis, referred myofascial pain, and even bursitis. For example, greater trochanteric pain syndrome is a common compensatory consequence of gluteus medius weakness and tendinopathy. This leads to inflammation of the greater trochanteric/subgluteus maximus bursa. Additionally, metastatic disease into the posterior ileum or sacrum may present with back or groin pain similar to sacroiliitis. Taken together, direct tumor

Table 6.3.1 Hip Cancer–Related Pain Etiologies

Musculoskeletal	Neurologic	Vascular	Bone	Other
• Osteoarthritis • Myofascial pain • Bursitis • Tendinopathy • Contractures • Muscular tumor invasion • Postsurgical pain • Labral damage • Hip joint capsulitis • Hip joint impingement	• Lumbosacral radiculopathy • Polyneuropathy (CIPN) • Radiation-induced plexopathy • Chemo/ immunotherapy-induced neuropathy • Leptomeningeal disease • Tumor invasion causing compression • Mononeuropathy/ mononeuritis multiplex • Paraneoplastic neuropathy • Complex regional pain syndrome • Central pain syndrome	• Avascular necrosis • DVT • Hematoma	• Primary bone tumors • Metastasis • Osteoporosis • Insufficiency fracture	• Fibromyalgia • Graft-versus-host disease • Radiation dermatitis • Radiation-induced fibrosis • Lymphedema • Infection • Anxiety

Table 6.3.2 Hip Cancer–Related Pain Treatment Algorithm

Survivorship Pain	Active Cancer	Treatment-Related
• Corticosteroids • Viscosupplementation • Peripheral nerve stimulation • Intraarticular nerve ablation • Regenerative medicine (for remission cases) • Neuroaxial options (spinal cord stimulation, dorsal root ganglion stimulation)	• Corticosteroids • Viscosupplementation • Intraarticular nerve ablation (if musculoskeletal tumor invasion) • Temporary peripheral nerve stimulation • Neuroaxial options (spinal cord stimulation, dorsal root ganglion stimulation) • Surgical (Dorsal root exit zone lesioning, cordotomy)	• Corticosteroids, viscosupplementation (musculoskeletal injury) • Neuromodulation before joint denervation (for nerve injury) • Follow survivorship (for remission cases) • Injection steroids vs. viscosupplementation if MSK injury

invasion or treatment with radiation/chemotherapy/immunotherapy have the potential to affect neurologic structures, such as the exiting L1–L3 or S1–S2 nerve roots, creating neuropathic pain in the hip regions.

Contraindications

While many contraindications for hip injections exist in the general population, a risk-versus-benefit analysis may be considered for end-of-life and extreme pain patients. For example, even though the hip injection is considered a low-risk procedure, consideration for performing injections in patients with thrombocytopenia and using anticoagulation is decided on a case-by-case basis. Infection remains a significant risk, especially within the joint. Another consideration is to use viscosupplementation and ablative procedure in an effort to avoid intra-articular corticosteroids, which can further worsen bone degradation and the immune system [Table 6.3.3].

Table 6.3.3 Contraindications to Hip Intra-Articular Injection and Radiofrequency Ablation

Contraindications	Related Types *(recommended intervention)*
Absolute	Refusal for the procedure Localized or systemic infection Severe coagulopathy
Relative	Thromboctyopenia *(smaller needle gauge size)* Anticoagulation *(smaller needle gauge size)* Immunocompromised patients *(viscosupplementation instead of corticosteroids)* Distorted anatomy *(modified injection approach, consider neuromodulation)* Prior nerve injury or damage *(neuromodulation)* Allergy to anesthetics *(saline with injection)* Implanted pacemaker *(intrathecal drug delivery)* Allodynia *(neuromodulation)* Inability to consent to the procedure

Critical Anatomy

The hip joint is the largest joint in the body and is known as a multiaxial ball and socket joint. There is a synovial articulation between the head of the femur and the deep acetabulum allowing for maximum stability. The acetabulum is a fossa where the femoral head articulates and is rimmed by the acetabular labrum, a fibrocartilaginous collar of tissue, which further deepens the joint allowing for greater stability. The labrum, when damaged, can be a common pain generator and may lead to accelerated formation of osteoarthritis.

The joint capsule is composed of the acetabular labrum, the intertrochanteric line of the femur, transverse acetabular ligament, and three fibrous capsular ligaments (iliofemoral, ischiofemoral, pubofemoral) (Figure 6.3.1). The capsule also includes the proximal two-thirds of the femoral neck. Primary or metastatic disease and subsequent surgical intervention all have the potential to distort any or all of these structures, leading to hip pain.

Another common source of pain is an inflamed trochanteric or subgluteus maximus bursa, which sits in between the gluteus maximus and medius as they converge over the greater trochanter. The iliotibial band is another common pain generator, which is found to insert on the lateral aspect of the knee running superior and lateral along the thigh originating from the pelvis. These injuries may be commonly seen as part of deconditioning, postural malalignment, and poor gait biomechanics as a result treatment interventions.

The gluteus medius, which originates from between the anterior and posterior gluteal lines on the lateral ilial surface and inserts on the posterosuperior and lateral portions of the greater trochanter of the femur, and the gluteus minimus, which originates from between the anterior and inferior gluteal lines on the lateral ilial surface and inserts on the anterior portion of the greater trochanter of the femur, are the main abductors of the hip. These structures can undergo tendinopathy and become pain generators as a result of changes in the kinetic chain and poor biomechanics.

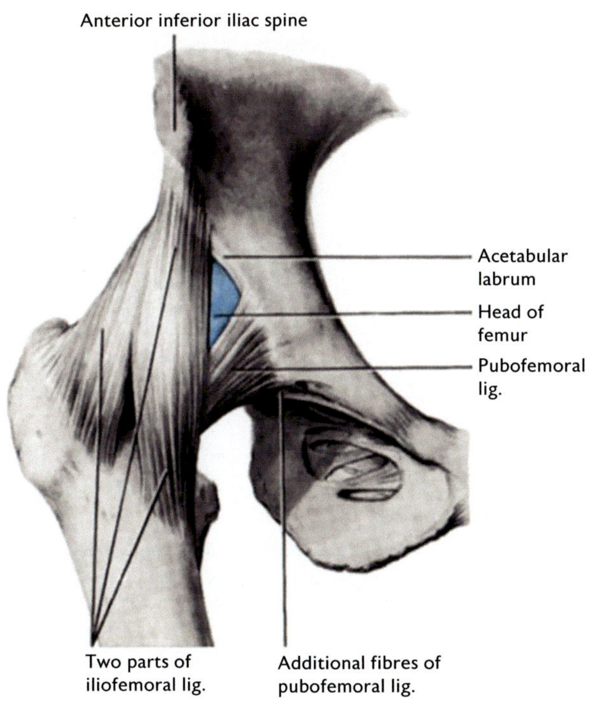

Figure 6.3.1 Dissection of the anterior hip joint and surrounding ligaments. (Reprinted with permission from Cunningham's Manual of Practical Anatomy: Upper and Lower Limbs, 16th Edition)

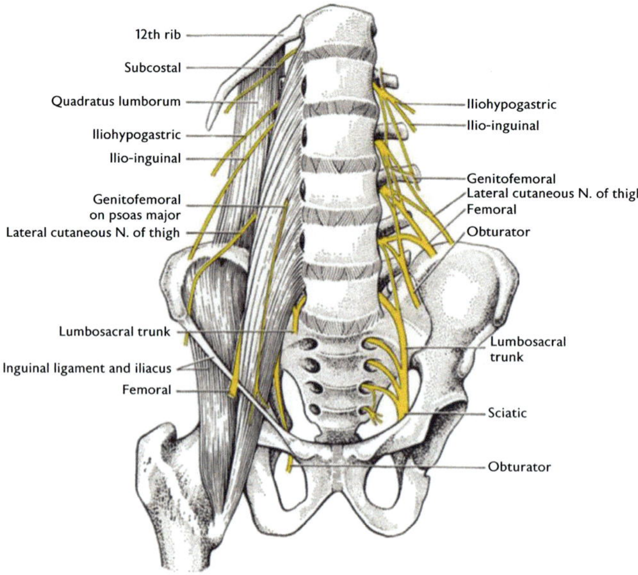

Figure 6.3.2 Lumbar plexus shown on the posterior abdominal wall revealing the femoral and obturator nerves. (Reprinted with permission from Cunningham's Manual of Practical Anatomy: Upper and Lower Limbs, 16th Edition)

Significant blood supply to the hip capsule includes the medial and lateral circumflex arteries branching off the deep branch of the femoral artery. The media circumflex artery can be found on the medial aspect of the femur, while the lateral circumflex artery runs anterior to the femoral neck. Loss of blood flow during chemotherapy treatments, systemic steroids, radiation, or surgical interventions may result in avascular necrosis, causing severe pain in this population.

Finally, the hip joint has multiple innervations. Anteriorly, the femoral nerve provides the main sensory innervation, while the anterior division of the obturator nerve serves the inferior aspect of the hip joint (Figure 6.3.2). The articular branch of the sciatic nerve serves the lateral portion of the hip joint, and the superior gluteal nerve innervates the posterior aspect of the joint. Neural injury may be seen uncommonly with certain chemotherapies, radiation therapy, tumor invasion, and surgical manipulation.

Equipment and Patient Preparation

1. Monitors and Sterility

a. No specific monitoring is required during this procedure. It is highly advised that vital signs, including blood pressure, heart rate, respiratory rate, and pulse oximetry, be obtained prior to starting the procedure to ensure the patient is hemodynamically stable. A set of vitals is often taken post procedure as well.

b. Strict antiseptic technique should be observed including sterile draping, probe cover, ultrasound gel, sterile gloves, and sterile gauze. Chlorhexidine or other skin prep agent should be used to clean the skin prior to commencing the procedure.

2. **Imaging modalities:**
   a. Ultrasound
      i. Probe: high-frequency linear array or low-frequency curvilinear array
3. **Needle type:**
   i. Local anesthetic: 27- or 30-gauge 1.5-inch needle
   ii. Hip joint injection: 22- to 25-gauge 2- to 3.5-inch spinal needle
   iii. Hip joint radiofrequency ablation: 50 to 100 mm needle with 5 or 10 mm active tip
4. **Patient position:** Supine
5. **Injectate:**
   a. Local anesthetic: lidocaine 1%–2%; ropivacaine 0.2%–0.5%; bupivacaine 0.25%–0.5%
   b. Adjuvant: particulate or nonparticulate steroid

Procedure Technique

Intra-Articular Hip Joint Injection—Anterior Approach (Figure 6.3.3)

1. **Ensure the patient is consented, positioned in supine, area prepped, and equipment is ready.**
2. **Place the probe in an axial plane below the ASIS in the groin region.** Identify the femoral artery and vein, then translate the probe laterally to visualize the femoral head and acetabulum.
3. **Oblique the lateral end of the probe to be in a longitudinal view of the femoral head–neck junction.** The target will be within the joint capsule at the head–neck junction. Of note, the joint capsule had redundant deep fibers laterally, which when targeted will cause injectate to flow extra-articularly.
4. **A small-gauge needle is used to make a wheal of local anesthetic** just lateral to the transducer, serving as the entry point.
5. **The injectate needle is inserted lateral to the probe.** As the needle is advanced, a palpable "pop" will be felt as it passes through the joint capsule and iliofemoral ligament.
6. **Once needle placement is confirmed, aspirate to ensure the needle is not inadvertently in a vascular structure and inject the anesthetic and steroid mixture slowly.** Once the injectate is fully immersed, the needle is slowly pulled out and disposed of appropriately.

Intra-Articular Hip Joint Injection—Lateral Approach (Figure 6.3.4)

1. **Ensure the patient is consented, positioned in lateral decubitus with legs slightly flexed, area prepped, and equipment is ready.**
2. **Place the probe in a coronal plane along the greater trochanter.** Then translate the probe slightly cranial to visualize the femoral head, neck, and acetabulum.
3. **Visualize the target, which will be within the joint capsule at the head–neck junction.** Of note, the joint capsule has redundant deep fibers closer to the greater trochanter, which when targeted will cause injectate to flow extra-articularly.
4. **A small-gauge needle is used to make a wheal of local anesthetic** just lateral to the transducer, serving as the entry point.

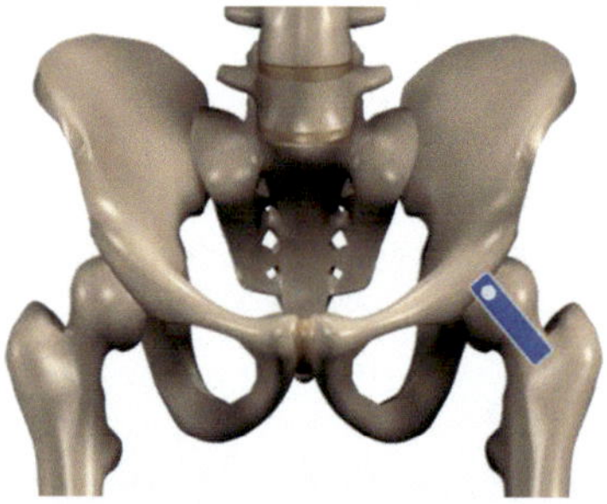

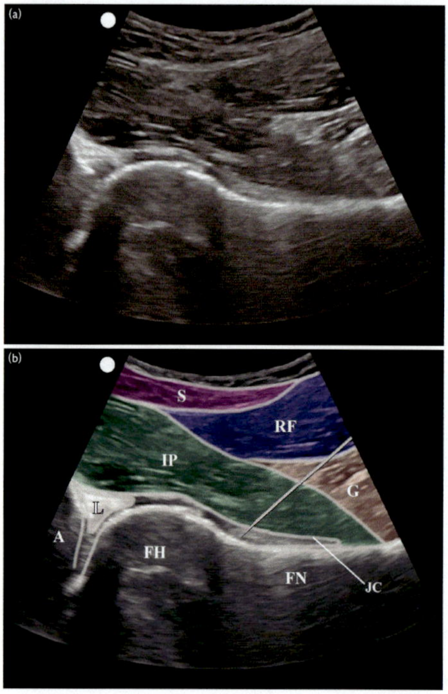

Figure 6.3.3 a, Ultrasound image of the anterior hip joint in an axial oblique plane. **b,** Labeled ultrasound image of in-plane needle placement for an anterior approach intra-articular hip joint injection. *S* sartorius, *RF* rectus femoris, *IP* iliopsoas, *G* gluteus muscle, *A* acetabulum, *L* anterior labrum, *FH* femoral head, *FN* femoral neck, *JC* hip joint capsule.

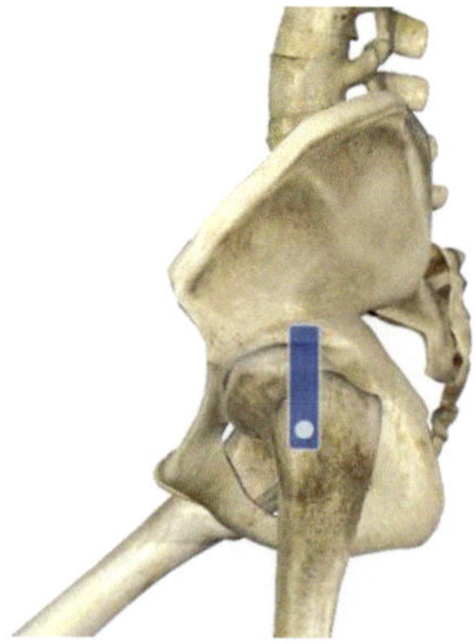

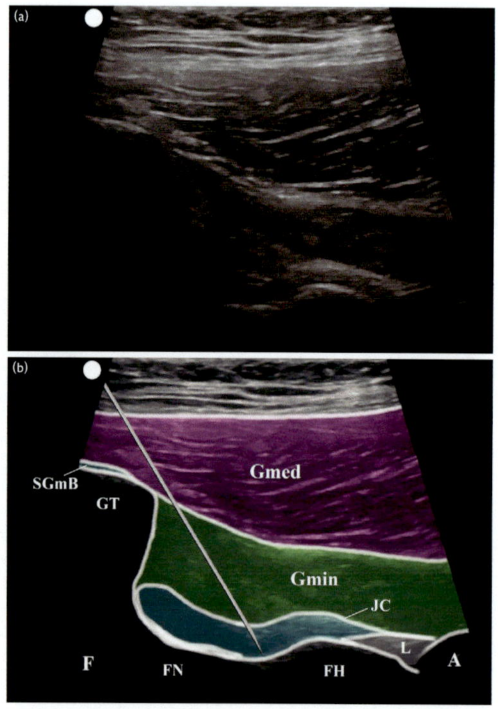

Figure 6.3.4 a, Ultrasound image of the lateral hip joint in a coronal plane. **b,** Labeled ultrasound image of in-plane needle placement for a lateral approach intra-articular hip joint injection. *Gmed* gluteus medius, *SGmB* subgluteus medius bursa, *GT* greater trochanter, *Gmin* gluteus minimus, *JC* hip joint capsule, *L* anterior labrum, *F* femur, *FH* femoral head, *FN* femoral neck, *A* acetabulum.

5. **The injectate needle is inserted lateral to the probe.** As the needle is advanced, a palpable "pop" will be felt as it passes through the joint capsule and iliofemoral ligament.
6. **Once needle placement is confirmed, aspirate to ensure the needle is not inadvertently in a vascular structure and inject the anesthetic and steroid mixture slowly.** Once the injectate is fully immersed, the needle is slowly pulled out and disposed of appropriately.

Tips

- Be sure to use doppler to search for and identify satellite vessels near the target area to avoid during procedures.

Greater Trochanteric/Subgluteus Maximus Bursa Injection

1. **Ensure the patient is consented, positioned in lateral decubitus with legs slightly flexed, area prepped, and equipment is ready.**
2. **Place the probe in an axial plane along the greater trochanter.** Then translate the probe cranial and caudal to identify the anterior and lateral facets that the gluteus minimus and medius attach to, respectively.
3. **Visualize the greater trochanteric or subgluteus maximus bursa**, which will lie between the gluteus maximus and gluteus medius muscles as shown in Figure 6.3.5.
4. **A small-gauge needle is used to make a wheal of local anesthetic** just posterior to the transducer, serving as the entry point.
5. **The injectate needle is inserted in a posterior-to-anterior direction** as it advances toward the target.
6. **Once needle placement is confirmed, aspirate to ensure the needle is not inadvertently in a vascular structure and inject the anesthetic and steroid mixture slowly.** Once the injectate is fully immersed, the needle is slowly pulled out and disposed of appropriately.
7. **The procedure may also be performed in a longitudinal/coronal plane by rotating the probe 90 degrees as shown in** Figure 6.3.6.
8. **The gluteus medius and minimus tendons may also be targeted for a tenotomy or a PRP injection.**

Tips

- Be sure to use doppler to search for and identify satellite vessels near the target area to avoid during procedures.

Hip Joint Capsule Ablation

1. **Ensure the patient is consented, positioned in supine, area prepped, and equipment is ready.**
2. **Place the probe in an axial plane below the ASIS in the groin region.** Identify the femoral artery and vein.
3. **Translate the probe cephalad and laterally to visualize the femoral head, anterior inferior iliac spine (AIIS), and iliopectineal eminence.** The target for the femoral component of the hip joint for an ablation will be at the bone just lateral to the AIIS (Figure 6.3.7).
4. **twist the medial end of the probe about 45–60 degrees, then translate the probe medially and inferiorly, the "teardrop of the pelvis" will be visualized.** The target for the obturator component of the accessory obturator nerve is just medial to the pelvic teardrop (Figure 6.3.8).

Tips

- Be sure to use doppler to search for and identify satellite vessels near the target area to avoid during procedures.

Postprocedure Management

After injection or radiofrequency (or cryoablation) neuroablation, there can be soreness near the injection entry points up to 2–3 weeks. Ice is recommended in the first few days after procedure

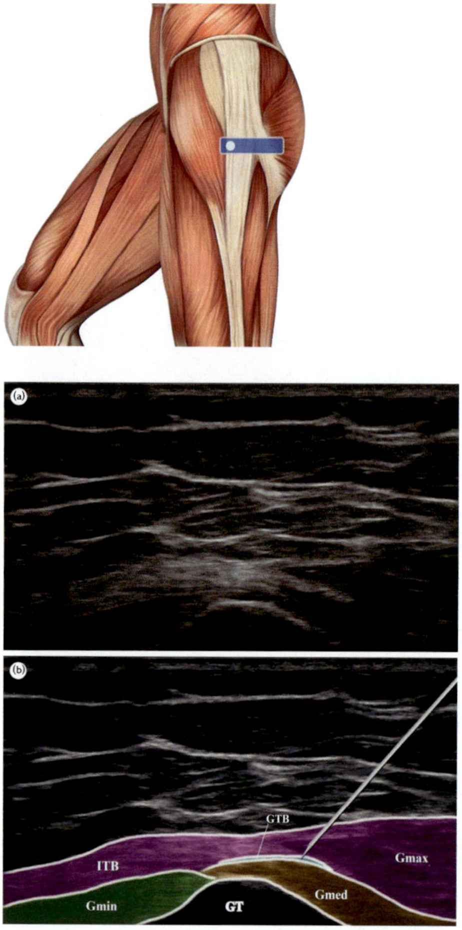

Figure 6.3.5 **a,** Ultrasound image of the lateral hip in an axial plane. **b,** Labeled ultrasound image of in-plane needle placement for a greater trochanteric (subgluteus maximus) bursa injection in short-axis. *ITB* iliotibial band, *GTB* greater trochanteric bursa, *Gmax* gluteus maximus, *Gmed* gluteus medius, *Gmin* gluteus minimus, *GT* greater trochanter.

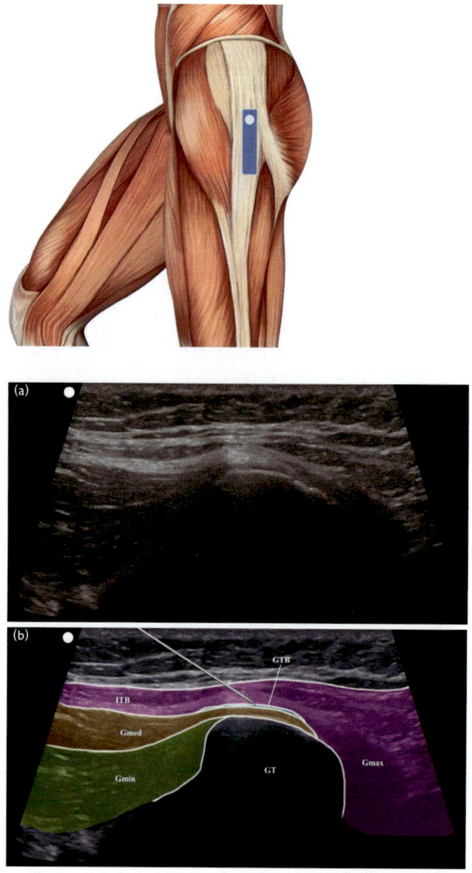

Figure 6.3.6 **a,** Ultrasound image of the lateral hip in a coronal plane. **b,** Labeled ultrasound image of in-plane needle placement for a greater trochanteric (subgluteus maximus) bursa injection in long-axis. *ITB* iliotibial band, *GTB* greater trochanteric bursa, *Gmax* gluteus maximus, *Gmed* gluteus medius, *Gmin* gluteus minimus, *GT* greater trochanter.

along with slow return to exercise after resting for 24 hours. It is possible to have bleeding, allergy, and infection as complications. Patients are usually observed up to 45 minutes with a blood pressure check before being discharged from the office. They can shower after procedure but should avoid submerging the needle sites for 48 hours. Patients who complain of sudden leg weakness, excessive redness, swelling, discharge, fever, or severe pain at the injection site are instructed to go to the emergency room. For hip intra-articular, tendon, or bursa injections, complications are rare but can include bleeding and infection. Severe cases may result in septic joint.

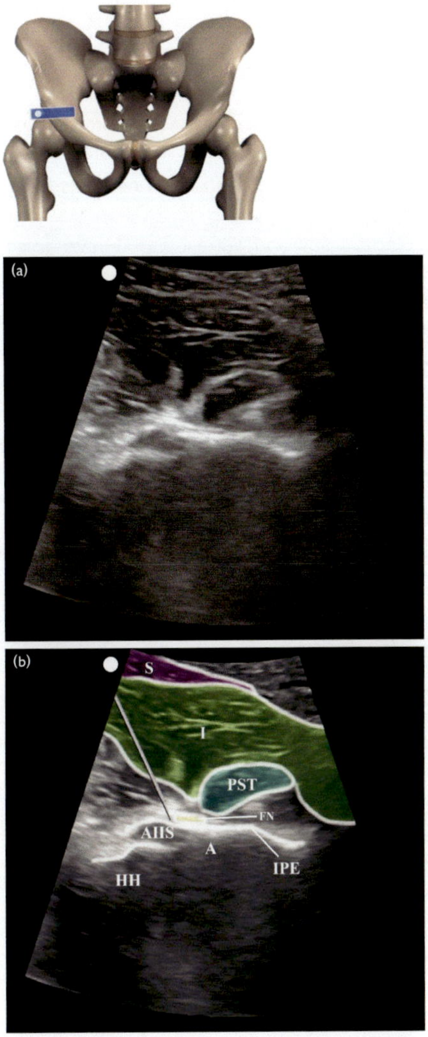

Figure 6.3.7 a, Ultrasound image of the anterior hip in an axial plane. **b,** Labeled ultrasound image of in-plane needle placement for a block of the sensory accessory branch of the femoral nerve of the hip joint capsule in short-axis. *S* sartorius, *IP* iliopsoas, *PST* psoas tendon, *FN* sensory accessory branch of the femoral nerve, *AIIS* anterior inferior iliac spine, *A* acetabulum, *IPE* iliopectineal eminence, *HH* femoral head.

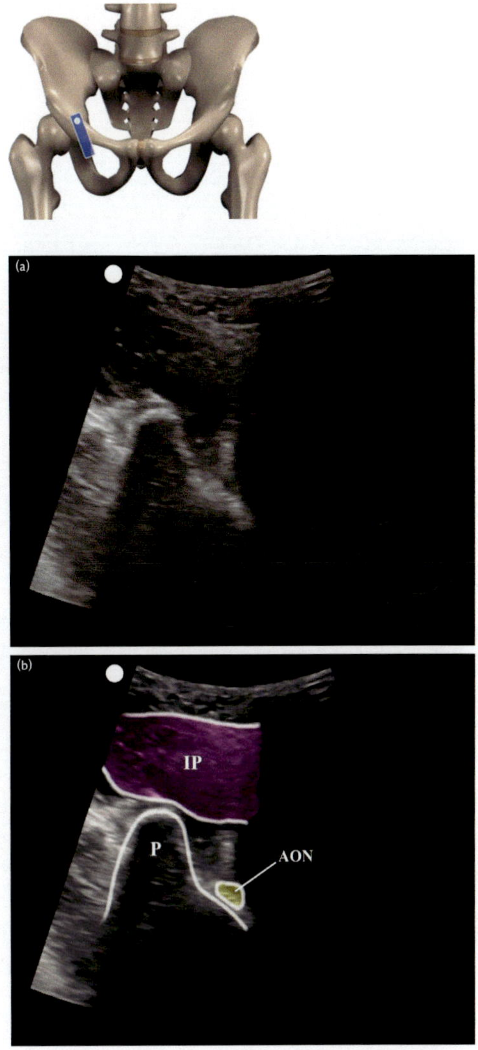

Figure 6.3.8 a, Ultrasound image of the anterior hip in a sagittal oblique plane. **b,** Labeled ultrasound image of in-plane needle placement for a block of the obturator nerve branch of the hip joint capsule *IP* iliopsoas, *P* pelvis, *AON* likely location of anterior branch of the accessory obturator nerve.

Further Reading

- Atchabahian A. Chapter 64: Obturator Nerve Block in: Diwan S, Staats P. *Atlas of pain medicine procedures*. New York, NY: McGraw-Hill Education; 2015: 600–610.
- Brown MA. Chapter 55: Intra-Articular Joint Injections in: Diwan S, Staats P. *Atlas of pain medicine procedures*. New York, NY: McGraw-Hill Education; 2015: 515–521.
- Balch R. Chapter 56: Tendon Injections in: Diwan S, Staats P. *Atlas of pain medicine procedures*. New York, NY: McGraw-Hill Education; 2015: 516–522.
- Solomon J, Roque-Dang C, Wyss J. Chapter 50: Fluoroscopy and Ultrasound-Guided Joint Injections in: Diwan S, Staats P. *Atlas of pain medicine procedures*. New York, NY: McGraw-Hill Education; 2015: 410–416.
- Thakur A, Staats PS. Chapter 80: Radiofrequency Neurolysis in: Diwan S, Staats P. *Atlas of pain medicine procedures*. New York, NY: McGraw-Hill Education; 2015: 750–755.
- Moore KL, Agur AMR. Essential clinical anatomy. Philadelphia, PA: Lippincott Williams & Wilkins; 2006.
- Magee DJ. *Orthopedic physical assessment*. 6th ed. St. Louis: Elsevier Saunders; 2014.
- Bhatia A, Peng PWP. Chapter 21: Ultrasound-Guided Peripheral Nerve Blockade in Chronic Pain Management in: *Atlas of ultrasound-guided procedures in interventional pain management*. S.N. Narouze (ed.) Springer Science and Business Media; 2011: 279–292.

References

1. Qvistgaard E, Christensen R, Torp-Pedersen S, Bliddal H. Intra-articular treatment of hip osteoarthritis: a randomized trial of hyaluronic acid, corticosteroid, and isotonic saline. *Osteoarthritis and Cartilage*. 2006;14(2):163–170.
2. Bhatia A, Hoydonckx Y, Peng P, Cohen SP. Radiofrequency procedures to relieve chronic hip pain: an evidence-based narrative review. *Reg Anesth Pain Med*. 2018;43(1):72–83.
3. Torres A, Fernandez-Fairen M, Sueiro-Fernandez J. Greater trochanteric pain syndrome and gluteus medius and minimus tendinosis: nonsurgical treatment. *Pain Manag*. 2018;8(1):45–55.
4. Zhang M, Pessina MA, Higgs JB, Kissin EY. A vascular obstacle in ultrasound-guided hip joint injection. *J Med Ultrasound*. 2018;26(2):77–80.
5. Cien-Leong C, Cheng-Leong L, Kang L, Ya-Wen C, Po-Chou L. Pulsed radiofrequency treatment of articular branches of femoral and obturator nerves for chronic hip pain. *Clin Interv Aging*. 2015;10:589–574.
6. Dodre E, Lefebvre G, Cockenpot E, et al. Interventional MSK procedures: the hip. *Br J Radiol*. 2016;89(1057):20150408.
7. Bloem J, Reidsma I. Bone and soft tissue tumors of hip and pelvis. *European Journal of Radiology*. 2012; 81(12):3793–801
8. Teo W, Peh W. Primary bone tumors of adulthood. *Cancer Imaging*. 2004;4(2): 74–83.
9. Rafiei A, Amiri A. Analysis of patients with post-chemotherapy arthralgia and arthritis in breast cancer. Indian Journal of Medical Sciences. 2010;64(5):197.
10. Kim MJ, Ye YM, Park HS, Suh CH. Chemotherapy-related arthropathy. *J Rheumatol*. 2006;33:1364–8.

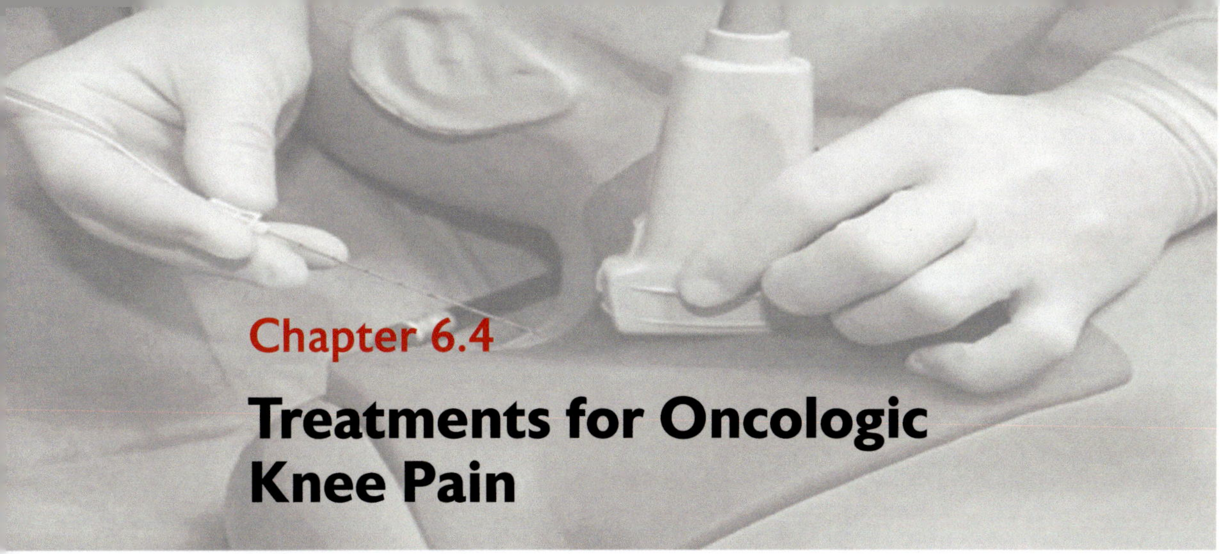

Chapter 6.4

Treatments for Oncologic Knee Pain

Frank V. Schirripa

Contents

Introduction

Knee pain in the cancer patient may arise from primary or metastatic tumors, and oncologic treatments (chemotherapy, radiation and surgery), as well as, post-treatment deconditioning and fatigue. In addition to physical therapy and bracing, corticosteroid, viscosupplementation, and, in rare cases, regenerative medicine injections may be chosen as a treatment modality.[1–4] Ultrasound guidance offers multiple approaches to inject into a knee joint and surrounding structures. Finally, in severe pain cases, consideration for denervation of the knee joint may be considered. Commonly, the "genicular" nerves may be targeted with ablative techniques under fluoroscopic and ultrasound guidance.[2–3] More recently, neuromodulation may provide pain relief for refractory cases. The following chapter discusses optimal techniques in managing knee pain for the cancer patient.

Indications

In patients younger than 20 years old, primary malignancy of bone is the third leading cause of death.[5] Benign lesions are more common and usually asymptomatic.[6,7] Besides exclusion of multifocal lesions, malignant bone tumors are most common seen in the femur, tibia, and pelvis, respectively. Femur, tibia, and humerus are the most common sites for benign bone tumors, respectively, excluding multifocal lesions.[8]

Pain is usually the most common symptom, with a palpable mass as a second presenting symptom.[9] Sometimes, tumors can impinge on the peroneal nerve, causing pain and weakness. In certain cases with fibular tumors, resections can still lead to foot drop and peroneal nerve pain.[10] Pediatric patients who undergo amputation secondary to a malignant bone tumor experience phantom limb pain 50%–90% of the time.[11,12]

Survivors of cancer may have accelerated osteoarthritic changes due to radiation and chemotherapy,[13,14] as well as deconditioning, fatigue, and disuse atrophy. When considering knee treatments in active cancer- or treatment-related pain, a careful assessment of anatomy and cause of the pain syndrome is needed before choosing the best treatment option (Tables 6.4.1, 6.4.2). In any case, collaboration with physical therapy and rehabilitation will be helpful in maximizing care for the oncologic patient.

Table 6.4.1 Knee Cancer–Related Pain Etiologies

Musculoskeletal	Neurologic	Vascular	Bone	Other
• Osteoarthritis • Myofascial pain • Bursitis • Tendinopathy • Contractures • Muscular tumor invasion • Postsurgical pain • Meninscal and ligamentous damage • Patellofemoral syndrome	• Lumbosacral radiculopathy • Polyneuropathy (CIPN) • Radiation-induced plexopathy • Chemo/immunotherapy-induced neuropathy • Leptomeningeal disease • Tumor invasion causing compression • Mononeuropathy/mononeuritis multiplex • Paraneoplastic neuropathy • Complex regional pain syndrome • Central pain syndrome	• Avascular necrosis • DVT • Hematoma	• Primary bone tumors • Metastasis • Osteoporosis • Insufficiency fracture	• Fibromyalgia • Graft-versus-host disease • Radiation dermatitis • Radiation-induced fibrosis • Lymphedema • Infection • Anxiety

Table 6.4.2 Knee Cancer–Related Pain Treatment Algorithm

Survivorship Pain	Active Cancer	Treatment-Related
• Corticosteroids • Viscosupplementation • Peripheral nerve stimulation • Genicular nerve ablation • Regenerative medicine (for remission cases) • Neuroaxial options (spinal cord stimulation, dorsal root ganglion stimulation)	• Corticosteroids • Viscosupplementation • Genicular nerve ablation (if musculoskeletal tumor invasion) • Temporary peripheral nerve stimulation • Neuroaxial options (spinal cord stimulation, dorsal root ganglion stimulation) • Surgical (Dorsal root exit zone lesioning, cordotomy)	• Corticosteroids, viscosupplementation (musculoskeletal injury) • Neuromodulation before joint denervation (for nerve injury) • Follow survivorship (for remission cases) • Injection steroids vs. viscosupplementation if MSK injury

Contraindications

The absolute contraindications to a knee joint injection and joint denervation are patient refusal for the procedure, localized/systemic infection, or severe coagulopathy.

The relative contraindications for intervention in the oncologic population include thrombocytopenia, anticoagulation, immunocompromised patients, distorted anatomy, prior nerve injury or damage, allergy to anesthetics, implanted pacemaker, allodynia, and inability to consent to the procedure. Table 6.4.3 outlines the contraindications and recommended treatment intervention to mitigate overall risk to the patient.

For active cancer patients, a discussion with the treatment team is needed prior to choosing the most appropriate intervention strategy. For example, in patients undergoing immunotherapy, it should be considered that viscosupplementation be used prior to corticosteroids for an injection. Choice of neuromodulation may depend on patients' needs for MRI surveillance and thus necessitate an understanding of the particular device's MRI conditionality.

Table 6.4.3 Contraindications to Knee Interventions

Contraindications	**Related Types** *(recommended intervention)*
Absolute	Refusal for the procedure Localized or systemic infection Severe coagulopathy
Relative	Thromboctyopenia *(smaller needle gauge size)* Anticoagulation *(smaller needle gauge size)* Immunocompromised patients *(viscosupplementation instead of corticosteroids)* Distorted anatomy *(modified injection approach, consider neuromodulation)* Prior nerve injury or damage *(neuromodulation)* Allergy to anesthetics *(saline with injection)* Implanted pacemaker *(intrathecal drug delivery)* Allodynia *(neuromodulation)* Inability to consent to the procedure

Critical Anatomy

The knee joint is composed of the femur, which articulates superiorly on the inferior/medial tibia and slightly on the inferior/lateral fibula. The patella lies within the femoral intercondylar groove, which is also known as the patellofemoral joint. The medial and lateral menisci increase the contact area, add congruency, and provide absorption of loading/rotational forces located at the tibiofemoral joint. The medial and lateral collateral ligaments connect the knee joint medially and laterally and serve as stabilizers in the coronal plane of motion. The anterior and posterior cruciate ligaments are intracapsular extra-articular structures that serve as stabilizers in the sagittal plane of motion. The joint capsule adds to knee stability and is described as thick and fibrous, running superficially, and a thin layer at a deeper plane. Lining the inside of the capsule, the synovial membrane produces nourishing fluid lubricating the joint. The ideal position to assess for a joint effusion is to flex the knee 15 to 25 degrees while lying supine. The joint capsule is under low tension in this position and can be visualized using an ultrasound with the probe focusing on the suprapatellar recess.

The quadriceps muscles (rectus femoris, vastus lateralis, vastus medialis, vastus intermedius) are all innervated by the femoral nerve. The femoral nerve continues distally to form the saphenous nerve to supply the medial surface of the lower leg and foot. Of note, the saphenous gives off the infrapatellar branch prior to reaching the knee joint and innervates the prepatellar skin. The knee joint is innervated by distal branches from the femoral nerve supplying the three vasti, genicular nerves (superlateral, supermedial, inferomedial) branched from the tibial, common fibular, and obturator nerves (Figures 6.4.1–3). The genicular nerves are the common targets for neuroablation addressing chronic knee pain, as they provide significant innervation to the anterior knee capsule. These nerves tend to be distal branches from the nerves discussed above and have consistent point of contact with the femur and tibia, allowing for a standard approach for neurotomy. Additionally, they travel very closely with genicular arteries, which may be identified under ultrasound guidance.

Equipment and Patient Preparation

1. **Monitors and Sterility**
   a. No specific monitoring is required during this procedure. It is highly advised that vital signs, including blood pressure, heart rate, respiratory rate, and pulse oximetry, be obtained prior to starting the procedure to ensure the patient is hemodynamically stable. A set of vitals is often taken post procedure as well.
   b. Strict antiseptic technique should be observed including sterile draping, probe cover, ultrasound gel, sterile gloves, and sterile gauze. Chlorhexidine or other skin prep agent should be used to clean the skin prior to commencing the procedure.
2. **Imaging modalities:**
   a. Ultrasound
      i. Probe: high-frequency linear array or low-frequency curvilinear array
3. **Needle type:**
   i. Local anesthetic: 27- or 30-gauge 1.5-inch needle
   ii. Nerve and joint injections: 22- to 25-gauge 1.5- to 3.5-inch spinal needle
   iii. Knee joint radiofrequency ablation: 50 to 100 mm needle with 5 or 10 mm active tip
4. **Patient position:** Supine with knee flexed to 20 degrees
5. **Injectate:**
   a. Local anesthetic: Lidocaine 1%–2%; Ropivacaine 0.2%–0.5%; Bupivacaine 0.25%–0.5%
   b. Adjuvant: particulate or nonparticulate steroid

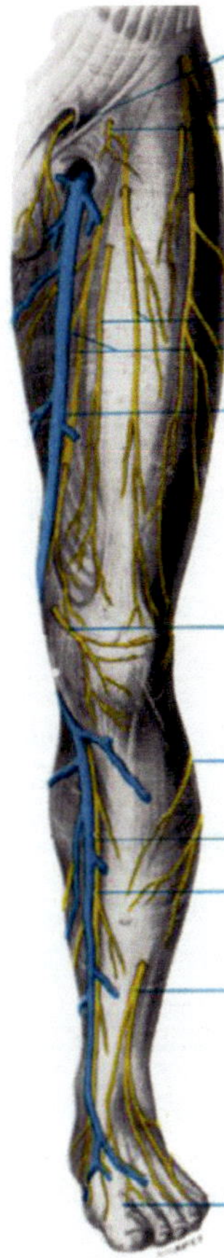

Figure 6.4.1 Cutaneous nerves on the front of the lower limb. (Reprinted with permission from Cunningham's Manual of Practical Anatomy: Upper and Lower Limbs, 16th Edition)

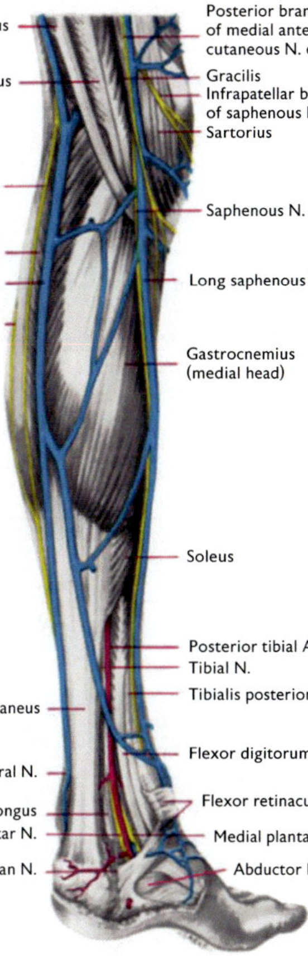

Figure 6.4.2 Superficial dissection of the leg, viewed from the posteromedial side, showing the veins and nerves. (Reprinted with permission from Cunningham's Manual of Practical Anatomy: Upper and Lower Limbs, 16th Edition)

Procedure Technique

Saphenous Nerve Block (Figure 6.4.4)

1. **The patient is positioned supine, area prepped, and equipment is ready;** the probe is placed in transverse axial plane on the medial aspect of the thigh midway between the anterior superior iliac spine (ASIS) and patella.
2. **The saphenous nerve can be visualized here in the adductor canal in the proximal, medial thigh.** Medial to this is the vastus medialis, lateral to the adductor muscles, and deep to the sartorius. The saphenous nerve proceeds under the sartorius as it runs distal from the adductor canal, with various branches of the nerve innervating the medial knee.
3. **An in-plane approach is utilized to deposit medication close to the saphenous nerve.** Local anesthetic is given for skin anesthesia, then a 22- or 25-gauge 1.5- to 3.5-inch needle is inserted. The target is the saphenous nerve deep the sartorius, and typically either superficial or lateral to the femoral artery.

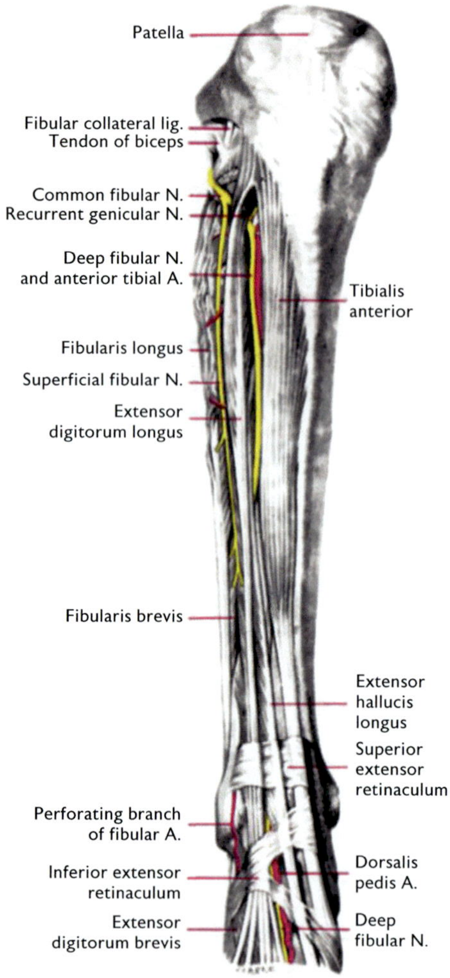

Figure 6.4.3 Dissection of the anterior and lateral sides of the leg. (Reprinted with permission from Cunningham's Manual of Practical Anatomy: Upper and Lower Limbs, 16th Edition)

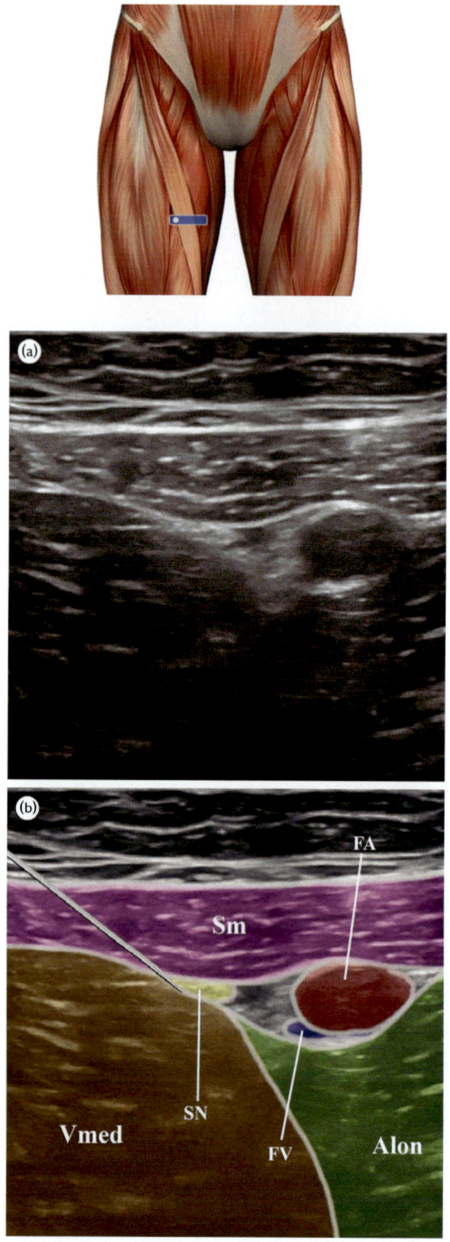

Figure 6.4.4 **a,** Ultrasound image of the anteromedial thigh. **b,** Labeled ultrasound image of in-plane needle placement for a saphenous nerve block. *Sm* sartorius, *Vmed* vastus medialis, *SN* saphenous nerve, *FV* femoral vein, *FA* femoral artery, *Alon* adductor longus.

Tips

- Be sure to use doppler to search for and identify femoral vessels near the target area to avoid during procedures.

Safety Considerations

- Avoid injecting to proximally, which will cause a femoral nerve block and motor weakness.

Intra-Articular Knee Joint Injection—Suprapatellar Recess Approach

1. **The patient is positioned supine with knee flexed to 15–25 degrees;** the probe is placed in a longitudinal sagittal plane over the distal thigh just superior to the superior pole of the patella.
2. **A joint effusion may be visualized in the suprapatellar recess.** It will be located directly deep to the quadriceps tendon and suprapatellar fat pad, as shown in Figure 6.4.5. The area of the largest amount of effusion is centered within the field of view.
3. **The probe is rotated 90 degrees into a transverse view.** This will reveal the suprapatellar recess in between the quadriceps tendon and the prefemoral fat pad.
4. **An in-plane approach is utilized to deposit medication into the knee joint.** Local anesthetic is given for skin anesthesia, then a 22- or 25-gauge 1.5- to 3.5-inch needle is inserted with the target being within the suprapatellar recess as shown in Figure 6.4.6.

Tips

- Be sure to use doppler to search for and identify satellite vessels near the target area to avoid during procedures.

Safety Considerations

- Avoid injecting into the prefemoral and suprapatellar fat pads, which can mimic the suprapatellar recess if not carefully identified beforehand.

Genicular Nerve Block—Short-Axis Approach (Figure 6.4.7)

1. **The patient is positioned supine, area prepped, and equipment is ready;** the probe is placed in longitudinal coronal plane on the distal medial aspect of the thigh.
2. **It is difficult to identify the superomedial genicular nerves**, but these can be seen near the genicular artery at the junction of the femoral condyle neck and femoral shaft. This can be your target for ablation of the knee joint near the medial superior genicular artery.
3. **An in-plane approach is utilized to deposit medication close to the superomedial genicular nerves, which is adjacent to the genicular artery.** Local anesthetic is given for skin anesthesia, then a 22- or 25-gauge 1.5- to 3.5-inch needle or a radiofrequency needle is insert. The target is the superomedial genicular compartment and the head junction of the femur.
4. **This procedure can be performed for the superolateral and inferomedial genicular nerves as well with the same technique.** The inferolateral compartment is avoided due to risk of involvement/damage to the common fibular nerve, medial collateral ligament and Pes Anserine.

Genicular Nerve Block—Long-Axis Approach (Figure 6.4.8)

1. **The patient is positioned supine, area prepped, and equipment is ready;** the probe is placed in longitudinal coronal plane on the distal medial aspect of the thigh.

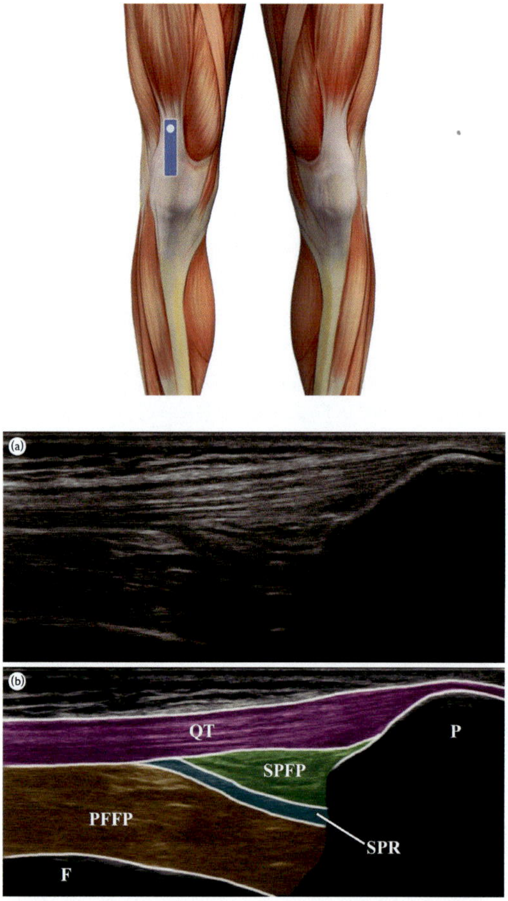

Figure 6.4.5 a, Ultrasound image of the anterior superior knee in longitudinal sagittal plane. **b,** Labeled ultrasound image of the suprapatellar recess in long-axis. *QT* quadriceps tendon, *P* patella, *SPFP* suprapatellar fat pad, *SPR* suprapatellar recess, *PFFP* prefemoral fat pad, *F* femur.

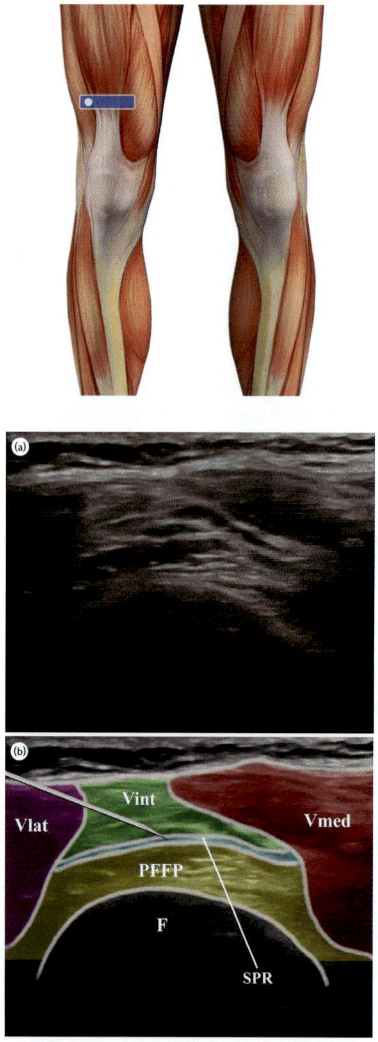

Figure 6.4.6 a, Ultrasound image of the anterior superior knee in a transverse axial plane. **b,** Labeled ultrasound image of in-plane needle placement for a suprapatellar recess intra-articular knee joint injection in short-axis. *Vlat* vastus lateralis, *Vint* vastus intermedius, *Vmed* vastus medialis, *SPR* suprapatellar recess, *PFFP* prefemoral fat pad, *F* femur.

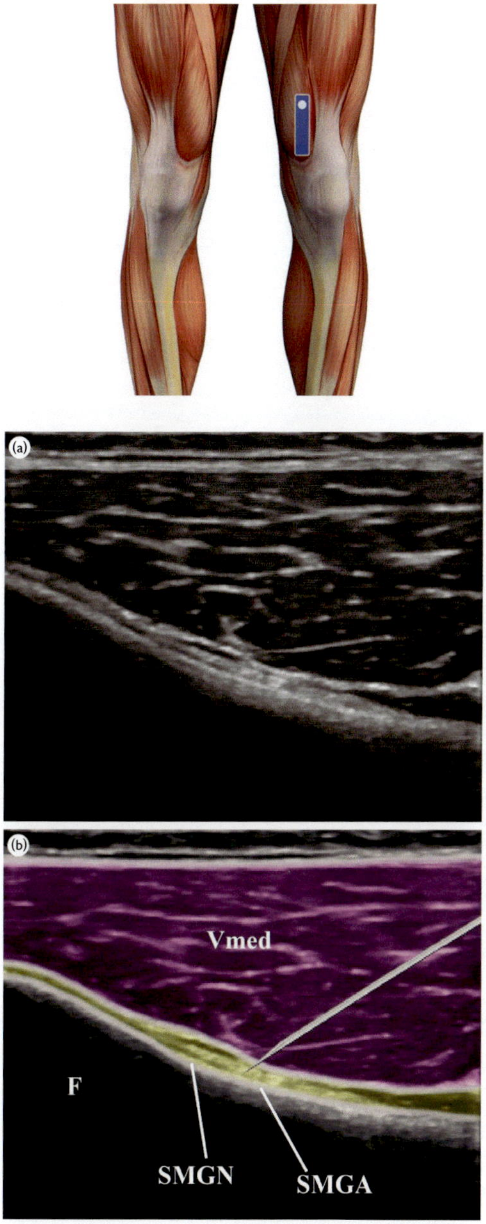

Figure 6.4.7 **a,** Ultrasound image of the anterior superomedial knee in short-axis. **b,** Labeled ultrasound image of in-plane needle placement for a superolateral genicular nerve block. *Vmed* vastus medialis, *SMGN* superomedial genicular nerve compartment, *SMGA* superomedial genicular artery compartment, *F* femur.

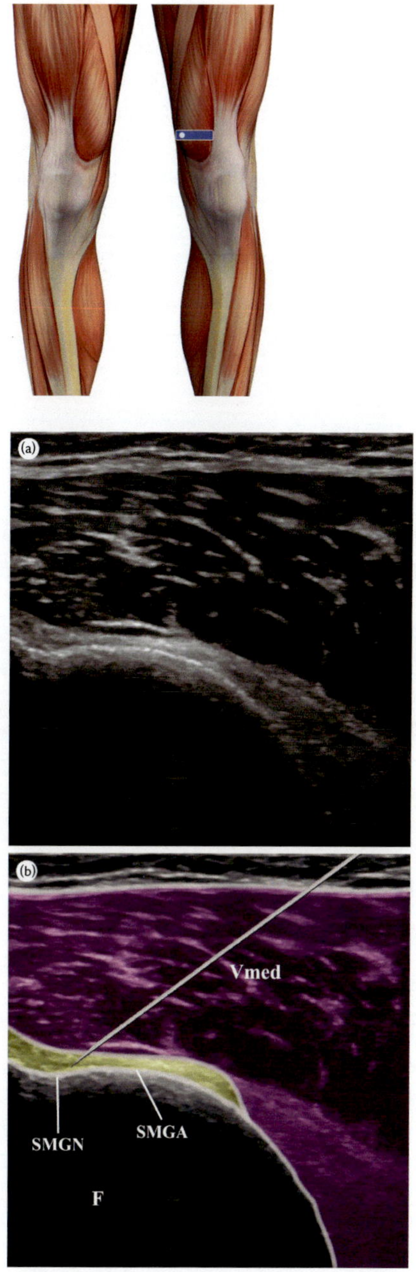

Figure 6.4.8 **a,** Ultrasound image of the anterior superomedial knee in a transverse axial plane. **b,** Labeled ultrasound image of in-plane needle placement for a superolateral genicular nerve block in long-axis. *Vmed* vastus medialis, *SMGN* superomedial genicular nerve compartment, *SMGA* superomedial genicular artery compartment, *F* femur.

2. **It is difficult to identify the superomedial genicular nerves**, but these can be seen near the genicular artery at the junction of the femoral condyle neck and femoral shaft. This can be your target for ablation of the knee joint near the medial superior genicular artery.
3. **The probe is rotated 90 degrees into a transverse view.**
4. **An in-plane approach is utilized to deposit medication close to the superomedial genicular nerves, which is adjacent to the genicular artery.** Local anesthetic is given for skin anesthesia, then a 22- or 25-gauge 1.5- to 3.5-inch needle or a radiofrequency needle is inserted. The target is the superomedial genicular compartment and the head junction of the femur.
5. **This procedure can be performed for the superolateral and inferomedial genicular nerves as well with the same technique.** The inferolateral compartment is avoided due to risk of involvement/damage to the common fibular nerve.

Tips

- Be sure to use doppler to search for and identify satellite vessels near the target area to avoid during procedures.

Genicular Nerve Radiofrequency Ablation

1. **This procedure can be performed in either the short- or long-axis approach as mentioned above.**
2. **Depending on the type of ablation, standard or bipolar, entry point for each cannula is marked.** For standard ablation, the distance between each cannula should be approximately 8–10 mm and 15 mm for bipolar ablation.
3. **The ultrasound transducer is placed in appropriate view over the marked region**. Each cannula is inserted at the marked location targeting near the periosteum.
4. **Once the cannula placement is confirmed under ultrasound, the ablation process can be initiated,** and once complete, each cannula is removed and disposed of appropriately.

Tips

- Be sure to use doppler to search for and identify satellite vessels near the target area to avoid during procedures.

Postprocedure Management Considerations

In the oncologic patient, evaluation for postinjection septic joint is recommended. For joint denervation procedures, it is possible to have a temporary increase in pain, bleeding, or allergy to anesthetic after procedure, with consideration for chronic hematoma and pseudoaneurysm.

Patients are usually observed up to 45 minutes with a blood pressure check before being discharged from the office. Patients who complain of sudden leg weakness, excessive redness, swelling or discharge at the needle site, fever, significant pain are instructed to go to the emergency room.

Further Reading

- Moore KL, Agur AMR. *Essential clinical anatomy*. Philadelphia, PA: Lippincott Williams & Wilkins; 2006.
- Solomon J, Roque-Dang C, Wyss J. Chapter 50: Fluoroscopy and Ultrasound-Guided Joint Injections in: Diwan S, Staats P. *Atlas of pain medicine procedures*. New York, NY: McGraw-Hill Education; 2015: 415–420.

- Brown MA. Chapter 55: Intra-Articular Joint Injections in: Diwan S, Staats P. *Atlas of pain medicine procedures*. New York, NY: McGraw-Hill Education; 2015: 445–451.
- Thakur A, Staats PS. Chapter 80: Radiofrequency Neurolysis in: Diwan S, Staats P. *Atlas of pain medicine procedures*. New York, NY: McGraw-Hill Education; 2015: 750–755.
- Bhatia A, Peng PWP. Chapter 21: Ultrasound-Guided Peripheral Nerve Blockade in Chronic Pain Management in: *Atlas of ultrasound-guided procedures in interventional pain management*. S.N. Narouze (ed.) Springer Science and Business Media; 2011: 279–292.

References

1. Kim SY, Le PU, Kosharskyy B, et al. Is genicular nerve radiofrequency ablation safe? A Literature Review and Anatomical Study. *Pain Physician*. 2016;19(5):E697–705.
2. Concoff A, Rosen J, Fu F, et al. A comparison of treatment effects for nonsurgical therapies and the minimum clinically important difference in knee osteoarthritis: a systematic review. *JBJS Rev*. 2019;7(8):e5.
3. Kidd VD, Strum, SR, Strum DS, et al. Genicular nerve radiofrequency ablation for painful knee arthritis: the why and the how. *JBJS Essent Surg Tech*. 2019;9(1):e10.
4. Ulasli AM, Ozcakar L, Murrei WD. Ultrasound imaging and guidance in the management of knee osteoarthritis in regenerative medicine field. *J Clin Orthop Trauma*. 2019;10(1): 24–31.
5. Siegel R, Naishadham D, Jemal A. Cancer statistics, 2013. *CA Cancer J Clin*. 2013;63(1):11–30.
6. Franchi A. Epidemiology and classification of bone tumors. *Clin Cases Miner Bone Metab*. 2012;9(2):92–95.
7. Wu JS, Hochman M. *Bone tumors: A practical guide to imaging*. New York, Dordrecht, Heidelberg, London: Springer; 2012.
8. Niu X, Xu H, Inwards CY, Li Y, Ding Y, Letson GD, Bui MM. Primary bone tumors: epidemiologic comparison of 9200 patients treated at Beijing Ji Shui Tan Hospital, Beijing, China, with 10 165 patients at Mayo Clinic, Rochester, Minnesota. *Archives of Pathology & Laboratory Medicine*. 2015;139(9): 1149–1155.
9. Arikan Y, Misir A, Gur V et al. Clinical and radiologic outcomes following resection of primary proximal fibula tumors: Proximal fibula resection outcomes. *Journal of Orthopaedic Surgery*. 2019;27(2).
10. Dieckmann R, Gebert C, Streitburger A. Proximal fibula resection in the treatment of bone tumours. *Int Orthop*. 2011;35(11):1689–1694.
11. Wilkins KL, McGrath PJ, Finley GA, Katz J. Phantom limb sensations and phantom limb pain in child and adolescent amputees. *Pain*. 1998;78:7–12.
12. Flor H. Phantom-limb pain: characteristics, causes, and treatment. *Lancet Neurol*. 2002;1:182–189.
13. Rafiei A, Amiri A. Analysis of patients with post-chemotherapy arthralgia and arthritis in breast cancer. *Indian Journal of Medical Sciences*. 2010;64(5):197.
14. Kim MJ, Ye YM, Park HS, Suh CH. Chemotherapy-related arthropathy. *J Rheumatol*. 2006;33:1364–1368.

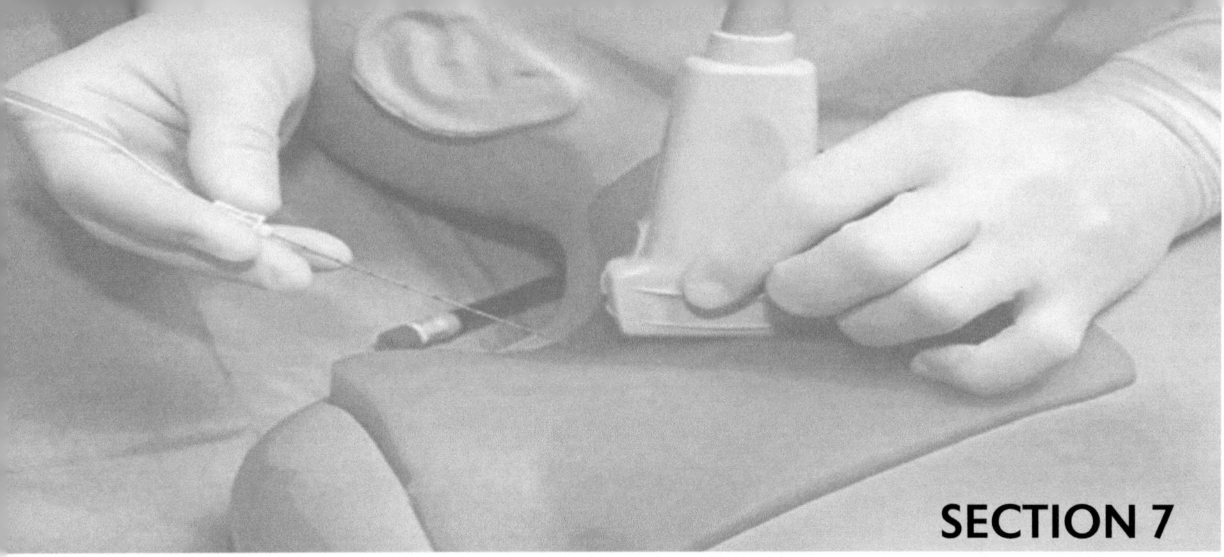

SECTION 7

ADVANCED PROCEDURES SECTION

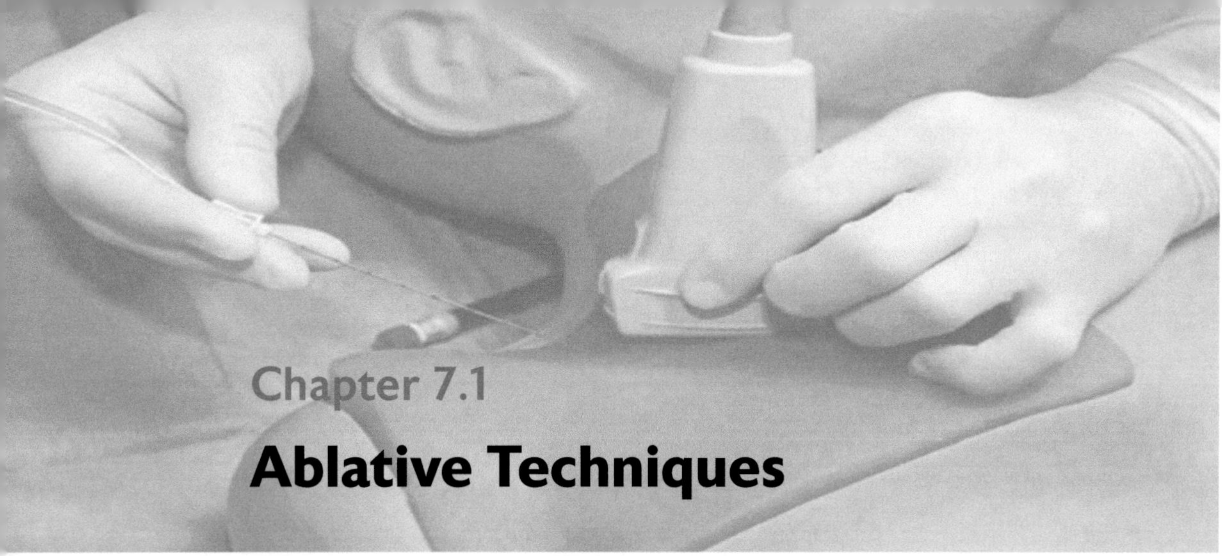

Chapter 7.1

Ablative Techniques

Andrew Mendelson and Storm Horine

Contents

Continuous Thermal Radiofrequency Ablation

Radiofrequency ablation (RFA) has been used in clinical practice since the early 1950s.[1] The RFA closed-loop circuit consists of a generator, an active electrode, a resistor (i.e., the patient), and a dispersive electrode (i.e., the grounding pad). The active electrode generates a high-frequency alternating current that produces a heat lesion. The current then reaches the dispersive electrode, which serves as a return pathway. Tissue heating results from radiofrequency (RF) ionic oscillation, and tissue destruction begins to occur at temperatures greater than 45°C.[1] The RF probe should lie adjacent to the nerve to create a lesion with the best chance of success of interrupting pain signal transmission. Lesion size depends on the duration of heat creation, electric field size, and temperature.[1] Once the RF probe is in the correct position, sensory and motor stimulation is tested to confirm correct probe placement. Ablation should then occur for 60–90 seconds with a target temperature of 65°C–90°C. Clinical applications of thermal RFA include image-guided tumor ablation and neuropathic pain states.

Cooled Radiofrequency Ablation

Cooled RFA uses an internally cooled probe to expose surrounding tissues to destructive temperatures.[2] The probe is cooled by circulating fluid that prevents the tip of the probe from reaching excessively high temperatures. This allows for continuous flow of radiofrequency energy and results in spherical thermal lesions that are larger than traditional RF lesions.[3] Cooled RFA produces a lesion that extends beyond the tip of the probe, allowing the probe to create a satisfactory lesion while oriented directly on top of and perpendicular to a target. This is a significant advantage over traditional RFA, which requires probes to be oriented parallel to a target nerve .[3] Lesion size depends on probe size, temperature, and duration of the current applied. Target temperature and duration for the cooled RFA is 60°C for 60–90 seconds. Cooled RFA has clinical applications similar to those of traditional continuous thermal RFA.

Pulsed Radiofrequency Ablation

Pulsed radiofrequency ablation (PRF) uses radiofrequency energy, which is delivered in 2-10 pulses per second (Hertz) with each pulse width between 20 to 50 miliseconds. The short pulse width allows time for heat to dissipate after each pulse is delivered. The total cycle can be applied for 4 to 20 minutes, with some studies showing longer duration associated with improved clinical effectiveness.[4] This alternating pattern keeps temperatures below 45°C, preventing complete tissue destruction. The mechanism of action of PRF remains unclear, but pain relief may be related to modulation of second-order neuron activity in the spinal cord.[5] Pulsed radiofrequency ablation is conducted in a similar manner to thermal RFA; however, it remains unknown if the orientation of the probe to the nerve affects outcome.[4] Clinical applications of PRF are broader than other ablative techniques, as it does not cause direct tissue destruction and is relatively painless. Pulsed radiofrequency ablation has shown benefit in various pain syndromes including sympathetically mediated pain, radicular pain, facial pain, and axial back pain.

Ethyl Alcohol Neurolysis

Ethyl alcohol causes nonselective nerve destruction. Neural cholesterol, cerebrosides, mucopeptides, and other essential components of the neural cellular membrane are extracted, leading to demyelination and cell death.[6] Ethyl alcohol comes in a variety of concentrations, but 50%–95% ethyl alcohol is typically used for neurolysis. Local anesthetics are commonly given before or concurrently with ethyl alcohol, which is painful on injection. Patient positioning must be considered during injection as ethyl alcohol is hypobaric compared to cerebrospinal fluid.[6] Although nerve injury from ethyl alcohol neurolysis can rarely cause paraplegia, the most common complication is neuritis, which can last from days to weeks.[7] Image guidance is recommended to visualize the spread of alcohol solution to minimize the risk of unintended neurolysis and paraplegia.

Phenol Neurolysis

Phenol is a benzene ring with one hydrogen atom replaced by a hydroxyl group.[6] Phenol, which is poorly soluble in water, is not commercially available and must be compounded by a pharmacy. It is typically mixed with glycerin to limit its spread from the injection site.[6] Concentrations of phenol for neurolysis range from 4% to 10%.[6] Phenol causes neurolytic destruction by diffusing directly into the axon and denaturing intracellular proteins.[8] Possibly due to their different mechanisms of action for neurolysis, nerves regenerate faster after phenol neurolysis than they do after ethyl alcohol neurolysis.[6] Unlike ethyl alcohol, phenol possesses local anesthetic properties and is usually not painful on injection.[8] Again, image guidance is recommended to visualize the spread of the phenol solution to minimize the risk of neurolysis in an unintended area. Viscous preparations of phenol diluted with glycerin are hyperbaric in relation to cerebrospinal fluid.

Cryoneurolysis

Cryoneurolysis causes cell ischemia by induction of cold temperatures. Studies have shown that temperatures between −5°C and −70°C damage the vasa nervorum, causing severe endoneurial damage and Wallerian degeneration while preserving the myelin sheath.[9] A cryoprobe is a hollow tube with a smaller inner tube. The smaller inner tube releases highly pressured gases (most commonly N_2O or CO_2) or supercooled liquid gases (liquid nitrogen) which expand quickly at the distal tip. Gaseous expansion decreases the temperature signficantly below zero, depending on the cyrogen to form an iceball.[9] The size of the cryoprobe correlates with the size of the iceball formed.[4] Commonly, a series of three freeze–thaw cycles is used for cryoneurolysis. Each cycle is composed of a 1- to 2-minute freeze followed by a 30-second thawing period. Benefits of cryoneurolysis include avoiding potential neuroma formation, as the endoneurium of the nerves remains intact. Cryoneurolysis is an effective treatment for facial pain, pelvic pain, abdominal pain, and both upper and lower extremity pain.

References

1. Cosman ER, Cosman ER (2009) Radiofrequency Lesions. In: Lozano AM, Gildenberg PL, Tasker RR (eds) Textbook of Stereotactic and Functional Neurosurgery. Springer, Berlin, Heidelberg. P1359–1382.
2. Cosman ER, Dolensky JR, Hoffman RA. Factors That Affect Radiofrequency Heat Lesion Size. *Pain Med Pain Med* 2014 Dec;15(12):2020–2036.
3. Zachariah C, Mayeux J, Alas G, et al. Physiological and functional responses of water-cooled versus traditional radiofrequency ablation of peripheral nerves in rats. *Regional Anesthesia & Pain Medicine* 2020;45:792–798.
4. Malik K (2018) Pulsed Radiofrequency, Water-Cooled Radiofrequency, and Cyroneurolysis. In: Benzon HT, Raja, SN, Liu SS, et al. (eds) Essentials of Pain Medicine. Elsevier, Philadelphia, PA. P619–626.
5. Byrd D, Mackey S. Pulsed radiofrequency for chronic pain. *Curr Pain Headache Rep*. 2008;12(1):37–41.
6. Saeed K, Adams MC, Hurley RW (2018) Central and Peripheral Neurolysis. In: Benzon HT, Raja, SN, Liu SS, et al. (eds) Essentials of Pain Medicine. Elsevier, Philadelphia, PA. P655–661.
7. Loh TH, Patel S, Mirchandani A, Eckmann M. Brachial Plexus Chemical Neurolysis with Ethanol for Cancer Pain. *Case Rep Med*. 2018 Jul 24;2018:8628645. doi:10.1155/2018/8628645. PMID: 30140288; PMCID: PMC6081596.
8. Koyyalagunta D, Burton A.W. The role of chemical neurolysis in cancer pain. *Curr Pain Headache Rep*. 2010;14:261–267.

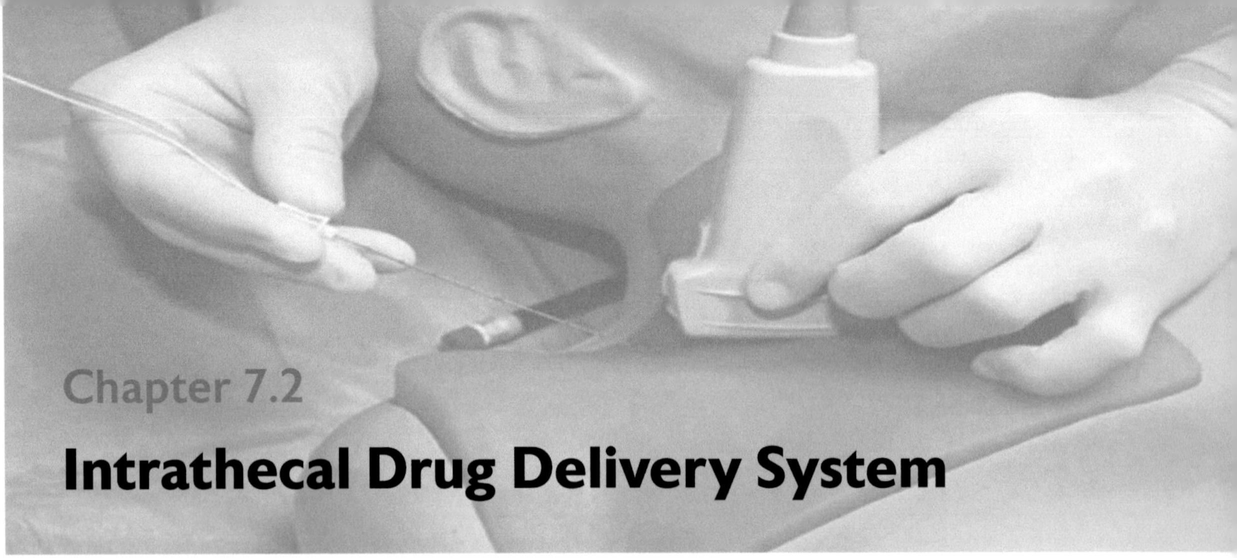

Chapter 7.2
Intrathecal Drug Delivery System

Storm Horine, Grant Chen, Shane Brogan, and Priyanka Ghosh

Contents

Introduction

August Bier published a paper in 1899 to show that local anesthetic in the spinal fluid can block the sensation of pain.[1] This technique was modified to using an implanted malleable needle in 1939 and then further modified to a catheter technique in 1944 by Dr. Tuohy.[2] In 1981, Onofrio implanted an intrathecal opioid delivery device for intractable malignant pain.[3] Intrathecal drug delivery techniques continued to advance, and modern Intrathecal drug delivery systems (IDDS) now consist of a medication reservoir, pump or propellant, catheter extending from the pump to the intrathecal space, and computer that can be wirelessly interrogated for information. Intrathecal drug delivery systems are approved by the US Food and Drug Administration (FDA) for chronic use in patients with moderate-to-severe pain from cancer or noncancer causes.

BOX 7.2.1 Disease Indications for Intrathecal Drug Delivery Systems

Primary or metastatic tumors causing pain from tissue invasion
Neuropathy or nerve irritation from chemotherapy or radiation therapy
Surgical pain secondary to resection or spinal fusion
Severe chronic pain in a cancer patient in remission, arthritis including osteoarthritis and rheumatoid arthritis
Peripheral neuropathy refractory to conservative treatments

Indications

Optimal patient selection for IDDS therapy is complex and requires evaluation of both patient-specific and disease-specific factors, which are listed in Boxes 7.2.1 and 7.2.2, respectively. Patient selection begins with evaluation of medical history, pain treatment history, and psychiatric comorbidities. Disease-specific considerations include the diagnosis of a pain etiology that could benefit from intrathecal medications, determination of which spinal level to place the IDDS, and identifying where to place the IDDS pump. Intrathecal pumps have been shown to decrease oral morphine–equivalent opioid doses as well as pain scores.[4–5] Cancer-related pain, either from active cancer or pathology due to cancer treatment, is one of the major indications for IDDS therapy.[6] Relief from the side effects of pain medications, such as nausea or fatigue, is often another powerful indication for IDDS implantation.

Trials

Therapeutic trials prior to permanent IDDS implantation are a contentious topic, although trials may be required by some insurances. Trial options include single bolus injections, multiple bolus injections, and temporary continuous infusions; each of which can be performed either intrathecally or epidurally.[7] Data regarding whether trials can accurately predict efficacy of IDDS therapy after implantation are very limited[8] and appropriate intrathecal drug dosing can be estimated without trials.[9]

Contraindications

Patient-specific contraindications include patient refusal, local or systemic infection, inability to implant the pump/reservoir 2.5 cm (1 inch) or less from the skin, insufficient body mass to accept pump bulk and weight comfortably, thrombocytopenia and other anticoagulation issues, and spinal anomalies making catheter placement impossible. Patients typically undergo psychological evaluations prior to IDDS placement, although this may be suspended for palliative cancer patients to expedite care. Psychological and psychosocial comorbidities affecting pain outcomes should be evaluated, and history of psychosis must be identified as it contraindicates ziconotide.[7]

BOX 7.2.2 Patient Selection Criteria

More conservative treatment options have failed, or other options are unacceptable or not indicated.
Oral or transdermal medications produce unacceptable side effects or an unacceptable level of relief.
The patient's spinal anatomy will allow for the placement of a spinal catheter.
The patient is medically stable with no untreated bleeding disorders, infectious processes, or disorders that would preclude implantation of an intrathecal catheter and a surgical foreign body.

Critical Anatomy

Intrathecal drug delivery systems implantation requires an in-depth understanding of relevant anatomy. Most of the time, the spinal column is composed of 33 vertebral bones that can be divided into five different regions based on structure: cervical, thoracic, lumbar, sacral, and coccygeal. The individual vertebrae can be further divided into an anterior vertebral body and a posterior vertebral arch. The posterior vertebral arch consists of pedicles, inferior and superior articulating processes, lamina, and a midline spinous process. Five ligaments support the spinal column: the supraspinous ligament, interspinous ligament, ligmentum flavum, posterior longitudinal ligament, and anterior longitudinal ligament. The spinal cord extends from the foramen magnum of the skull to its termination at the L1 or L2 level, where it becomes the cauda equina. The spinal cord is encased within the posterior vertebral arch and three meninges: the dura, arachnoid mater, and pia mater. The epidural space is a potential space between the ligamentum flavum and dura. Between the arachnoid mater and pia mater is referred to as the subarachnoid space. Deep to the pia mater is intrathecal space, which contains the spinal cord and cerebrospinal fluid and is the location for the catheter of the pump. The needle entry site for IDDS placement is typically at the L2/L3 interspace; however, the final position of the IDDS catheter tip should be at the spinal level of the pain syndrome. Table 7.2.1 identifies ideal catheter tip location for various regions of pain.[10]

Initial Medications Calculation

Intrathecal pumps tend to run well between 0.2 and 0.5 mL per day. For cancer patients, pump reservoirs are usually 40 mL, as opposed to 20 mL, to minimize the number of necessary trips to the clinic for pump refills. Here is an outline of how to set up initial settings for an intrathecal pump regimen with an example patient who has abdominal pain from an unresectable pancreatic tumor.

1. Choose the intrathecal opioid dose based on oral morphine equivalent.
    a. Patient received relief of pain symptoms at 200 mg/day of oral morphine.
    b. A ratio of 100:1 oral:intrathecal dose would be used to convert the oral morphine–equivalent dose to intrathecal morphine dose. In this case, this would be 2 mg/day of intrathecal morphine.

Table 7.2.1 Catheter tip Location for Specific Regions of Pain (adapted from Chen 2020 [10])

Region of Pain	IDDS Catheter Location
Brachial Plexus	C3–C5
Arm	C3–C5
Breast	T1–T2
Upper Chest Wall	T3–T4
Visceral Abdomen	T5–T6
Lower Chest Wall	T6–T7
Abdominal Wall	T6–T7
Pelvis	T9–T12
Leg	T10
Sacral	Vertebral body level corresponding to conus or sacral nerve roots

Table 7.2.2 Recommended Bupivacaine Dosage Based on Catheter Location (adapted from Chen 2020 [10])

Catheter Tip Level	Initial Bupivacaine Dose (mg/day)
Cervical	5
T1–T4	8
T5–T8	10
T9–T12	8
Lumbar	8

2. Choose the bupivacaine dose for the patient based on the chart of where the catheter tip will be located.
   a. For this patient with visceral abdominal pain, the catheter tip will be at T5–T6, which means the dose of bupivacaine will start at 10 mg/day [Table 7.2.2].
3. Choose the concentration of the medication—generally start at the lowest rate and then progressively increase.
   a. This often depends on the compounding pharmacy limitation of how concentrated the medication compound can be. At a flow rate of 0.25 mL/day, this concentration would be morphine 8 mg/mL + bupivacaine 40 mg/mL.
4. Consider addition of clonidine.
   a. Clonidine can augment the pain relief provided by the IDDS. At our institution, clonidine is added at 100 mcg/day for neuropathic pain or if intrathecal morphine dose is too high to create the compounded medication.
5. Ziconotide and baclofen may also be considered as intrathecal adjuvants in the cancer pain population.

Equipment

Monitors and Patient Preparation

Patients should be placed in lateral decubitus position and continuously monitored with pulse oximetry, electrocardiography, noninvasive blood pressure measurements, and capnography. Patients should be given supplemental oxygen, and a peripheral intravenous line should be established. Patients typically require moderate sedation or general anesthesia.

Sterility

IDDS placement is a sterile procedure. Skin at the procedure site should be sterilized with a skin preparation agent such as chlorhexidine. Antibiotic prophylaxis of cefazolin 2 grams or clindamycin 600 mg may be given intravenously prior to skin incision.

Fluoroscopy and Procedural Equipment

IDDS placement requires:

1. Intrathecal catheter
2. Intrathecal pump
3. #11 or #15 blade scalpel
4. Tunneling device
5. Anchoring device

6. Sutures
7. Lidocaine 1%–2% or bupivacaine 0.25% for local infiltration
8. Spinal needle

Many of these supplies are provided by the manufacturer.

Procedural Technique

1. **Mark the intended pump implantation site while the patient is awake and sitting upright.** Ensure the pump is away from bony prominences, such as the iliac crest and ribs. Consideration should be given regarding which side the patient sleeps on to avoid pressure on the pump while asleep. There should be sufficient subcutaneous fat for comfortable pump placement while still allowing the pump to be accessed. Marking while the patient is sitting upright avoids inadvertent placement below the beltline.
   a. Note: If abdominal placement is not possible, consider moving the insertion site to the superior gluteal region or using the smaller 20 mL reservoir size.
2. **Position the patient in lateral decubitus position (**Figure 7.2.1**).**
3. **Obtain anteroposterior fluoroscopic image of lumbar spine (**Figure 7.2.2**).** Visualize both the site of entry and target location of final catheter tip placement.
4. **Anesthetize the entry site with local anesthetic and insert spinal needle (Figure 7.2.3**). The spinal needle should be at a 30–45 degree angle using a paramedian approach. Contact the lamina of the vertebral level caudal to the target interlaminar space. Withdraw the needle and "walk off" the lamina until engaging ligament in the interlaminar space. Use loss of resistance technique to access the epidural space. Use anterior and lateral fluoroscopy imaging to monitor needle depth and advance into the intrathecal space (Figure 7.2.4).
   a. Note: If possible, patients should be responsive during this step to communicate any discomfort when advancing the needle intrathecally. This safeguards against inadvertent nerve damage.
5. **Confirm free flow of cerebrospinal fluid (CSF).** Troubleshoot if needed by rotating the bevel of the needle or advancing further with fluoroscopic guidance. After obtaining free CSF flow, re-stylet the needle to avoid excessive CSF drainage.
6. **Turn the needle bevel cephalad, withdraw stylet, and thread catheter.** Ensure the catheter guidewire is fully in the catheter. Use live lateral fluoroscopic imaging and thread the catheter to the target spinal level on the posterior portion of the spinal cord.
   a. Note: Refer to Table 7.2.1 for recommended catheter tip location based on pain pathology.

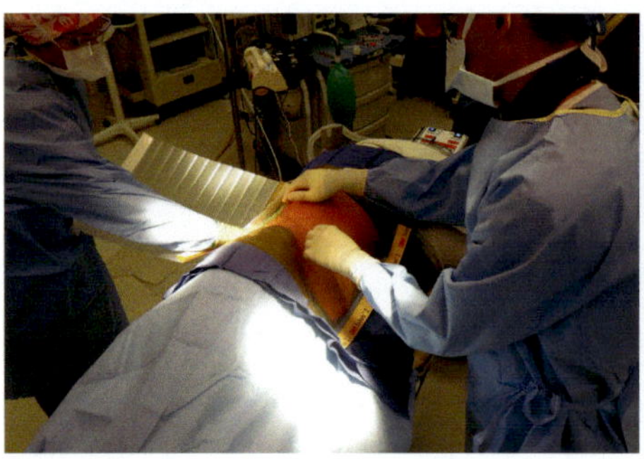

Figure 7.2.1 Patient position in lateral decubitus position for intrathecal pump placement.

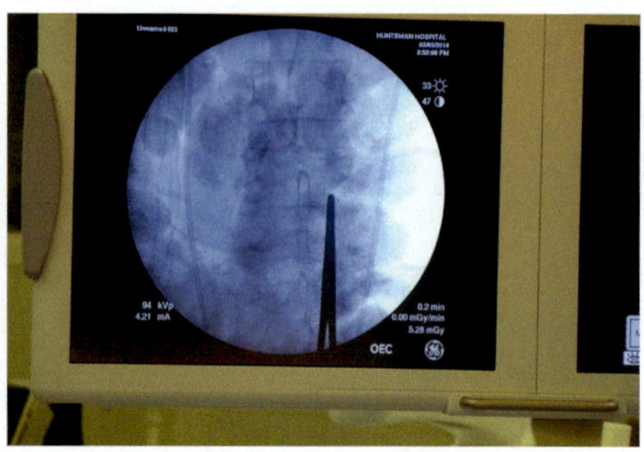

Figure 7.2.2 Anterior-posterior fluoroscopic image of lumbar spine to plan for entry site location.

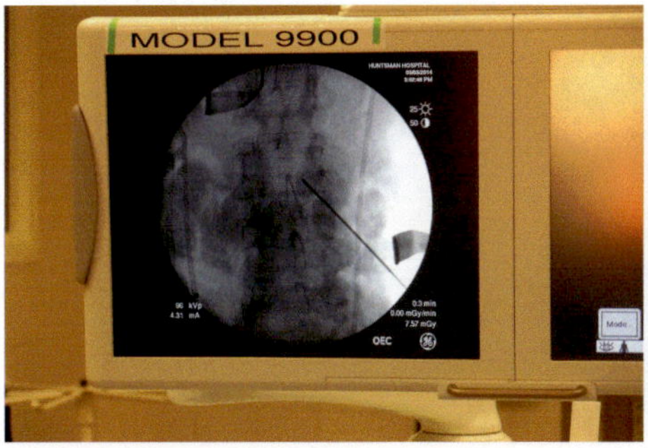

Figure 7.2.3 Anterior-posterior fluoroscopic image of spinal needle using a paramedian approach.

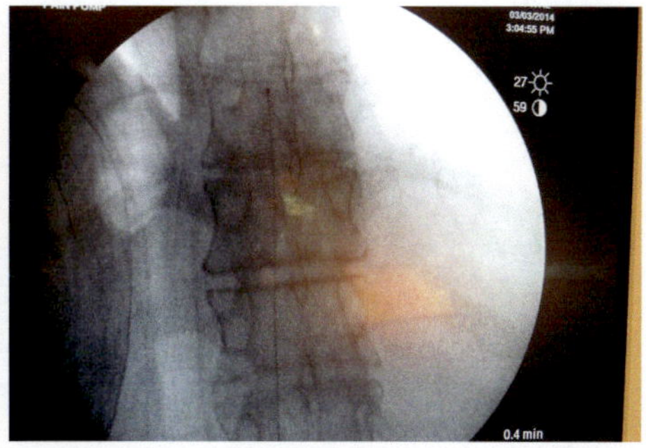

Figure 7.2.4 Anterior-posterior fluoroscopic image of intrathecal catheter tip.

7. **Withdraw the spinal needle out of intrathecal space and into the subcutaneous tissue.** With the needle protecting the catheter in the subcutaneous tissue, make a 5–8 cm sagittal incision over the spinous processes, extending cephalad and caudal from the entry site of the needle. Bluntly dissect down to the lumbar paravertebral fascia. Anchor the catheter to the fascia using either sutures or a company-specific anchoring device (Figure 7.2.5a).
    a. Note: An alternative technique is to dissect down to the fascia prior to inserting the spinal needle. This often simplifies spinal needle and catheter placement, but commits to having an incision and dissection at a spinal level prior to establishing intrathecal access.
8. **Remove the spinal needle and catheter stylet.** Reconfirm free CSF flow. Create a loop with the catheter to relieve strain with patient movement.
9. **Anesthetize the pocket site with local anesthetic.**
10. **Use a #11 or #15 blade to make a 10–12 cm transverse incision at the pocket site.** Dissect down 1–3 cm to the abdominal fascial plane. Create a pocket in the subcutaneous tissue caudally by bluntly dissecting a space slightly larger than the pump (Figure 7.2.6). Test the size of the pocket with company-specific sizers.
    a. Note: Avoid cephalad pocket creation, as the weight of the pump would rest on the incision and cause discomfort.
11. **Tunnel the catheter from the catheter site to the pocket site using a company-specific tunneling device** (Figure 7.2.7). Palpate the tunneling device while advancing to ensure it remains in the superficial subcutaneous tissue.

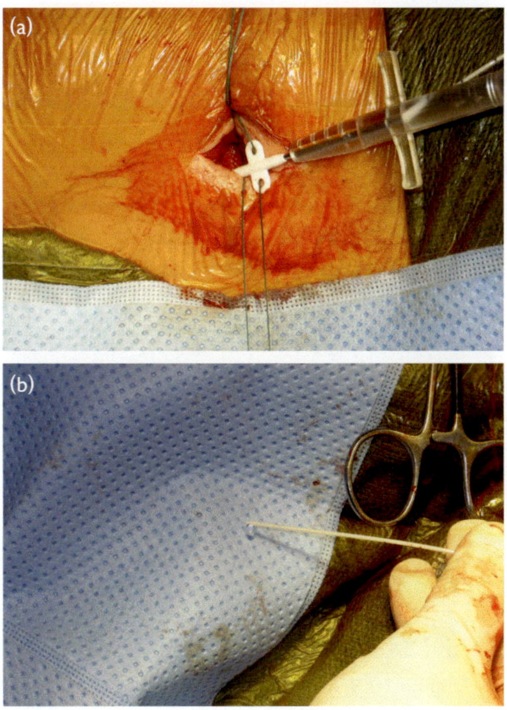

Figure 7.2.5 a, Intrathecal catheter anchored to the fascia. **b,** Confirmation of free CSF flow from the catheter.

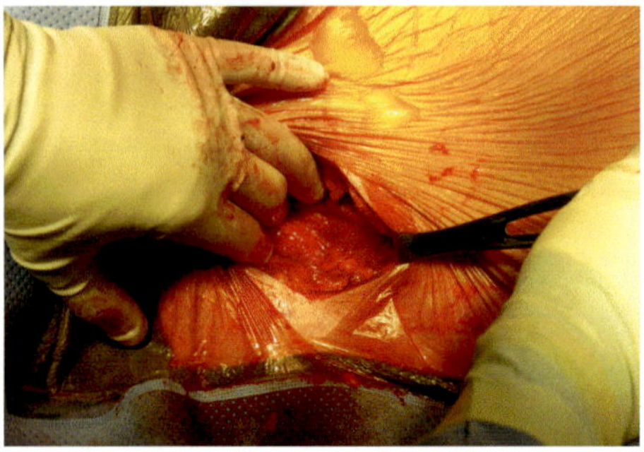

Figure 7.2.6 Creation of a pocket in the subcutaneous tissue by blunt dissection.

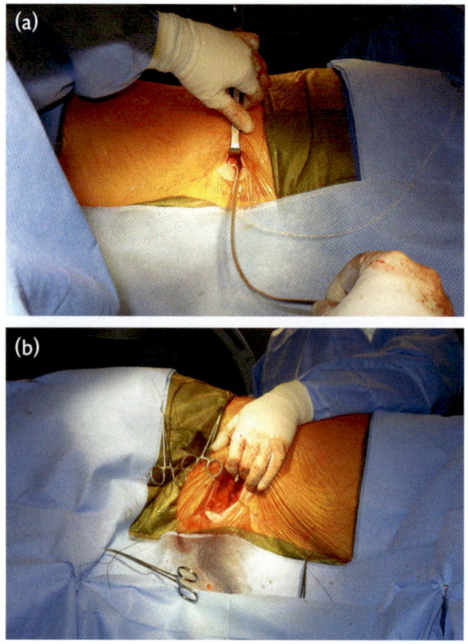

Figure 7.2.7 a & b, Demonstrating the catheter being tunneled from the catheter site to the pocket site.

12. **Reconfirm CSF flow from the catheter (Figure 7.2.8) and attach the catheter to the pump (Figure 7.2.9)**. Create a second loop with the catheter behind the pump to accommodate strain with movement.
    a. Note: The catheter may need to be trimmed prior to attachment to the pump.
13. **Place the pump in the pocket and suture the pump to the abdominal fascia (Figure 7.2.10)**. Ensure the pump reservoir port lies superficially to allow access for medication refills. Take final fluoroscopic images to evaluate the final locations of the catheter and pump.

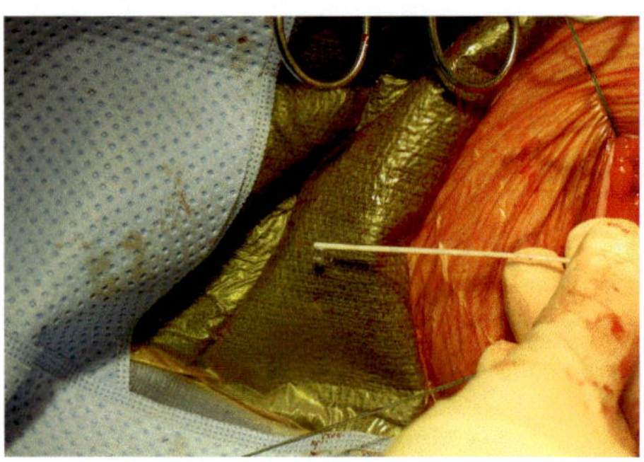

Figure 7.2.8 Reconfirmation of the free CSF flow from the catheter after tunneling.

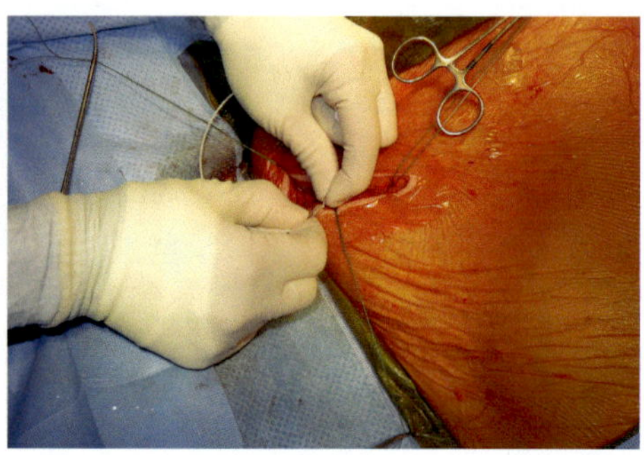

Figure 7.2.9 Attaching the intrathecal catheter to the pump.

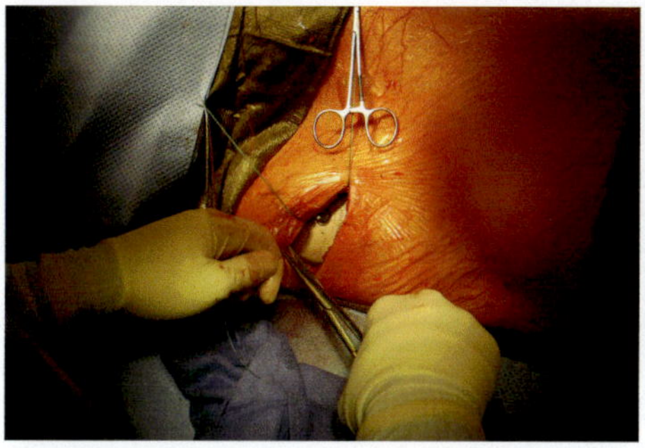

Figure 7.2.10 Placement of the pump in the pocket and then sutured to the abdominal fascia.

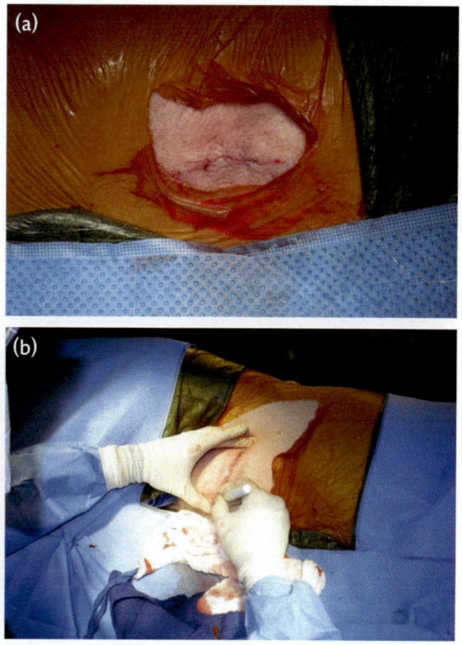

Figure 7.2.11 **a,** Closure of the surgical sites with both subcutaneous and dermal suture layers. **b,** Final closure layer with Dermabond application.

14. **Ensure hemostasis and close incision sites with both subcutaneous and dermal suture layers (**Figure 7.2.11**).** Meticulous pocket closure includes both hemostasis and tight tissue approximation during closure to avoid hematoma and seroma, respectively.

Postoperative Management and Complications

Patients should have a thorough neurologic exam following IDDS placement to evaluate for nerve or spinal cord injury. The pump can be filled with intrathecal medications on the day of implantation or normal saline can be used temporarily. Complications shared with all surgical procedures include bleeding, infection, and injury to adjacent structures. Bleeding can present at the catheter site as an epidural hematoma, possibly leading to spinal cord compression. Bleeding at the pump site may lead to hematoma filling the pump pocket. Infections may be superficial or deep, including neuraxial infection and meningitis. Spinal cord or spinal nerve injury can occur during catheter placement. This risk can be minimized by having a responsive patient during catheter placement. Cerebrospinal fluid leak can occur and lead to postdural puncture headache. Other complications related to the pump and pocket include wound dehiscence, pump migration/turning, and seroma formation. These risks can be mitigated with meticulous wound closure, pump securement, and pocket sizing.

References

1. Bier A. Experiments regarding the cocainization of the spinal cord. Surv Anesth. 1962;6(3):352–358.
2. Denny NM, Selander DE. Continuous spinal anaesthesia. Br J Anesth. 1998;81:590–597.
3. Onofrio, BM, Yaksh TL, Arnold PG. Continuous low-dose intrathecal morphine administration in the treatment of chronic pain of malignant origin. Mayo Clin Proc. 1981;56(8):516–520.

4. Spiegel MA, Chen GH, Solla AC, Hingula LP, Legler A, Gulati A. Evaluation of an intrathecal drug delivery protocol leads to rapid reduction of systemic opioids in the oncological population. J Palliat Med. 2021 Mar;24(3):418–422. doi: 10.1089/jpm.2020.0206.
5. Brogan SE, Winter NB. Patient-controlled intrathecal analgesia for the management of breakthrough cancer pain: a retrospective review and commentary. Pain Med. 2011;12(12):1758–1768.
6. Deer TR, Smith HS, Burton AW, et al.; Center For Pain Relief, Inc. Comprehensive consensus based guidelines on intrathecal drug delivery systems in the treatment of pain caused by cancer pain. Pain Phys. 2011;14(3):E283–E312. PMID: 21587338.
7. Deer TR, Smith HS, Cousins M, et al. Consensus guidelines for the selection and implantation of patients with noncancer pain for intrathecal drug delivery. Pain Phys. 2010;13(3):E175–E213. PMID: 20495597.
8. Khimani N, Narang S. Intrathecal drug delivery system trialing for cancer pain management. In: Gulati A, Puttanniah V, Bruel B, Rosenberg W, Hung J (eds), Essentials of Interventional Cancer Pain Management. Springer, Cham; 2019: 273–276. https://doi.org/10.1007/978-3-319-99684-4_30
9. Malhotra VT, Root J, Kesselbrenner J, et al. Intrathecal pain pump infusions for intractable cancer pain: an algorithm for dosing without a neuraxial trial. Anesth Analg. 2013;116(6):1364–1370. doi: 10.1213/ANE.0b013e31828d670e. Epub 2013 Apr 4. PMID: 23558833; PMCID: PMC5529040.
10. Chen GH, Spiegel MA, Magram YC, Baig E, Clement K, Laufer I, Gulati A. Evaluation of fixed intrathecal bupivacaine infusion doses in the oncologic population. Neuromod. 2020;23(7): 984–990. doi: 10.1111/ner.13161. Epub 2020 Apr 28.

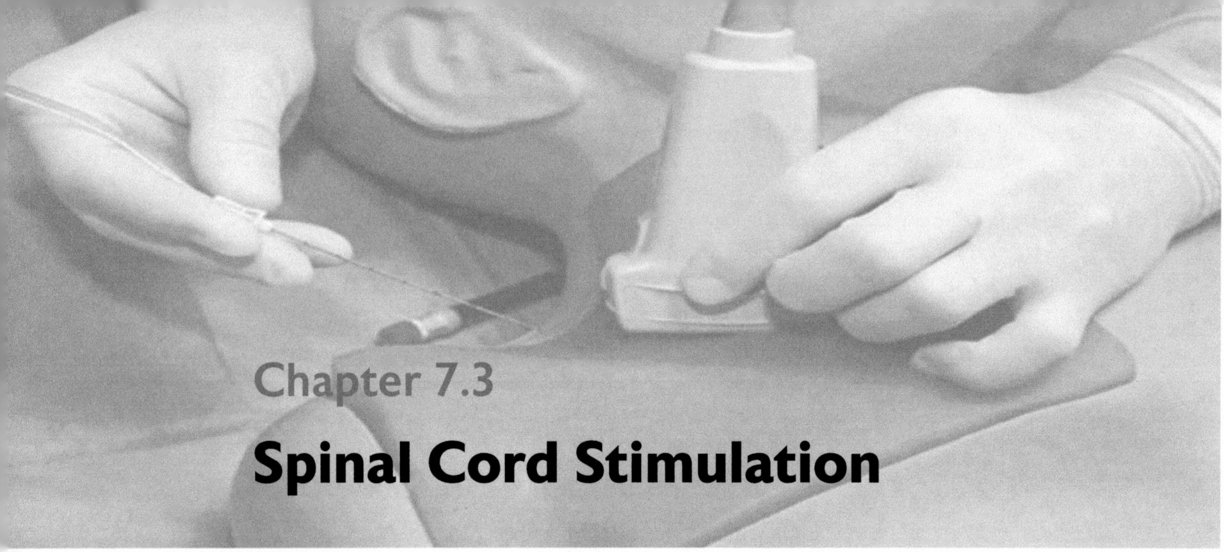

Chapter 7.3

Spinal Cord Stimulation

Aron Legler and Priyanka Ghosh

Contents

Introduction

The first known application of a spinal cord stimulator (SCS) device was in 1967 for a terminal patient suffering with chronic chest and abdominal pain secondary to an inoperable lung cancer that had metastasized to pleura and liver.[1] Since then, the techniques and indications have evolved substantially; however, the basic principle of applying an alternating electric current to the dorsal column of the spinal cord has cemented itself as an indispensable and cost-effective modality in the treatment of certain painful conditions.

Initially, the primary mechanism of pain relief from the SCS was hypothesized to act via the "gate control theory" to inhibit nociceptive input to the spinal cord.[2] Current hypotheses paint a much more complex picture, including central mechanisms for cortical reorganization, inhibition of neural conduction at the dorsal horn and the supraspinal structures, GABAergic and endogenous opioid receptor activation, attenuation of neuronal excitability, and inhibition of glial cell activation.[3]

In the United States, SCS therapy is used less frequently for cancer pain than it is for typical indications including failed back surgery syndrome, complex regional pain syndrome, painful radiculopathies, painful peripheral vascular disease, and neuropathy.[4] Refractory angina is another well studied indication in Europe; however, this is not currently approved for use in the United States.

Spinal cord stimulator systems continue to evolve as breakthroughs in basic science, hardware technology, and programming options continue to advance. Although the downsides of the technology and surgical implantation are not trivial, the incidence of complications is decreasing, likely due to the culmination of improving technology and advancement in surgical technique.[5]

Indications in the Cancer Patient

Spinal cord stimulator therapy holds great promise for various malignancy-related pains as well as iatrogenic pain resulting from cancer treatment. Spinal cord stimulators may benefit patients with inadequate relief despite standard medical management including opiate therapy, nonopiate adjuvants, injections, and others. The goal of the device is not to replace traditional management but rather to supplement it. Patients with intractable pain who undergo SCS implantation have shown significant reductions in their pain medication consumption.[6]

The use of SCS for neuropathic pain is well established in the literature. Sham-controlled studies show significance for this use in this population.[7] and, although the preponderance of this data does not focus on oncologic population, some of this could be generalizable to other etiologies of neuropathic pain. For example, chemotherapy-induced peripheral neuropathy (CIPN) and diabetic peripheral neuropathy are both axonal sensorimotor neuropathies that often present with similar symptoms.[8–9] While SCS has demonstrated benefit for diabetic peripheral neuropathy.[10] there is still a paucity of data for SCS use for CIPN. Given the similarities between the two neuropathies, SCS may be a valid avenue for treatment for patients with CIPN who have failed conservative measures.

Visceral pain remains difficult to treat in the oncologic population, but SCS therapy has shown promise in early studies.[11–13] Examples of SCS therapy in oncologic cases related to visceral pain are presented in Figures 7.3.1–2. In our experience, SCS implants have been helpful in managing both cancer pain of the lumbosacral spine and pelvis and treatment-related pain syndromes, such as radiation neuritis.

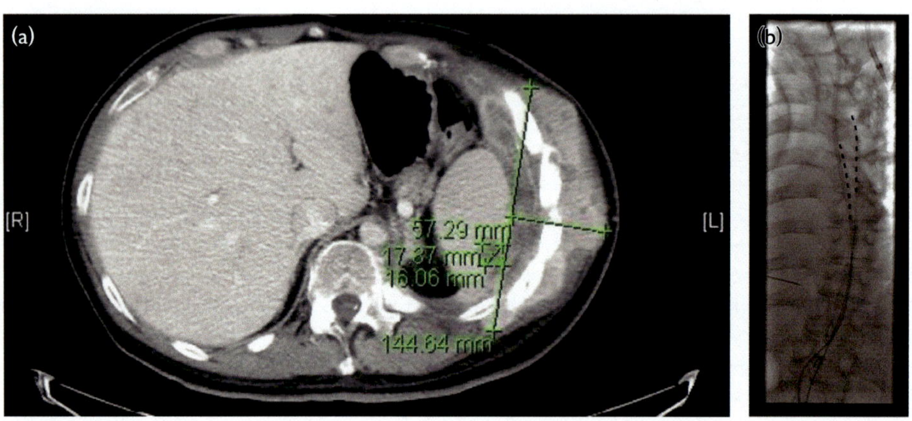

Figure 7.3.1 a, 48-year-old male with active lung cancer and extra pleural metastasis—this is on hospice care with severe chest wall paresthesia presented with uncontrolled pain. Intrathecal drug delivery was used to manage upper lung pain but did not control chest wall pain. **b,** SCS leads were placed in upper thoracic spine with following settings: frequency—500 Hz, pulse width—500 μs. He had significant decrease in pain sensation and passed away comfortably two months post-implant.

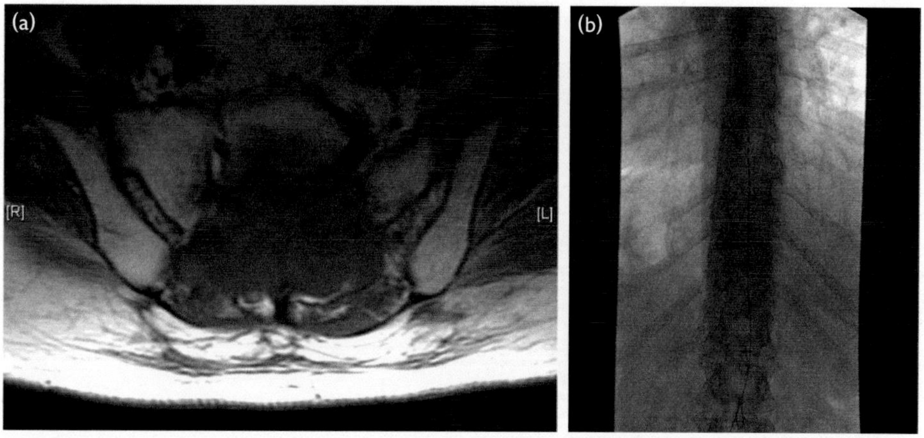

Figure 7.3.2 **a,** 62-year-old female with metastatic chordoma presented with sacral back and bilateral leg pain. A chordoma was radiated in the past but continued to slowly grow post-treatment, causing worsening pain. **b,** Leads were placed covering the T9–T10 interspace, using paresthesia free settings led to pain relief of 2 points on a Numerical Rating Scale.

Trials

Performing a trial with percutaneous leads is a vital step in the patient selection process prior to undergoing permanent implantation. This is important for practical reasons—proving efficacy before implantation—and financial reasons given are required for most insurers to cover the implantable system. The trial involves percutaneous placement of one or two leads for up to one week to allow the patient to gain familiarity with this modality and to assess its efficacy.

A binary question is frequently asked at the end of the trial: "Did you experience at least 50% pain relief?" While this seemingly arbitrary cutoff may be important to documentation for insurance approval, for the cancer patient and particularly those considering undergoing a palliative procedure several other domains should be evaluated prior to deciding to proceed with an implant. The magnitude of pain relief is important but should be considered simultaneously with other potential benefits from the trial including quality of life improvements, change in functional status, psychological impact on the patient, analgesic-sparing effect (and potential decrease in adverse effects from these medications), patient satisfaction, and healthcare cost containment.[3]

The lead placement for the trial is nearly identical to the lead placement for the implant. Both are performed with strict aseptic technique as described below. At the conclusion of the trial period, the percutaneous leads are withdrawn and a washout period begins in order for the patient to compare overall satisfaction with the therapy both during and after its cessation. If the trial is successful and the patient opts to proceed with permanent implantation, the radiographic imagery taken during trial lead placement helps to direct the permanent lead positioning.

We recommend a pretrial MRI to determine ease of placement of trial and subsequent permanent leads. Additionally, the MRI should be recent (1 month or less) for active disease patients to determine whether the neuraxial space has been compromised with disease burden or infection. Finally, if the spine has been radiated in the past, determine which levels were irradiated and place the leads above those levels if possible. Table 7.3.1 presents starting locations for percutaneous lead placement. Of note, these settings are meant for paresthesia stimulation

Table 7.3.1 Percutaneous Lead Placement Recommendations for Given Region of Pain Symptoms

Region of Pain	Electrode Tip Location
Neck	Above C3 (optimal stimulation usually C1–C2).
Shoulder	C2–C4
Hand	C5–C6
Chest/Abdominal Wall	T1–T4 (chest), T4–T6 (abdomen)** Lateral or anterior chest or abdominal pain place lateral epidural space at level of intercostal neuralgia
Anterior Thigh	T9–T11
Posterior Thigh	T9–T12
Foot	L1
Perineum	T11–L1*** (Conus of spinal cord)
Low Back	T8–T10
Buttock	T11–T12

** Both sensory and motor stimulation are often found at the same threshold. Thus, more difficult to obtain therapeutic benefit.
*** Difficult to stimulate. Leads should be placed closer to midline.

Table Adapted from McKenzie-Brown 2020 and Barolat 1993 (14–17).

and paddle lead placement. Newer waveforms may necessitate alternative locations for pain control.[14–17]

Contraindications

Patients who should not be considered for this device include those with metastases in the intrathecal and/or epidural space locally, systemically infected patients, patients unable to tolerate sedation, patients who are unable to consent to or refuse the procedure, or coagulopathies posing an undue risk of epidural hematoma.

Relative contraindications include psychiatric comorbidities, not exhausting conservative management, and significant spinal abnormalities (e.g., hardware disrupting epidural space).

Equipment

Monitors and Patient Preparation

Prior to proceeding with the implant, the clinician should mark an appropriate pocket site for the pulse generator. Care should be taken in this selection in order to avoid areas of pressure (e.g., against skeletal protuberances such as the iliac crest and ribs) or areas of potential cutaneous friction (e.g., the belt-line). Permanent implantation is typically performed under moderate sedation, however in rare circumstances this will need to be tailored to fit the patient's needs.

After obtaining intravenous access, the patient should be placed in the prone position (or less commonly, in the lateral decubitus position) with standard ASA monitors used. Supplemental oxygen will likely be required depending on the depth of sedation.

Antibiotics are recommended and should be tailored toward skin flora. Cefazolin is a commonly chosen agent, but this may need to be modified in case of patient specific factors such as allergies or known antibiotic resistance (e.g., colonization with MRSA).

Fluoroscopy and Procedural Equipment

Spinal cord stimulator trial placement requires:

1. Lidocaine 1%–2% or bupivacaine 0.25% for local infiltration with a small cutaneous needle
2. Loss-of-resistance syringe
3. Spinal needle 3.5" or 5" (optional)
4. Spinal cord stimulator lead(s)
5. 14-gauge needle (curved and/or straight, typically supplied by manufacturer in same kit as the leads)
6. Anchoring device and/or sutures

Implantation requires the above, plus:

1. #11 or #15 blade scalpel
2. Bovie (for hemostasis)
3. Tunneling device
4. Implantable pulse generator

Procedural Technique for Standard Lead Placement

1. **Sterilely prep and drape the patient in accordance with institutional policy.**
2. **Obtain anteroposterior fluoroscopic image of thoracolumbar spine.** Appropriate visualization will include the site of needle entry and the site of epidural access.
3. **Administer subcutaneous local anesthetic.**
4. **(Optional) Use a 25-gauge spinal needle to anesthetize the anticipated path of the larger 14-gauge needle.** Fluoroscopic images of the spinal needle will also help with determining the appropriate angle of approach for the epidural needle.
5. **Insert the epidural needle at least one level below the planned epidural entry site**. Needle insertion is typically performed at a 30–45 degree angle, depending on habitus, and with a paramedian approach. Many practitioners prefer to make contact with lamina below the level of entry and "walk off" the lamina until engaging in ligament. Loss of resistance technique is then used to identify the epidural space. Fluoroscopic images can be obtained intermittently between AP and lateral views to assist in the guidance of the needle.
6. **(Optional) Use of the kit dilator can help ensure smooth entrance of the lead into the epidural space.**
7. **Place the lead a few centimeters into the epidural space.** Confirm using a lateral fluoroscopic image that the lead is proceeding in the dorsal aspect of the epidural space and has not progressed around the cord into the ventral space.
8. **Using live fluoroscopy, drive the lead to the desired target level, approximately 2–3 mm off midline toward the laterality of the patient's pain.** Ensure the lead remains in the dorsal space during this process.
9. **(Depending on manufacturer) Test the lead on a paresthesia setting to ensure the patient has adequate coverage.** This may require a lessening of the depth of sedation in order to allow patient participation. If the patient is under general anesthesia, this may require neuromonitoring of somatosensory evoked potentials to determine accurate placement.
10. **Withdraw epidural needle under live fluoroscopy, with care taken to avoid any lead tip migration during this process.**

Additional Procedural Steps For Implantation

11. **Secure the anchoring device onto the lead(s) and suture in place to the fascial layer.**
12. **Administer subcutaneous local anesthesia and predetermined location of pocket placement.**

13. **Use a #11 or #15 scalpel to make skin incision. Dissect the pocket wide enough to allow for placement of the implantable pulse generator (IPG).** Use of the size-model supplied with most kits can be helpful here, as overly large pockets have an increased risk of seroma formation among other complications.
14. **Using the manufacturer provided tunneling device, bring the tail of the leads into the newly dissected pocket.**
15. **Securely attach the leads to the IPG.** Leave enough slack in the lead to prevent tension from pulling the lead during patient movements.
16. **Place the IPG into the pocket and suture the device to the thoracolumbar fascia.** Take final fluoroscopic images to evaluate the final locations of lead positioning.
17. **Ensure hemostasis and close incision sites with multilevel closure approach including both subcutaneous and dermal layers.** Careful attention to hemostasis, accurate skin approximation, and maintaining sterility is critical to reduce perioperative complications.

Postoperative Management and Complications

Upon arrival into the postanesthesia care unit, patients should have a thorough neurologic exam to evaluate for potential complications. Immediate diagnosis of rare but severe complications such as epidural hematoma or spinal cord injury and appropriate mitigation can help reduce the likelihood of complications including long-term disability. Other periprocedural complications include bleeding (in addition to aforementioned epidural hematoma, this can include bleeding within the tunneling location and/or pocket), surgical site infection, epidural abscess formation, lead migration, IPG disconnection from the leads, hardware failure, and seroma within the pocket. Dural puncture can be particularly symptomatic given increased likelihood of larger dural defect caused by the 14-gauge needle. In the case of severe postdural puncture headaches, conservative measures should be attempted first but epidural blood patch at the level below the entry site can be used. Meticulous attention to detail can help reduce the incidence of these complications and also allow for more rapid diagnosis and treatment.

References

1. Shealy, C. N., J. T. Mortimer, and J. B. Reswick. 1967. "Electrical Inhibition of Pain by Stimulation of the Dorsal Columns: Preliminary Clinical Report." *Anesthesia and Analgesia* 46 (4): 489–91.
2. Melzack, R., and P. D. Wall. 1965. "Pain Mechanisms: A New Theory." *Science* 150 (3699): 971–79.
3. Mekhail, Nagy, Ogi Visnjevac, Gerges Azer, Diana Sue Mehanny, Priya Agrawal, and Victor Foorsov. 2018. "Spinal Cord Stimulation 50 Years Later: Clinical Outcomes of Spinal Cord Stimulation Based on Randomized Clinical Trials; A Systematic Review." *Regional Anesthesia and Pain Medicine* 43 (4): 391–406.
4. Parekh, Raj N. 2017. "Clinical Indications for Spinal Cord Stimulation." *Seminars in Spine Surgery* 29 (3): 147–49.
5. Deer, Timothy R., Nagy Mekhail, David Provenzano, Jason Pope, Elliot Krames, Michael Leong, Robert M. Levy, et al. 2014. "The Appropriate Use of Neurostimulation of the Spinal Cord and Peripheral Nervous System for the Treatment of Chronic Pain and Ischemic Diseases: The Neuromodulation Appropriateness Consensus Committee." *Neuromodulation: Journal of the International Neuromodulation Society* 17 (6): 515–50; discussion 550.
6. Pollard, E. Morgan, Tim J. Lamer, Susan M. Moeschler, Halena M. Gazelka, W. Michael Hooten, Markus A. Bendel, Nafisseh S. Warner, and M. Hassan Murad. 2019. "The Effect of Spinal Cord Stimulation on Pain Medication Reduction in Intractable Spine and Limb Pain: A Systematic Review of Randomized Controlled Trials and Meta-Analysis." *Journal of Pain Research* 12 (April): 1311–24.

7. Duarte, Rui V., Sarah Nevitt, Ewan McNicol, Rod S. Taylor, Eric Buchser, Richard B. North, and Sam Eldabe. 2020. "Systematic Review and Meta-Analysis of Placebo/Sham Controlled Randomised Trials of Spinal Cord Stimulation for Neuropathic Pain." *Pain* 161 (1): 24–35.
8. Zajączkowska, Renata, Magdalena Kocot-Kępska, Wojciech Leppert, Anna Wrzosek, Joanna Mika, and Jerzy Wordliczek. 2019. "Mechanisms of Chemotherapy-Induced Peripheral Neuropathy." *International Journal of Molecular Sciences* 20 (6): 1451. https://doi.org/10.3390/ijms20061451.
9. Azhary, Hend, Muhammad U. Farooq, Minal Bhanushali, Arshad Majid, and Mounzer Y. Kassab. 2010. "Peripheral Neuropathy: Differential Diagnosis and Management." *American Family Physician* 81 (7): 887–92.
10. Vos, Cecile C. de, Kaare Meier, Paul Brocades Zaalberg, Harold J. A. Nijhuis, Wim Duyvendak, Jan Vesper, Thomas P. Enggaard, and Mathieu W. P. M. Lenders. 2014. "Spinal Cord Stimulation in Patients with Painful Diabetic Neuropathy: A Multicentre Randomized Clinical Trial." *Pain* 155 (11): 2426–31.
11. Hunter, Corey, Nimish Davé, Sudhir Diwan, and Timothy Deer. 2013. "Neuromodulation of Pelvic Visceral Pain: Review of the Literature and Case Series of Potential Novel Targets for Treatment." *Pain Practice: The Official Journal of World Institute of Pain* 13 (1): 3–17.
12. Kapural, Leonardo, Hassan Nagem, Heather Tlucek, and Daniel I. Sessler. 2010. "Spinal Cord Stimulation for Chronic Visceral Abdominal Pain." *Pain Medicine* 11 (3): 347–55.
13. Baranidharan, Ganesan, Karen H. Simpson, and Karthikeyan Dhandapani. 2014. "Spinal Cord Stimulation for Visceral Pain: A Novel Approach." *Neuromodulation: Journal of the International Neuromodulation Society* 17 (8): 753–58; discussion 758.
14. McKenzie-Brown, Anne Marie. 2020. "Spinal Cord Stimulation: Placement and Management." In *UpToDate*, edited by Scott Fishman and Marianna Crowley. Waltham, MA: UpToDate.
15. Barolat, G., F. Massaro, J. He, S. Zeme, and B. Ketcik. 1993. "Mapping of Sensory Responses to Epidural Stimulation of the Intraspinal Neural Structures in Man." *Journal of Neurosurgery* 78 (2): 233–39.
16. Taghva, Alexander, Edward Karst, and Paul Underwood. 2017. "Clinical Paresthesia Atlas Illustrates Likelihood of Coverage Based on Spinal Cord Stimulator Electrode Location." *Neuromodulation: Journal of the International Neuromodulation Society* 20 (6): 582–88.
17. Yang, Michael I. 2017. "Anatomy for Traditional Spinal Cord Stimulation and Barolat Map." In *Treatment of Chronic Pain Conditions: A Comprehensive Handbook*, edited by Jason E. Pope and Timothy R. Deer, 207–8. New York, NY: Springer.

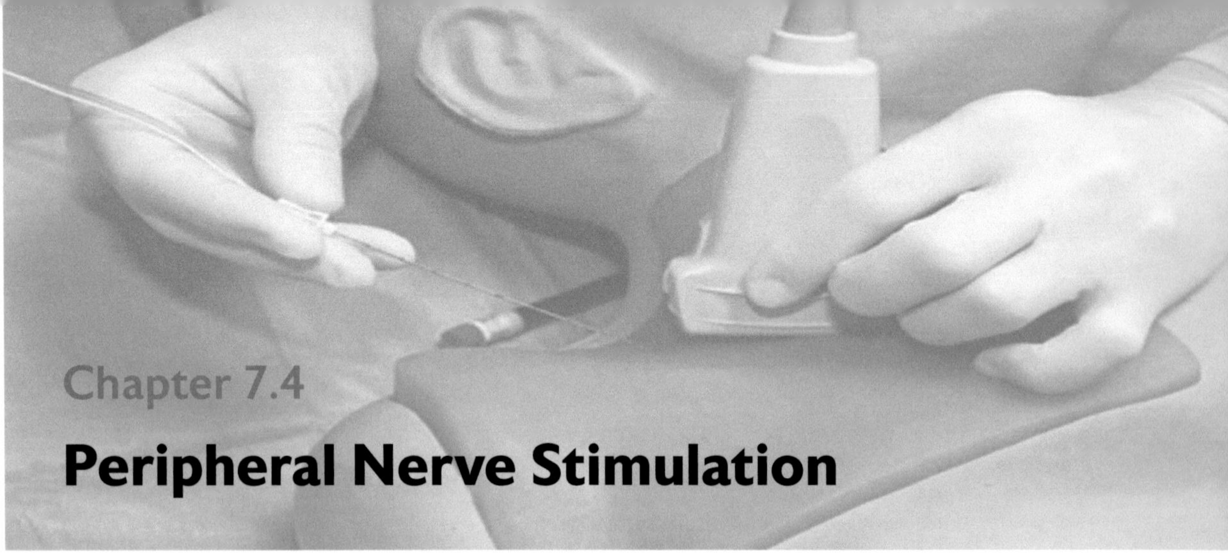

Chapter 7.4

Peripheral Nerve Stimulation

Ojas Mainkar and Grant Chen

Contents

Introduction

Oncologic patients suffer from pain syndromes originating directly from the neoplasm on adjacent structures and nerves, from side effects of treatments, and from causes unrelated to malignancy.[1] This chapter discusses applications of peripheral nerve stimulation (PNS) to treat pain caused directly by neoplasm as well as the treatment side effects. These side effects include postsurgical pain, chemotherapy and immunotherapy-induced neuropathy, and radiation-induced neuritis.[2]

Peripheral nerve stimulation has been used for decades. The earliest versions used invasive paddles and devices that needed to be surgically placed adjacent to neural targets. Later, percutaneous techniques were designed for dorsal column stimulation. More recently, several percutaneous devices have entered the market that are specifically designed for PNS, improving efficacy and reducing complications such as infection and lead migration. Unfortunately, studies focusing on the oncologic population are limited to a few case series published in 2020. These studies demonstrated approaches targeting the brachial plexus, suprascapular nerve, sciatic nerve, femoral nerve, and proximal spinal nerves.[2–3] In addition, this chapter highlights several novel techniques and neural targets in oncologic patients based on neural targets studied in nononcologic patients.

There are multiple proposed theories for the mechanism of action of PNS. One is the gate control theory, which postulates that orthodromic activation of A-beta fibers leads to inhibition of pain signals from A-delta and C nerve fibers due to finite limitations in bandwidth that can be transmitted. This inhibition is thought to be carried out by the inhibitory interneurons in the dorsal horn. Another theory focuses on the local, peripheral effects of PNS. Studies have shown that PNS alters local levels of chemical mediators, such as neurotransmitters and endorphins, which may increase latency of nociceptive nerve fibers creating an analgesic effect.[2]

General Technique

The procedure can be performed using either ultrasound guidance and/or fluoroscopy depending on the specific neural target. Ultrasound guidance allows for efficient placement of leads without the need for a fluoroscopy suite. It has been demonstrated that these leads can be placed with an average time of about 20 minutes per lead.[3] The general technique is listed below with the understanding that each PNS manufacturer provides a slight variation to their device.

1. The neural target or bony landmark location should be visualized using an appropriate ultrasound probe. Generally, a linear probe is used for extremities, femoral nerve, brachial plexus, and paravertebral targets, while a curvilinear probe is used for sciatic nerves and spinal nerves.
2. In most cases depending on the manufacturer, a manufacturer-provided stimulating finder needle is advanced within 1–1.5 cm of the target nerve. This is felt to be the appropriate distance to avoid nerve damage while still achieving "comfortable sensations" in the distribution of the target nerve.
3. Testing is then done with the finder needle in place to determine whether the nerve stimulator covers the location of pain.
4. Once the location is satisfactory, the finder needle is replaced with a manufacturer-provided introducer needle that facilitates deployment of the PNS lead using a Seldinger technique though the initial finder needle.
5. The external portion of the stimulating lead is then connected to a dermally mounted pulse generator.[2–3]

Each company's device is slightly different. The devices vary in the location of the pulse generator and power source as well as the duration of implantation. All the devices on the market at this time use perceptible paresthesias although future devices may incorporate subthreshold paresthesias similar to newer spinal cord stimulators.

Neural Targets

Peripheral Mononeuropathies

Peripheral nerve stimulation can be used to treat peripheral mononeuropathies, which will often manifest as localized extremity or somatic truncal pain. This type of pain can be more difficult to target with typical dorsal column stimulation. In the upper extremity, PNS can be placed by the brachial plexus, suprascapular nerve, and any of the individual nerves of the arms. In the truncal region, the ilioinguinal, genitofemoral, or intercostal nerves can be targeted. In the lower extremity, the femoral nerve, sciatic nerve, lateral femoral cutaneous nerve, or any of the more distal nerves in the lower extremities including the ankle and foot can be targeted. The specific target should be determined by the location of the patient's pain and symptoms. Prior to implanting a PNS, many providers perform a peripheral nerve block with local anesthetic as a trial to predict responsiveness to PNS. The use of a trial block prior to PNS is an area of ongoing research.[4]

Oncologic patients are at increased risk of extremity pain for a variety of reasons. A majority of oncologic PNS case reports treated patients with pain associated with extremity tumors or pain as a sequela of resection.[2] Additionally, these patients are at risk of developing pain related to chemotherapy-induced peripheral neuropathy or complex regional pain syndrome.

One other popular target for PNS has been medial branches of the dorsal rami to treat axial back pain from facet arthropathy. With this technique, the stimulator leads will classically lead to activation of the multifidus muscle.[4] Although facet arthropathy is not an oncologic pathology, it is often a comorbid chronic pain pathology in oncologic patients and an increasingly popular application of PNS.[4]

Spinal Nerve Targets

Targeting the spinal nerve for stimulation is a relatively new technique that has been used to treat a variety of dermatomal pain syndromes. A technique similar to regional anesthesia is used to access the paravertebral space or erector spinae plane. Next, the stimulation lead is positioned near the spinal nerve, just lateral to where the nerve exits the intervertebral foramen. At this point, paresthesias will be triggered in the dermatomal distribution in both the ventral and dorsal rami. Potential indications for this target include postmastectomy pain, complex regional pain syndrome, post-thoracotomy pain, postherpetic neuralgia, and lumbar radiculopathy. Peripheral nerve stimulation has been successfully performed at the cervical, thoracic, and lumbar levels. A key advantage of this technique is that it provides a less invasive alternative for the treatment of dermatomal pain compared to dorsal column or dorsal root ganglion stimulation. It can be performed under ultrasound guidance without the need for a fluoroscopy suite depending on clinician comfort with ultrasound anatomy.[3]

Special Considerations in Oncology Patients

MRI Compatibility

Magnetic resonance imaging is considered the standard of care for routine surveillance and monitoring in cancer patients because it provides superior soft tissue image quality without exposure to radiation.[5] Most patients receive several MRIs during their first two years after diagnosis. A study on pediatric neurologic soft-tissue tumors showed patients typically received 2–4 MRI scans within the first year, 1–2 scans in the second year, and annually thereafter.[6] Pain providers need to consider the patient's need for MRI prior to implantation. Like other implanted devices, PNS devices usually have restrictions on MRI compatibility.

Fractured Leads

One of the most common complications with PNS is retained, fractured leads. This can occur spontaneously or during device extraction.[7–9] A recent study on some PNS leads showed a 7.5% incidence of lead fracture on extraction.[9] A majority of fractured leads do not need any further treatment, but the patient should be made aware of the complication in case they develop symptoms. Additionally, the leads may place permanent restrictions on MRI compatibility. Our literature review showed one case report of a patient who had to have removal of a PNS due to an urgent MRI.[2]

Risk of Infection

As with implantation of any foreign body, infection is always a concern and this is heightened in cancer patients suffering from immunosuppression as a consequence of myelosuppressive chemotherapy or hematopoietic stem cell transplantation. Neutropenic patients are unable to mount an immunologic response to infectious agents and often present with febrile neutropenia as the only presenting sign of infection. Febrile neutropenia is a medical emergency requiring hospitalization and aggressive intravenous antibiotic treatment.[10] The incidence of febrile neutropenia in patients undergoing their first chemotherapy cycle is about 5%–6%.[11]

Management of Anticoagulation and Hypercoagulability

Cancer patients are at 6.5-fold higher risk of venous thromboembolism (VTE) compared to the average population. One in 200 cancer patients will develop a VTE, which is the second-leading cause of death in this patient population, only behind the malignancy itself.[12] Implementing PNS while patients are on systemic anticoagulation is considered intermediate-to-high risk depending on the vascularity and compressibility of the targeted area, according to recent American Society of Regional Anesthesia guidelines. Based on this risk stratification, all patients should hold anticoagulants for five half-lives until full resolution of their anticoagulant effect prior to performing the procedure and should restart novel oral anticoagulants 24 hours after the procedure.[13]

Chemotherapy-Induced Wound-Healing Impairment

Bevacizumab is an anti–vascular endothelial growth factor (VEGF) monoclonal antibody used for neoadjuvant or adjuvant chemotherapy. It is approved for use in metastatic colorectal cancer, renal cell carcinoma (RCC), glioblastoma multiforme (GBM), and non–small cell lung cancer (NSCLC). Bevacizumab has been shown to impair wound healing due to impaired angiogenesis when used to treat metastatic colorectal cancer. No increase in wound healing was found with RCC or NSCLC. No prior studies have looked at the incidence specifically in GBM. However, this is based on limited evidence and further studies will be needed to confirm the malignancy-specific association of this side effect. As bevacizumab has a half-life of 20 days, surgery is not recommended within 60 days of initiation and bevacizumab should not be restarted until 28 days after surgery or until the surgical incision has fully healed. The most common complications seen were incisional hernias and dehiscence.[14] This risk of impaired wound healing needs to be considered in choosing the appropriate treatment options for oncologic patients.

Conclusion

PNS is a new field that has the potential to have many applications for treating pain in oncologic patients. Interest in this field has been spurred by the introduction of several percutaneously implanted devices to the market over the past decade. These techniques have several unique advantages compared to more invasive forms of neuromodulation pertaining to specific challenges encountered in oncologic patients, including risk of infection, anticoagulation, and ability to tolerate invasive procedures. As of now, there is a limited but growing body of literature in the use of PNS in oncologic patients. Potential uses that should be considered include postmastectomy pain, complex regional pain syndrome, postherpetic neuralgia, chronic postsurgical pain from nerve transection, post-thoracotomy pain, or chemotherapy-induced neuropathy.

References

1. K. D. Candido, T. M. Kusper, and N. N. Knezevic, "New Cancer Pain Treatment Options," *Curr. Pain Headache Rep.*, vol. 21, no. 2, p. 12, 2017, doi: 10.1007/s11916-017-0613-0.
2. O. Mainkar, C. A. Sollo, G. Chen, A. Legler, and A. Gulati, "Pilot Study in Temporary Peripheral Nerve Stimulation in Oncologic Pain," *Neuromod.*, vol. 23, no. 6, pp. 819–826, 2020, doi: 10.1111/ner.13139.
3. O. Mainkar, H. Singh, A. Gargya, J. Lee, A. Valimahomed, and A. Gulati, "Ultrasound-GuidedPeripheral Nerve Stimulation of Cervical, Thoracic, and Lumbar Spinal Nerves for Dermatomal Pain: A Case Series," *Neuromodulation Technol. Neural Interface*, vol. 24, no. 6, pp. 1059–1066, 2021, doi: 10.1111/ner.13334.
4. C. A. Gilmore, J. Patel, L. G. Esebua, and M. Burchell, "A Review of Peripheral Nerve Stimulation Techniques Targeting the Medial Branches of the Lumbar Dorsal Rami in the Treatment of Chronic Low Back Pain," *Pain Med.*, vol. 21, no. 1, pp. S41–S46, 2020, doi: 10.1093/pm/pnaa084.

5. S. Radhakrishna *et al.*, "Departments of 1 Medical Oncology, 5 Radiology, 6 Surgery and 7 CT Scan and MRI, Sir Ganga Ram Hospital," 2018, doi: 10.4103/sajc.sajc_104_18.
6. S. P. Stevens *et al.*, "The Utility of Routine Surveillance Screening with Magnetic Resonance Imaging (MRI) to Detect Tumour Recurrence in Children with Low-Grade Central Nervous System (CNS) Tumours: A Systematic Review," *J. Neurooncol.*, vol. 139, pp. 507–522, 2018, doi: 10.1007/s11060-018-2901-x.
7. B. M. Ilfeld *et al.*, "Ultrasound-Guided Percutaneous Peripheral Nerve Stimulation: Neuromodulation of the suprascapular Nerve and Brachial Plexus for Postoperative Analgesia Following Ambulatory Rotator Cuff Repair: A Proof-of-Concept Study," *Reg. Anesth. Pain Med.*, vol. 44, no. 3, pp. 310–318, Mar. 2019, doi: 10.1136/rapm-2018-100121.
8. B. M. Ilfeld *et al.*, "Ultrasound-Guided Percutaneous Peripheral Nerve Stimulation for Analgesia Following Total Knee Arthroplasty: A Prospective Feasibility Study," *J. Orthop. Surg. Res.*, vol. 12, no. 1, pp. 506–507, Jan. 2017, doi: 10.1186/s13018-016-0506-7.
9. B. M. Ilfeld *et al.*, "A Feasibility Study of Percutaneous Peripheral Nerve Stimulation for the Treatment of Postoperative Pain Following Total Knee Arthroplasty," *Neuromodulation*, vol. 22, no. 5, pp. 653–660, Jul. 2019, doi: 10.1111/ner.12790.
10. J. Crawford, D. C. Dale, and G. H. Lyman, "Chemotherapy-Induced Neutropenia Risks, Consequences, and New Directions for Its Management," *Cancer*, vol. 100, pp. 228–265, 2004, doi: 10.1002/cncr.11882.
11. T. Aagaard *et al.*, "Development and Validation of a Risk Score for Febrile Neutropenia After Chemotherapy in Patients with Cancer: The FENCE Score," *JNCI Cancer Spectr.*, vol. 2, no. 4, p. pky053, 2018, doi: 10.1093/jncics/pky053.
12. A. A. Khorana *et al.*, "Duration of Anticoagulant Therapy and VTE Recurrence in Patients With cancer," *Support Care Cancer.*, vol. 27, no. 10, pp. 3833–3840, 2019, doi: 10.1007/s00520-019-4661-3.
13. S. Narouze *et al.*, "Interventional Spine and Pain Procedures in Patients on Antiplatelet and Anticoagulant Medications (Second Edition): Guidelines from the American Society of Regional Anesthesia and Pain Medicine, the European Society of Regional Anaesthesia and Pain Therapy, the American Academy of Pain Medicine, the International Neuromodulation Society, the North American Neuromodulation Society, and the World Institute of Pain," *Reg. Anesth. Pain Med.*, vol. 43, no. 3, pp. 225–262, 2018, doi: 10.1097/AAP.0000000000000700.
14. H. Zhang, Z. Huang, X. Zou, and T. Liu, "Bevacizumab and Wound-Healing Complications: A Systematic Review and Meta-Analysis of Randomized Controlled Trials," *Oncotarget.*, vol. 7, no. 50, pp. 82473–82481, 2016

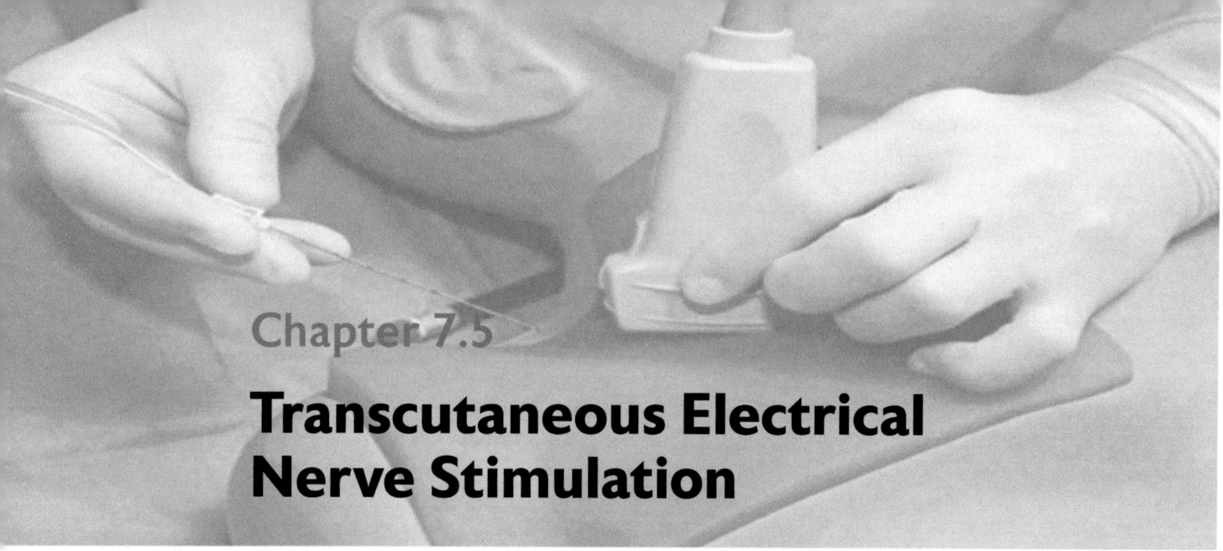

Chapter 7.5

Transcutaneous Electrical Nerve Stimulation

Kelly Leap

Contents

Introduction

Transcutaneous electrical nerve stimulation (TENS) is a noninvasive, nonpharmacologic intervention used for both acute and chronic pain. Given its low risk and low side-effect profile, TENS serves as a safe adjunctive intervention for multimodal pain management. The most common TENS applications include conventional TENS (low intensity, high frequency), acupuncture-like TENS (high intensity, low frequency), and pulsed/burst TENS (low intensity, high frequency bursts).[1–4] Of the three applications, conventional TENS remains the preferred technique in the oncologic population due to its targeted effect on sensory nerve stimulation.[4] Whereas conventional TENS does not incite a painful response during use, acupuncture-like TENS may be quite painful and, thus, less tolerated in the oncologic population.[1,5] However, TENS does not typically produce long-lasting pain relief; therefore, frequent and repeated use is recommended, particularly during painful episodes. Because TENS is intended for self-administration after proper patient education, this intervention provides patients with great control and autonomy over their pain management. The mechanism of action for conventional TENS can be understood by the gate control theory, whereby TENS stimulates large-diameter (A-beta) fibers and inhibits small-diameter (A-delta and C-fiber) fibers in the substantia gelatinosa of the spinal cord to ultimately decrease pain perception.[1,6–7]

Indications

Debate exists regarding the clinical efficacy of TENS for cancer pain, as many of the current studies lack power or sufficient sample sizes. The most updated Cochrane review that evaluated the effectiveness of TENS for cancer-related pain in adult patients found insufficient evidence supporting the use of TENS for cancer pain, as it only identified three RCTs, with contradictory results.[1] Of the three RCTs, Bennett et al. was the only study that observed a statistically significant reduction in pain, specifically bone metastasis-related pain, with high-frequency TENS (80 Hz).[1,8]

Because conventional TENS is preferred for the oncologic population, this chapter will specifically identify studies that used high-frequency, low-intensity settings. Since Hurlow and colleagues' systematic review, several studies have demonstrated either a clinically or statistically significant benefit with conventional TENS. Whereas some studies broadly explored the effect of TENS on cancer pain without differentiating specific oncologic diagnoses,[5,9] most studies focused on one specific cancer subpopulation. Of the two studies that observed more general populations with various cancer diagnoses, Loh and Gulati found statistically significant reductions in pain with high-frequency TENS (>80 Hz), whereas Siemens et al. did not observe a significant improvement in pain with high-frequency TENS (80Hz).[5,9] The bulk of studies exploring conventional TENS in the oncologic setting focused more specifically on a single cancer subpopulation such as head and neck cancer patients with mucositis pain secondary to radiation therapy,[6] cancer patients with advanced disease-related pain,[10] sarcoma patients with bone pain secondary to tumor resection,[11] lung cancer patients with post-thoracotomy pain,[12] and cancer patients with chemotherapy-induced peripheral neuropathy.[13] The studies used TENS with varying frequencies, ranging from 60 to 125 Hz. Lee and colleagues used the highest frequency of 125 Hz in their randomized crossover pilot study and observed significantly reduced oral mucositis resting pain in head and neck cancer patients.[6] Nakano and colleagues used a slightly lower frequency of 100 Hz in their randomized crossover pilot study and found a statistically significant reduction in pain scores immediately after TENS as compared to prior, as well as a statistically significant reduction in average pain scores during the day.[10] Loh and Gulati similarly found a reduction in sarcoma-related pain in their case series using variable frequencies of at least 80 Hz.[11] Fiorelli and colleagues used 80 Hz with each participant in their randomized prospective study and found a statistically significant reduction in post-thoracotomy pain.[12] Lastly, Gewandter and colleagues used a frequency range of 60–100 Hz and found a statistically significant reduction in peripheral neuropathy pain in their feasibility study.[13]

Though not commonly practiced due to limitations in this population, acupuncture-like and pulsed/burst TENS have also shown promising results in cancer pain populations, specifically breast cancer patients with postmastectomy pain.[14] Silva and colleagues conducted a randomized clinical trial that observed a decrease in postmastectomy intercostobrachial nerve pain with both acupuncture and pulsed/burst TENS.[14]

Contraindications

Absolute contraindications to TENS include patients with cardiac pacemakers, metal implants on electrode sites, and implantable cardioverter defibrillators.[2,9] Additional precautions include arrhythmias, pregnancy, epilepsy, active malignancy, deep-vein thrombosis, nonintact skin, and a history of allergy to electrodes or adhesives.[2,9] Transcutaneous electrical nerve stimulation should not be used over the carotid sinuses due to risk of hypotension, the anterior neck due to risk of laryngospasm, directly over sites of active disease, or areas of sensory impairment due to risk of unintentional burns.[3] Lastly, TENS should be used cautiously in patients with either a spinal cord stimulator or intrathecal pump due to risk of device interactions.[3]

Critical Anatomy

Transcutaneous electrical nerve stimulation can be applied to the skin several ways—directly over the site of pain, in a dermatomal or neurotomal pattern that corresponds to the painful area or organ, over nerve bundles proximal to the site of pain, on trigger points, or on acupuncture sites.[1,4] The pads should be placed no further than three inches from each other as greater distances are not conducive to the low-intensity settings.

Equipment and Patient Preparation

- Monitors:
  - No special monitors are needed for this procedure.
- TENS Unit: 1 or more electrical-signal generators, 1 battery, 1 set of electrodes with adhesive pads.
  - Pad sizes vary based on anatomical location.
- Patient position: patients are encouraged to change positions during therapy and perform normal activities such as walking, standing, or sitting to observe benefit.

Procedure Technique

1. Set the amplitude (mA), frequency/pulse rate (Hz), and duration/pulse width (ms). Typical amplitude ranges from 0 to 100 mA; typical frequency/pulse rate ranges from 1 to 250 Hz; and typical duration/pulse width ranges from 10 to 1000 ms.[4]
   a. Conventional TENS Settings: Frequency/pulse rate: 40–150 Hz; Amplitude: 10–30 mA; duration/pulse width: <50 ms.[3]
   b. Acupuncture TENS Settings: frequency/pulse rate: 1–10 Hz; amplitude: as high as tolerated by patient.[3]
   c. Pulsed/Burst TENS Settings: burst frequency/pulse rate: 1–2 Hz; impulses within burst frequency/pulse rate: 100 Hz.[3]
2. Clean the skin with a mild soap and thoroughly dry the skin prior to pad placement.
3. Apply the electrode pads approximately 1–3 inches apart on the skin.
4. Set the amplitude (mA) to a strong, but comfortable, intensity as tolerated by the patient.
5. Treatment duration: 20–60 mins.[6,8,10,11,15]
6. Treatment frequency: up to 6 times daily.[8,11,15]

Tips

- Given the numerous options for TENS settings, patients are encouraged to trial various options to ultimately achieve optimal pain relief.[3–4]
- Patients are encouraged to include a caregiver in the education process, as the caregiver may help apply the pads to otherwise inaccessible areas.
- Patients are encouraged to use TENS when experiencing pain and to continue with normal activities while using TENS, such as walking, standing, or sitting.[11]
- The use of caffeine prior to TENS may decrease TENS efficacy.[4]
- If TENS is used frequently throughout the day, patients do not need to remove pads between use, but rather disconnect/reconnect the pads to the device as needed.

Safety Considerations

- Setting the amplitude too high may cause discomfort.[4]
- Setting the duration/pulse width too high (>100 ms) may cause muscle contraction.[4]
- High electrical intensity may cause skin burns or irritation.[4]
- The adhesive on the electrical pads may cause skin sensitivity or irritation. Pads should be regularly replaced as needed and removed by pulling in the direction of the patient's hair.
- TENS is associated with a theoretical risk of cancer recurrence at the site of stimulation due to increased muscle activity and blood flow.[5] However, maintaining TENS settings at a level below motor threshold greatly reduces this risk.[4] Loh and Gulati recommend high frequency (>80 Hz) as a safe setting for the oncologic population.[5] Direct stimulation over a tumor should be avoided.[10]

Postprocedure Management

No special postprocedure management considerations are associated with this procedure.

References

1. Hurlow A, Bennett MI, Robb KA, Johnson MI, Simpson KH, Oxberry SG. Transcutaneous electric nerve stimulation (TENS) for cancer pain in adults. Cochrane Database Syst Rev. 2012;2012(3):CD006276. Published 2012 Mar 14. doi:10.1002/14651858.CD006276.pub3
2. Johnson MI, Jones G, Paley CA, Wittkopf PG. The clinical efficacy of transcutaneous electrical nerve stimulation (TENS) for acute and chronic pain: a protocol for a meta-analysis of randomised controlled trials (RCTs). BMJ Open. 2019;9(10):e029999. Published 2019 Oct 28. doi:10.1136/bmjopen-2019-029999
3. Kaye V, Brandstater ME. Transcutaneous electrical nerve stimulation. Medscape. https://emedicine.medscape.com/article/325107-overview#a1. Published November 12, 2019. Accessed January 28, 2021.
4. Loh J. Transcutaneous electrical nerve stimulation for cancer pain. In Gulati A, Puttanniah V, Bruel BM, Rosenberg WS, Hung JC (Eds.). 2019:261–265. Essentials of Interventional Cancer Pain Management. Springer International Publishing.
5. Loh J, Gulati A. The use of transcutaneous electrical nerve stimulation (TENS) in a major cancer center for the treatment of severe cancer-related pain and associated disability. Pain Med. 2015;16(6):1204–1210. doi:10.1111/pme.12038
6. Lee JE, Anderson CM, Perkhounkova Y, Sleeuwenhoek BM, Louison RR. Transcutaneous electrical nerve stimulation reduces resting pain in head and neck cancer patients: a randomized and placebo-controlled double-blind pilot study. Cancer Nurs. 2019;42(3):218–228. doi:10.1097/NCC.0000000000000594
7. Melzack R, Wall PD. Pain mechanisms: a new theory. Science. 1965;150(3699):971–979. doi:10.1126/science.150.3699.971
8. Bennett MI, Johnson MI, Brown SR, Radford H, Brown JM, Searle RD. Feasibility study of transcutaneous electrical nerve stimulation (TENS) for cancer bone pain. J Pain. 2010;11(4):351–359. doi:10.1016/j.jpain.2009.08.002
9. Siemens W, Boehlke C, Bennett MI, Offner K, Becker G, Gaertner J. Transcutaneous electrical nerve stimulation for advanced cancer pain inpatients in specialist palliative care-a blinded, randomized, sham-controlled pilot cross-over trial. Support Care Cancer. 2020;28(11):5323–5333. doi:10.1007/s00520-020-05370-8
10. Nakano J, Ishii K, Fukushima T, et al. Effects of transcutaneous electrical nerve stimulation on physical symptoms in advanced cancer patients receiving palliative care. Int J Rehabil Res. 2020;43(1):62–68. doi:10.1097/MRR.0000000000000386

11. Loh J, Gulati A. Transcutaneous electrical nerve stimulation for treatment of sarcoma cancer pain. Pain Manag. 2013;3(3):189–199. doi:10.2217/pmt.13.15
12. Fiorelli A, Morgillo F, Milione R, et al. Control of post-thoracotomy pain by transcutaneous electrical nerve stimulation: effect on serum cytokine levels, visual analogue scale, pulmonary function and medication. Eur J Cardiothorac Surg. 2012;41(4):861–868. doi:10.1093/ejcts/ezr108
13. Gewandter JS, Chaudari J, Ibegbu C, et al. Wireless transcutaneous electrical nerve stimulation device for chemotherapy-induced peripheral neuropathy: an open-label feasibility study. Support Care Cancer. 2019;27(5):1765–1774. doi:10.1007/s00520-018-4424-6
14. Silva JG, Santana CG, Inocêncio KR, Orsini M, Machado S, Bergmann A. Electrocortical analysis of patients with intercostobrachial pain treated with TENS after breast cancer surgery. J Phys Ther Sci. 2014;26(3):349–353. doi:10.1589/jpts.26.349
15. Gadsby JG, Franks A, Jarvis P, Dewhurst F. Acupuncture-like transcutaneous electrical nerve stimulation within palliative care: a pilot study. Compliment Therap Med. 1997;5(1):13–18.

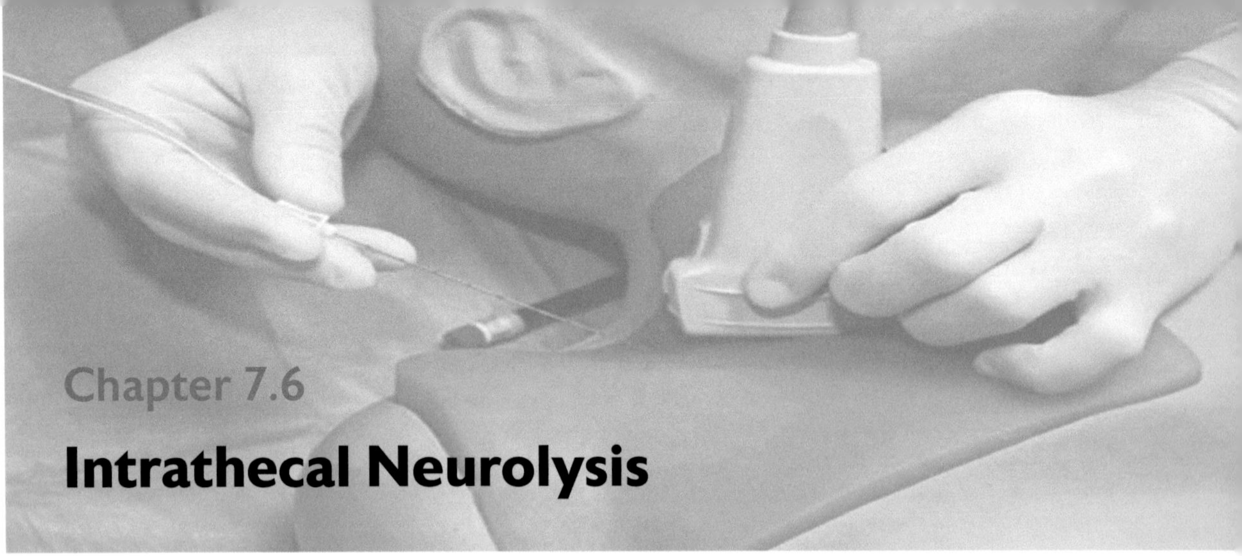

Chapter 7.6

Intrathecal Neurolysis

B. Carolina Hernández-Porras, Ricardo Plancarte, Angel Manuel Juárez-Lemus, Marcela Sámano-García, Rocío Guillén-Nuñez, and Ale Ismael García-Cazares

Contents

Introduction

As cancer rates are increasing worldwide, cancer pain is similarly increasing and is of great concern given its severe impact on quality of life.[1] Disruption of pain pathways through injections of neurolytic agents is a well-established modality in cancer pain treatments.[2] Intrathecal neurolysis is considered when cancer pain is intractable despite medical and interventional therapies.[3,4] The anatomical separation of the sensory and motor roots of the spinal nerves within the spinal canal allows this technique to selectively disrupt sensory transmission while preserving motor function.[5]

Clinical Anatomy

The relevant clinical anatomy for intrathecal neurolysis includes the vertebral column and its contents: the spinal cord, ligaments, and meninges. The vertebral column consists of 33 vertebrae divided into 5 segments based on the curvature of the vertebral column: 7 cervical, 12 thoracic, 5 lumbar, 5 sacral (fused to form the sacrum), and usually 4 coccygeal (fused to form the coccyx) [6]. Each vertebral level is uniquely shaped while still sharing characteristics with the other vertebrae in its spinal segment. These defining characteristics include transverse foramina in the cervical spine, rib articulation in the thoracic spine, and vertebral fusion in the sacrum. In general, vertebrae grow larger caudally to accommodate increased weight bearing until becoming smaller in the coccyx. These anatomic differences have an important impact on optimal needle placement for intrathecal neurolysis, which will be detailed later in the chapter.[7]

Each vertebra has an anterior vertebral body and posterior vertebral arch. The posterior arch consists of pedicles, transverse processes, lamina, superior and inferior articular processes, and a spinous process. The vertebral column is stabilized by the anterior longitudinal ligament, posterior longitudinal ligament, ligamentum flavum, interspinous ligament, and supraspinous ligament. The posterior arches of each vertebra combine to create the spinal canal from the foramen magnum to the sacral hiatus.[6,8] The spinal canal varies in shape and size depending on the segment of the vertebral column. It is smallest in the thoracic segments and largest in the lumbar segments. The spinal canal contains the spinal cord, spinal nerves, meninges, and vasculature (Figure 7.6.1). The spinal cord extends from the brainstem to its termination, called the filum terminal. At the filum terminal, the spinal cord divides within the thecal sac into spinal nerves called the cauda equina. The location of the filum terminal is variable, but typically is at L1 in adults and L3 in infants.[9=10] The thecal sac typically ends at the S2 level.[11]

The spinal cord and cauda equina are covered by three meninges: the dura mater, arachnoid and pia mater.[12] The pia mater adheres directly to spinal cord and spinal nerve roots, ending at the dorsal root ganglia. The pia membrane is a fragile vascular membrane. The space between arachnoid and pia space is known as the intrathecal or subarachnoid space. This intrathecal space is 2–3 mm in depth and contains cerebrospinal fluid (CSF).[12]

New methods calculate the total CSF volume to be between 250 and 400 mL in healthy adults.[12] About 75% of CSF is intracranial and 25% intraspinal.[10] The choroid plexus in the cerebral ventricles creates about 500 mL of CSF daily, which is then reabsorbed into the venous system. The volume of CSF is regulated by the hydrostatic and osmotic forces between the CSF and neural tissues.[6,7]

The behavior of any substance administered in the intrathecal space depends on CSF characteristics. The CSF volume accounts for 80% of spinal drug behavior.[2,3] The CSF dynamics is another factor that affects the behavior of intrathecal substances. Cerebrospinal fluid oscillates in synchrony with

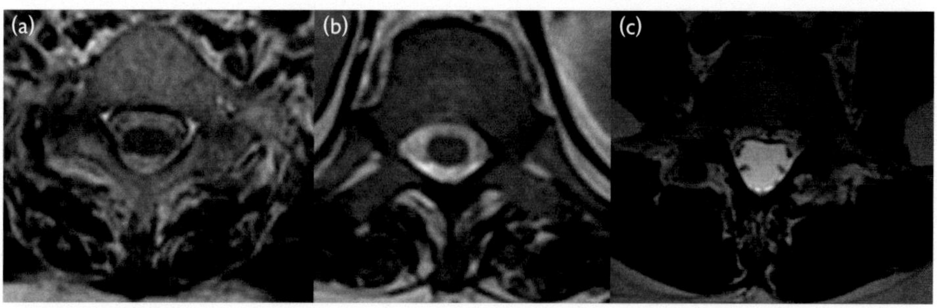

Figure 7.6.1 Spinal canal variation in shape and size that is dependent on the segment of the vertebral column. **a,** cervical; **b,** thoracic; **c,** lumbar.

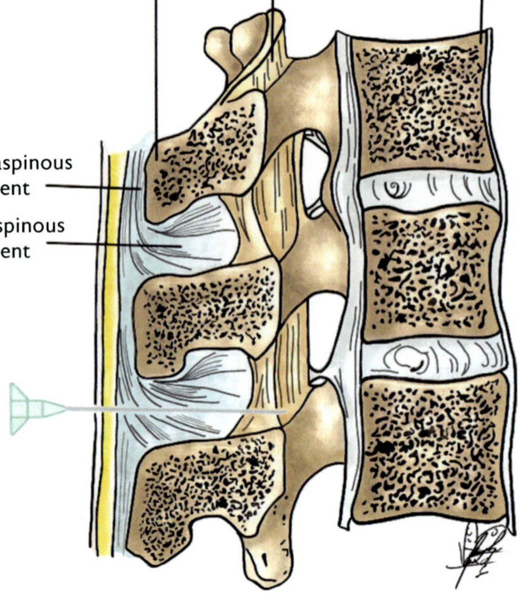

Figure 7.6.2 Illustration of the ligamentum flavum is an anatomical reference point prior to entrance of the epidural space with a needle.

the pulsations of arteries, creating a wavelike movement. The amplitude of CSF movement is 9 mm per cycle in the cervical segment and 4 mm in the thoracolumbar segments.[6] These oscillations in CSF affect the distribution of any substance in the intrathecal space.[8,10]

The arachnoid membrane is composed of overlapping layers of epithelial cells connected by tight junctions. This anatomic arrangement creates the main meningeal barrier in the blood-brain barrier.[8,10] The outermost membrane is the dura, which is a fibroelastic tube that ends at the inferior border of S2. The dura mater is surrounded by the epidural space that contains segmental nerve roots, fat, areolar tissue, lymphatics, and blood vessels like Baston's venous plexus. The epidural space's depth varies depending on the segment of the vertebral column. It is approximately 1–1.5 mm in the cervical segment, 2–3 mm in the thoracic segment, and 5–6 mm in the lumbar segment.[6] Midline and paramedian approaches often lead to larger depths, especially in the lumbar area, due to the triangular shape of the epidural space.[6] Posterior to the epidural space is the ligamentum flavum. The flavum ligament is an anatomical reference point and in healthy adults can be felt as a pop or loss of resistance with a needle as it is punctured (Figure 7.6.2).

Indications

Intrathecal administration of phenol or alcohol has been documented to provide adequate and prolonged pain relief in selected cases with an average benefit time of 3 months to even 1 year [13].

Advantages of This Technique Include

1. Simple technique that uses equipment standardly found in an interventional pain clinic
2. Can be repeated if necessary
3. Option for elderly and debilitated patients
4. Prolonged duration of pain relief

Risks of This Technique Include

1. Infection at skin or neuraxis
2. Bleeding at skin or neuraxis, including epidural hematoma
3. Unintended tissue injury or tissue necrosis
4. Unintended neural injury leading to fecal or urinary incontinence
5. Unintended neural injury leading to weakness or numbness, including paresis

General Indications for Performing This Technique Are

Patient selection is the most important part of the procedure, as it influences its success (Box 7.6.1). This procedure should be performed as an alternative option only after other treatment modalities have failed and in patients with life expectancies of no more than 12 months [14]. The pain must be localized and preferably without a neuropathic component.

Lynch[5] et al. performed intrathecal neurolysis in nine patients for the treatment of perineal and perianal cancer pain with the following inclusion criteria:

a. Pain limited to the perianal region with somatic origin
b. Inadequate control of pain after definitive surgery or radiotherapy with consumption of high doses of opioids complicated by intolerable adverse events
c. Ineligible for intrathecal or epidural opioid analgesic treatment
d. Pain relief of at least 75% after a diagnostic intrathecal block with hyperbaric bupivacaine 0.5% 0.2–0.5 mL.
e. Had a colostomy and urethrostomy or urinary catheter prior to performing intrathecal neurolysis. In the absence of colostomy or nephrostomy, it is essential that the patient is aware of the risk of postprocedure urinary incontinence and accepts it.
f. No radiological evidence (CT or MRI) of tumor infiltration into the medullary canal, or, in the event that there is suspicion of medullary infiltration, it is necessary to have a myelogram
g. An expected survival of 3 to 12 months

Lynch et al. reported a significant incidence of serious side effects, with two patients having permanent urinary retention.[5] The average daily oral morphine dose was reduced by approximately 20% during this time, and only two out of nine patients stopped opioids completely for a period of four weeks.

Even when performed by an expert, true sensory selectivity is rarely achieved with intrathecal neurolysis [16-19]. Therefore, this block can result in disturbances of the motor and autonomic

BOX 7.6.1 General Indications for Performing Intrathecal Neurolysis

Refractory pain in cancer
Intolerable adverse effects from standard pain treatment
Unilateral pain
Pain in 1 to 4 dermatomes
Somatic or visceral pain
Absence of intraspinal tumor or mass
Positive response to a diagnostic block with local anesthetic
Localized to the chest or abdomen *

Modified from: Candido K, Stevens R. Intrathecal neurolytic blocks for the relief of cancer pain. Best Practice & Research Clinical Anaesthesiology 2003;17 (3):407–428.

* Saeed K, Adams M, Hurles R. Chapter 72: Central and Peripheral Neurolysis. Editor (s): Honorio T, Benzon, Srinivasa N. Raja, Spencer S. Lui, Elsevier; 2018:655–662.

nervous systems as well. Patients must understand potential problems associated with the procedure including inadequate pain relief, short duration of effect, weakness of the limb muscles, and bowel or bladder incontinence [20]. The patient must understand that these procedures are not supported by prospective, randomized, controlled clinical trials to validate their use. In fact, the use of these blocks is based purely on anecdotal and observational reports [21-23].

Finally, the patient should expect systemic side effects after intrathecal neurolysis including a subjective feeling of "sickness" (nausea, headache, burning, or dysesthesia or paresthesia) that can persist from 1 day to 2–3 weeks [24].

Contraindications

Contraindications for this technique are listed in Table 7.6.1.

Equipment and Patient Preparation

1. **Monitors and Sterility:**
   a. It is highly advised that vital signs, including blood pressure, heart rate, respiratory rate, and pulse oximetry, be obtained prior to starting the procedure to ensure the patient is hemodynamically stable. A set of vitals is often taken post procedure as well.
   b. Strict antiseptic technique should be observed including sterile draping, sterile gloves, and sterile gauze. Chlorhexidine or another skin prep agent should be used to clean the skin before the procedure.
   c. The procedures are performed with the patient awake.
2. **Imaging modalities:**
   a. Fluoroscopy
3. **Needle type:**
   i. Local anesthetic: 25-gauge 1.5-inch needle
   ii. Intrathecal access: 20- to 25-gauge spinal needle

Table 7.6.1 Contraindications for Performing Intrathecal Neurolysis

Absolute	Relative
Severe coagulopathy (thrombocytopenia, Disseminated intravascular coagulation)	Poorly localized pain
Skin infection at the approach site pain	Neuropathic pain
Patient refusal	Sympathetic maintenance pain
	Pain poorly described
	Disseminated tumor where the blockage will only cover a part of the affected anatomical area
	Depression, anxiety
	Do not accept the possible adverse events associated with the technique
	Intraspinal mass
	2 failed prognostic or diagnostic blocks with local anesthetic

Table with information taken from: Candido K, Stevens R. Intrathecal neurolytic blocks for the relief of cancer pain. Best Practice & Research Clinical Anaesthesiology 2003;17(3):407-428.

4. **Patient position:** Lateral decubitus or seated
5. **Injectate:**
   a. Local anesthetic: lidocaine 1%–2%; ropivacaine 0.2%–0.5%; bupivacaine 0.25%–0.5%
   b. Neurolytic: phenol (hyperbaric) or dehydrated alcohol (hypobaric)

Technique

Cervical Subarachnoid Neurolysis—Fluoroscopy Approach

1. **Position the patient in lateral decubitus with the neck flexed.** The painful procedural side should be up if using hypobaric ethanol. The procedural side should be down if using hyperbaric phenol. A pillow can be placed under the chest for comfort.
2. **Identify the target at C6/7 or C7/T1 with an AP fluoroscopy image.** The intrathecal space should be accessed midline between the spinous processes or paramedian just lateral to the spinous processes.
3. **Anesthetize the skin at the needle insertion site.**
4. **Insert the procedural needle via a paramedian approach at the desired level.** Use a 22- or 25-gauge spinal needle.
5. **Obtain a lateral image to determine the depth of the needle**. Do not advance the needle tip beyond the spinolaminar line.
6. **Advance a few millimeters at a time until encountering CSF**. Puncturing the dura may be felt as a loss of resistance.
7. **Inject neurolytic medications.**
8. **After the desired dermatomes are treated, flush and withdraw the spinal needle, introducer, and syringe as one.** Ensure hemostasis and place a dressing.
9. **Maintain the patient in lateral decubitus position for at least 45 minutes after the procedure.**

Cervical Subarachnoid Neurolysis—Blind/Landmark Approach

1. **Position the patient in lateral decubitus with the neck flexed.** The painful procedural side should be up if using hypobaric ethanol. The procedural side should be down if using hyperbaric phenol. A pillow can be placed under the chest for comfort.
2. **Locate the C6/7 interspinous space via palpation.**
3. **Anesthetize the skin at the needle insertion site.**
4. **Insert a 10 cm, 22-gauge needle in the interspinous space** directed toward the midline (Figure 7.6.3).
5. **Advance slowly until a loss of resistance is felt, indicating dural puncture. (Figure 7.6.4**). Remove the stylet to see CFS flow from the needle.
6. **Attach the syringe with neurolytic injectate and aspirate to reconfirm free flowing CSF.**
7. **Inject 0.5 mL of the injectate.**
8. **Evaluate pain sensation in the targeted dermatomes by puncturing the skin with 25-gauge needles to provoke pain (Figure 7.6.4).** The patient's responses will determine whether additional small aliquots of neurolytic injectate are required.
9. **Repeat neurological evaluations and small injectate aliquots as required.**
10. **After the desired dermatomes are treated, flush and withdraw the spinal needle, introducer, and syringe as one.** Ensure hemostasis and place a dressing.
11. **Maintain the patient in lateral decubitus position for at least 45 minutes after the procedure.**

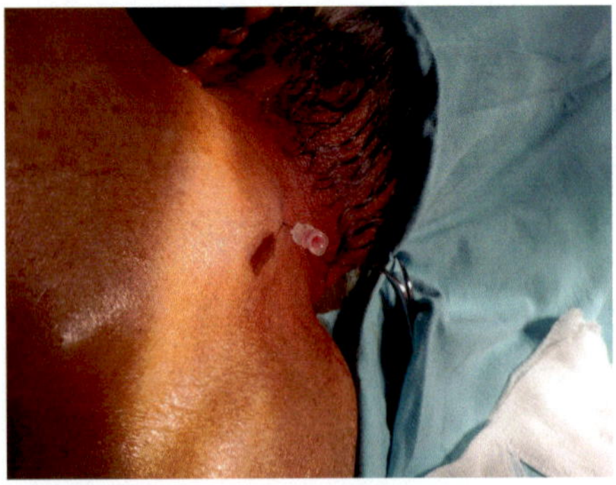

Figure 7.6.3 Insertion of at spinal need at the C6–7 interspace directed toward the midline via the landmark technique.

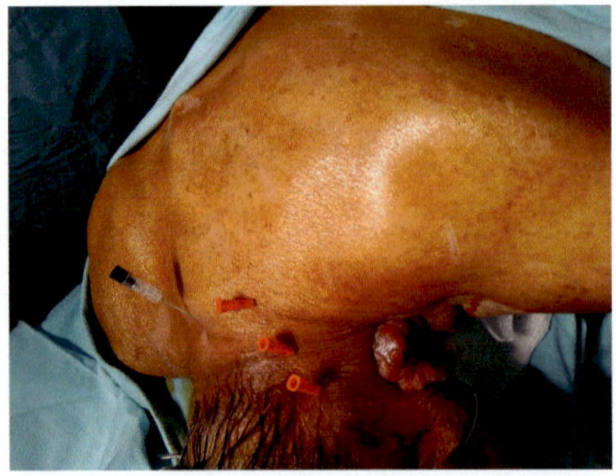

Figure 7.6.4 Needle advanced in the cervical interspace until a loss of resistance is felt, which would indicate a dural puncture. Additionally, 25-guage needles are utilized to assess for whether pain is covered based on associated dermatomes.

Thoracic Intrathecal Neurolysis—Blind/Landmark Approach

Accessing the thecal sac in the thoracic spine is frequently more difficult than in the cervical or lumbar spine due to enlarged and acutely angled posterior spinous processes. Here a paramedian approach is used to minimize difficulty.

1. **Position the patient in partial lateral decubitus at a 45-degree angle with the neck flexed.** The painful procedural side should be up if using hypobaric ethanol. The procedural side should be down if using hyperbaric phenol. A pillow can be placed under the chest for comfort.
2. **Locate the desired interspinous space via palpation.**
3. **Anesthetize the skin at the needle insertion site.**
4. **Insert a 20- to 22-gauge spinal needle using a paramedian approach until reaching the intrathecal space.** A loss of resistance may be felt after puncturing the dura (Figure 7.6.5).
5. **Inject 0.3 mL of neurolytic.**
6. **Evaluate pain sensation in the targeted dermatomes by puncturing the skin with 25-gauge needles to provoke pain.** The patient's responses will determine whether additional small aliquots of neurolytic injectate are required.
7. **After the desired dermatomes are treated, flush and withdraw the spinal needle and syringe as one.** Ensure hemostasis and place a dressing.
8. **Keep the patient in lateral decubitus for at least 45 minutes after the injection.**

Lumbar Intrathecal Neurolysis—Blind/Landmark Approach

1. **Position the patient in a sitting position with mild thoracolumbar flexion.** A 45-degree inclination increase the chances for the injectate to be deposited only along the sensory dorsal roots.
2. **Identify the L5–S1 interspinous space via palpation.** A common landmark is the iliac crest, which is typically at the L4–L5 level (Figure 7.6.6).
3. **Anesthetize the skin at the needle insertion site.**
4. **Insert a 20- to 22-gauge spinal needle using a midline approach until reaching the intrathecal space.** A loss of resistance may be felt after puncturing the dura.
5. **Redirect the bevel of the needle caudally and ensure free flow of CSF.**

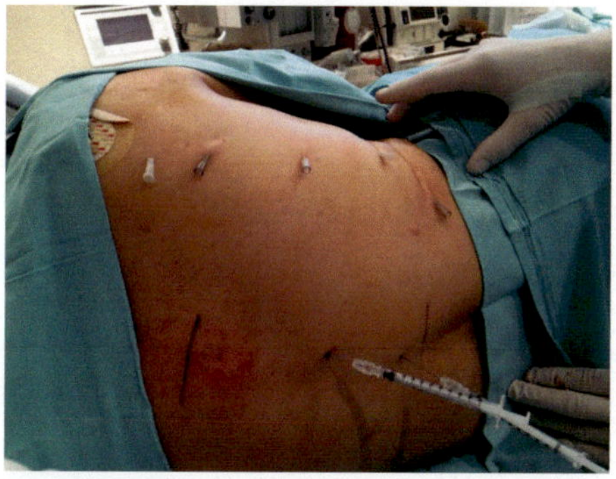

Figure 7.6.5 Insertion of a spinal need at the thoracic interspace using a paramedian approach until reaching the intrathecal space. Additionally, 25-gauge needles are utilized to assess for whether pain is covered based on associated dermatomes.

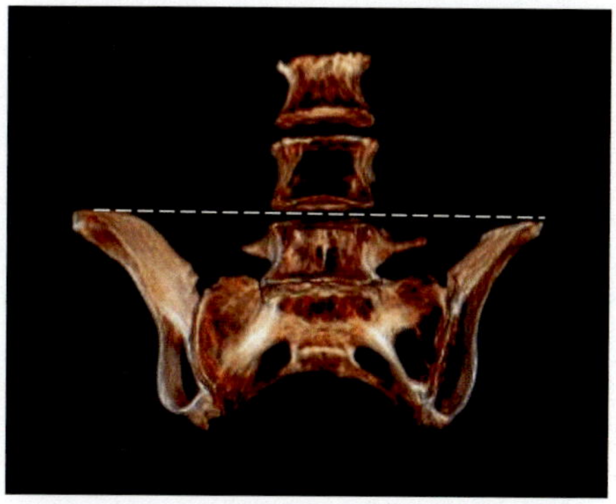

Figure 7.6.6 Illustration of the iliac crest as landmark denotes the L4–5 level.

6. **Connect a 1 mL syringe with** neurolytic injectate and inject 0.5 mL. Ethanol neurolysis can cause an intense pain along the affected dermatomes. This can be mitigated with local anesthetics injected immediately prior to neurolysis. While sensitivity trials are ideally performed, they are often difficult to assess at the perineal levels in a seated position. Nonetheless, pain relief occurs reliably in nearly every case after a single neurolytic dose.
7. **Flush and withdraw the spinal needle and syringe as one.** Ensure hemostasis and place a dressing. Stop the administration of alcohol when the patient's pain is relieved or lower motor strength diminishes.
8. **Keep the patient in the flexed seated position for at least 45 minutes after the injection.**

Safety Considerations

Neurologic examinations should be performed during the procedure whenever possible to evaluate which dermatomes have been affected [24]. This is more easily performed with the collaboration of a partner, allowing the proceduralist to continue titrating neurolysis until the desired dermatomes are treated. Ethanol neurolysis can cause intense pain along the affected dermatomes. This can be mitigated by an intrathecal local anesthetic injection prior to neurolysis. Finally, the needle must be flushed prior to removal. This prevents accidental deposit of neurolytic agents into other tissues, which can lead to injury and backache [24].

Tips

- Phenol concentration must be used between 4% to 10%, diluted in glycerol.
- Phenol is hyperbaric and ethanol is hypobaric. Therefore, positioning to target dorsal spinal roots depends on which compound is used.
- Do not perform this procedure where intrathecal tumors are present. Instrumenting a tumor could lead to tumor spread. The friability of tumor tissue could lead to bleeding, hematoma, and neurologic injury.
- In dorsal neurolysis, three needles can be used to distribute less volume and cover the chosen areas.

Epidural Neurolysis

A high percentage of pain relief, after epidural neurolaysis is performed, is reported in many studies, with a reported average of 3.3 months of significant pain relief after the procedure is completed.[14,15] The National Institute of Cancer in Mexico developed an alternative technique to intrathecal neurolysis: epidural neurolysis. This technique uses an epidural catheter directed to the desired position via fluoroscopy. Epidurography is then used to determine the volume of contrast required to cover the desired extension of the block. The same volume of phenol is then used for the epidural neurolysis. Three percent phenol is injected in aliquots of 2–4 mL until the total target volume is reached. The patient is asked to remain still in the prone position for 15 minutes, then spends 45 minutes with free movement supine in bed. Later a neurologic and pain evaluation is performed. If pain persists and there is no neurologic injury, the procedure can be repeated using 4% or 5% phenol with the same volume.

Literature Review

Dogliotti injected alcohol intrathecally first time in 1931.[23] and after that similar reports followed with a high incidence of reported complications. Maher introduced intrathecal phenol in 1955, claiming more predictable results.[16] In his original paper, Dogliotti described 45 patients with pain in the lower back, pelvis, and legs due to various nonmalignant conditions.[23] Of these 45 patients, 27 (60%) obtained good pain relief after intrathecal neurolysis.

In 1936, Tureen and Gitt described two cases of ethanol intrathecal neurolysis causing bladder disturbances that persisted for over a year.[24] They also found that intrathecal alcohol afforded only transient pain relief. Workers also noted that problems with bowel or bladder incontinence and motor paralysis of the lower extremities resulted after injections in the lumbar region, where mixed sensorimotor nerves were affected by the neurolysis.[17]

Lynch et al. reported nine patients with perianal or perineal cancer related pain had a short duration of pain relief (17.8 days) after IT neurolysis but two patients had permanent urinary retention. Given the high rate of urinary retention, intrathecal or epidural opiates may be preferable to neurolysis for patients with pelvic or perineal pain and intact bladder and/or bowel function.[5]

In 1959, Kelley et al. reported using intrathecal neurolysis with 10% phenol in various cases of painful spasticity.[2] Racz, Heavener, and Haynsworth reported the epidural administration of phenol for chronic pain and spasticity.[18]

Candido and Stevens reported four cases of cancer patients whose intractable pain was treated with intrathecal neurolysis with mixed results. One patient had an 80% reduction of her overall pain and was weaned off opioid and anticonvulsant medications until her death 4 months later. Another patient's pain returned just 6 weeks after the block despite having weakness and impaired bladder/rectal function for over 8 months.[3] A different patient required repeated injections at higher doses (reaching 5 mL of 6% phenol) before having a sustained 75% reduction in his original pain. However, he developed weakness and new hypoesthesia of his feet, which did not resolve. Another patient required 2 blocks using 0.5 mL of 6% phenol to achieve about 50% pain relief. At the patient's request, the same injection was repeated 1 week later and provided analgesia acceptable to the patient. No motor block or complications were encountered.

Butler et al. reported on pain relief in 15 cases of alcohol intrathecal neurolysis and 12 cases of phenol neurolysis. The study showed alcohol neurolysis gave good pain relief in 60%, fair relief in 22%, and poor relief in 18% of patients. Phenol neurolysis gave good pain relief in 58%, fair relief in 16%, and poor relief in 25% of patients.[19]

Among the most frequent complications reported by Gerbershagen[14] in 1981 after alcohol intrathecal neurolysis were bladder dysfunction (7.2%), paresis (5.2%), and bowel disorders (0.5%). The permanent complications were paresis or paralysis (0.8%), bladder dysfunction (0.8%), and bowel disorders (0.1%). Complications reported with phenol or intrathecal alcohol were: bladder dysfunction (9%), rectal sphincter dysfunction (2%), headache (3%), paresis (12.9%), and dysesthesias (8%).[3,20]

Hernandez-Porras[15] and the group of National Institute of Cancer reported a total of 27 patients and 32 procedures for cancer pain treatment. The mean baseline pain score was 7.46. The mean pain scores at a week, a month, and two months after the intervention were 4.70 ± 2.43, 4.93 ± 2.81, and 4.85 ± 1.95 respectively ($p < 0.005$). Intrathecal neurolytic block reduced pain and morphine daily dose mainly the first two months after the intervention for intractable cancer pain.

Recently, a randomized trial was performed on 40 patients with pelvic malignancies and intractable pain. Patients were randomized for thermal radiofrequency of S3 to S5 nerve roots or for phenol intrathecal neurolysis at L5/S1 with a maximum volume of 0.7 mL of 6% phenol administered. They reported similar results in both procedures and incidence of specific procedure-related adverse outcomes was also equivalent. However, the phenol group developed more major complications such as dysesthesias of lower limbs, paresis, bladder dysfunction, and fecal incontinence.[22]

References

1. Van den Beuken-Van Everdingen M, Hochstenbach L, Joosten E, et al. (2016) Update on prevalence of pain in patients with cancer: systematic review and meta-analysis. Journal of Pain and Symptom Management 1(6):1070–1090.
2. Swerdlow M (1989) The history of neurolytic block. In: Racz GB (ed.), Techniques of Neurolysis. Springer Science + Business Media: 1–2.
3. Candido K, Stevens R. (2003) Intrathecal neurolytic blocks for the relief of cancer pain. Best Practice and Research Clinical Anaesthesiology 17(3):407–428.
4. Saeed K, Adams M, Hurles R (2018) Chapter 72: Central and peripheral neurolysis. In: Benzon HT, Raja SN, Lui SS, et al. (eds.), Essentials of Pain Medicine, 4th edition. Elsevier: 655–662.
5. Lynch J, Zech D, GErond S (1992) The role of intrathecal neurolysis in the treatment of cancer-related perianal and perineal pain. Palliative Medicine 6:140–145.
6. Halaszynsky TM, Hartmaannsgruber WB (1998) Anatomy and physiology of spinal and epidural anesthesia. Seminars in Anesthesia Perioperative Medicine and Pain 17(1):24–37.
7. Macfarlane A, Brull R, Drasner K, Chan V (2015) Spinal, epidural and caudal anesthesia. In: Miller RD (ed.), Miller's Anesthesia. Elsevier Health Science: 1684–1820.
8. Halaszynsky TM, Hartmaannsgruber WB (1998) Anatomy and physiology of spinal and epidural anesthesia. Seminars in Anesthesia Perioperative Medicine and Pain 17(1):24–37.
9. Macfarlane A, Brull R, Drasner, K, Chan V (2015) Spinal, epidural and caudal anesthesia. In: Miller RD (ed.), Miller's Anesthesia. Elsevier Health Science: 1684–1820.
10. Lui SS, Mc Donald SB (2001) Current issues in spinal anesthesia. Anesthesiology 94:888–906.
11. Hogan Q (1998) Anatomy of spinal anesthesia: some old and new findings. Regional Anesthesia and Pain Medicine 23(4):340–243.
12. Martin BA, Pahlavian SH (2019) Anatomy and physiology of cerebrospinal fluid dynamics. In: Lanser R, Sarntinoranoht M (eds.), Nervous System Drug Delivery. Academic Press: 73–89.
13. Plancarte-Sanchez R, Guajardo-Rosas J, Guillén-Nuñez MDR. (2006) Neurolytic techniques for cancer pain management. In: Oscar DeLeon Casasola (ed), Cancer Pain. WB Saunders: 501–507.
14. Gerbershagen HU (1981) Neurolysis: subarachnoid neurolytic blockade. Acta Anaesthesiology Belgium. 32(1):45–57.
15. Hernández-Porras C (2012). Abstracts of the 6th World Congress of the World Institute of Pain, WIP 2012. Miami Beach, Florida, USA. February 4–6, 2012. Pain Pract 12(Suppl 1):1–199.
16. Lloyd JW (1989). Subarachnoid and other clinical uses of phenol. In: Techniques of Neurolysis. Eds Racz GB, Noe CE Springer: 33–44.

17. Blanchard J., Ramamurthy S (1989) Subarachnoid alcohol block. In: Techniques of Neurolysis. Racz GB, Noe CE Springer: 45–56.
18. Racz GB, Heavner J, Haynsworth R (1985) Repeat epidural phenol injections in chronic pain and spasticity. In: Lipton S, Miles J (eds.), Persistent Pain: Modern Methods of Treatment, vol. 5. Grune & Stratton: 157–179.
19. Bulter SH, Charlton JE (2001) Intrathecal neurolysis In: Loeser JD (ed.), Bonica's Management of Pain, Lippincott, Williams & Wilkins: 1988–1989.
20. Ferrer-Brechner T (1981) Epidural and intrathecal phenol neurolysis for cancer pain. Anesthesiology Reviews 8:14–32.
21. Korevaar WC (1988) Transcatheter thoracic epidural neurolysis using ethyl alcohol. Anesthesiology 69:989–993.
22. Reyad RM, Hakim SM, Abbas DN, Ghobrial HZ, Mansour E (2018) A novel technique of saddle rhizotomy using thermal radiofrequency for intractable perineal pain in pelvic malignancy: a pilot study. Pain Physician 21(6):E651–E660.
23. Dogliotti AM (1933) Segmental peridural spinal anesthesia. American Journal of Surgery 20(1):107–118. doi:10.1016/s0002-9610(33)91041-7
24. Tureen LL (1936) Cauda equina syndrome following subarachnoid alcohol injection. Journal of the American Medical Association 106(18):1535. doi:10.1001/jama.1936.02770180009003 25.

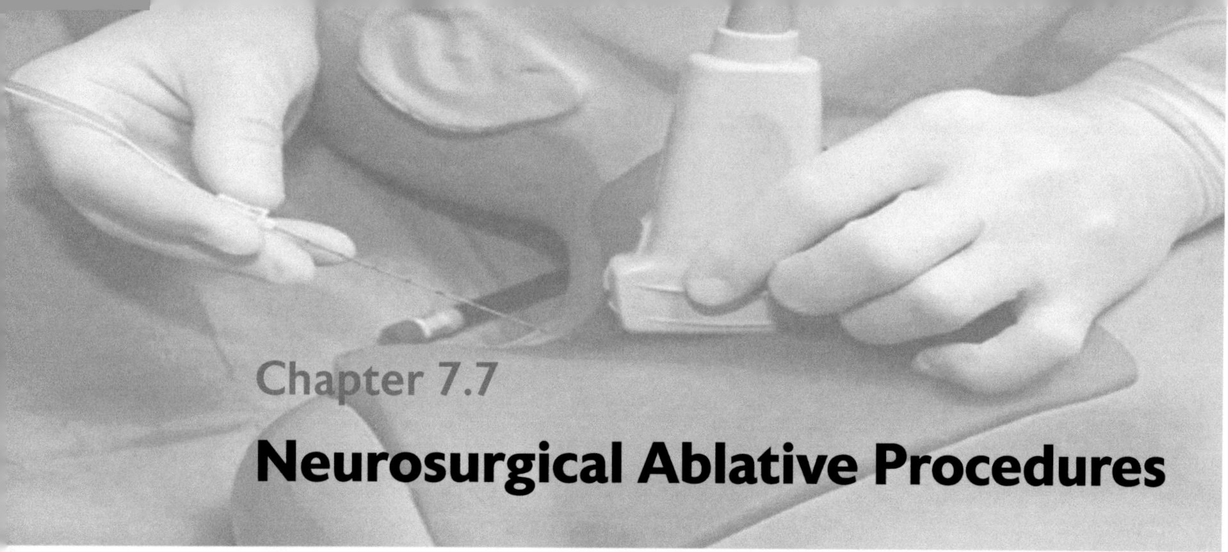

Chapter 7.7

Neurosurgical Ablative Procedures

Ido Straus

Contents

Introduction

Pain is one of the most common symptoms among cancer patients, particularly in those who suffer from advanced metastatic disease.[1] Most cancer pain patients can be effectively treated using the World Health Organization guidelines ("WHO Pain Ladder"), which were developed to treat cancer pain in a stepwise approach depending on the pain level reported by the patient.[1] Still, a small but significant proportion of cancer patients, estimated at 5%–10%, fail to respond to conventional medical treatment and may be deemed "refractory".[2] Therefore, one of the major challenges in the care of these advanced cancer patients is pain management, which can greatly influence quality of life and functional status.

The neurosurgical armamentarium for treating pain is extensive and includes both ablative and neuromodulatory therapies. The most commonly applied interventions are intrathecal or epidural drug delivery systems or spinal cord stimulators. These neuromodulatory techniques, although non-destructive and reversible, require ongoing maintenance and carry infectious risk, especially in immunocompromised and cachectic patients.

Advanced cancer patients require procedures that are minimally invasive, can be performed without general anesthesia, and achieve immediate and long-lasting pain relief. Therefore, selected patients suffering from refractory pain may benefit from targeted neurosurgical procedures that selectively intervene along the central pain pathways. Ablative procedures such as cordotomy, myelotomy, trigeminal tractotomy, stereotactic mesencephalotomy, and cingulotomy can be tailored to the patient's specific pain syndrome. This chapter gives an overview of available neurosurgical ablative procedures and describes our approach to the selection of the appropriate neurosurgical procedure by an interdisciplinary team (Figure 7.7.1).

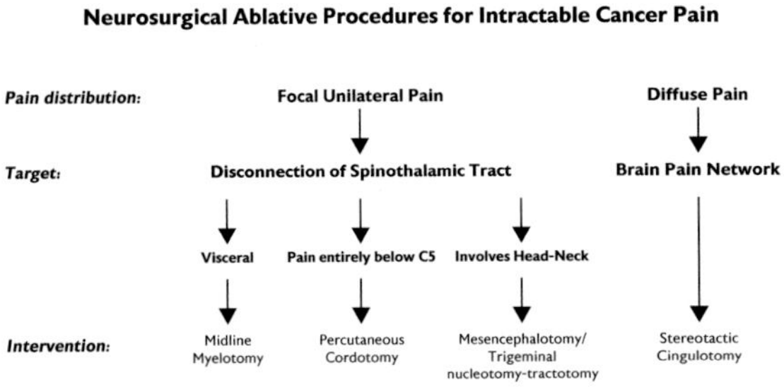

Figure 7.7.1 Selection algorithm for neurosurgical ablative procedures for intractable cancer pain.

Our treatment algorithm first distinguishes between patients suffering from unilateral localized pain and patients with diffuse, bilateral, or midline pain. Patients with unilateral localized pain should be preferably considered for disconnection of the spinothalamic pain and temperature pathway. The spinothalamic tract (STT) can be lesioned along the entire tract, from the thoracic level and up to the midbrain. Axons ascending in the STT are of second order neurons located in the contralateral dorsal horn of the spinal cord. The advantage of these procedures is that immediate and complete pain relief can be achieved in carefully selected patients.[2]

As pain fibers enter the spinal cord, they can ascend 1–2 segments in the Lissauer tract before synapsing on dorsal horn neurons.[3] Therefore, a STT lesion will provide pain control corresponding to a spinal level three levels below the lesion. For pain in a dermatome below the shoulder (C4) the most commonly used procedure to disconnect the STT is percutaneous cervical cordotomy (PCC). This is a minimally invasive procedure that involves insertion of a radiofrequency (RF) electrode through the lateral C1–C2 interspace into the anterolateral quadrant of the spinal cord (Figure 7.7.2). The procedure is performed under imaging guidance with either 2D-fluoroscopy or more recently 3D-computed tomography. Percutaneous cervical cordotomy is usually performed under local anesthesia and requires patient cooperation for intraoperative neurophysiological verification of the optimal ablation target. This can be challenging, as the procedure requires patients to lie supine for about one hour, which can be difficult with specific pain syndromes. We try to avoid sedation as much as possible while using remifentanil to control pain and allow patients to lie still during the procedure. Percutaneous cervical cordotomy can be relatively quickly mastered by neurosurgeons or pain specialists, who have the appropriate neuroanatomical knowledge and expertise to interpret intraoperative neurophysiological findings. Pain relief can be immediate, and postoperative recovery in most cases is relatively quick.

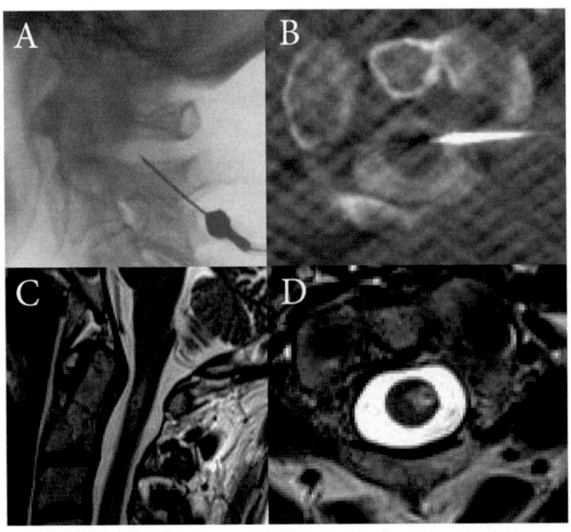

Figure 7.7.2 Images showing the C1–2 level percutaneous cordotomy. **a,** Sagittal fluoroscopy image showing the needle as it advances toward the C1–2 level. **b,** Axial myelographic CT image acquired using an O-arm, showing the tip of the electrode in the anterolateral quadrant of the spinal cord at the C1–2 level. **c–d,** Postoperative sagittal and axial MR images showing the lesion in the left anterolateral quadrant at the C1–2 level.

In modern series using computerized tomography (CT) guidance, significant morbidity in the form of respiratory complications or permanent paresis is rare.[2,4]

Common side effects include positional headaches, temporary ataxia, and contralateral limb pain.[2,4] Most of these side effects are usually mild and transient. Contraindications include uncorrectable coagulopathies and inability to cooperate during the procedure.

Other options for disconnection of the STT are available for patients who are not willing or cannot undergo PCC. Open thoracic cordotomy is a microsurgical anatomical operation that requires experience in intraoperative electrophysiological neuromonitoring. The procedure can be performed through a single-level laminectomy and has been previously described by several authors.

For patients suffering from head and neck pain above C4 level, two options are available depending on the exact pain distribution and available expertise. For craniofacial pain in the trigeminal distribution, trigeminal tractotomy-nucleotomy (TR-NC) is an option. The advantage is that, like PCC, it performed under local anesthesia using a CT-guided percutaneous approach as described by Kanpolat.[5–6] The patient is placed in the prone position and an RF electrode is introduced through a posterior approach between the occiput and C1 into the cervicomedullary junction, about 6–8 mm lateral to the midline. The technique targets the descending trigeminal tract and the nucleus caudalis of the spinal trigeminal nucleus conveying ipsilateral pain and temperature sensations. The procedure is performed on the side of the pain. The most common complications that have been reported so far are transient ataxia and motor dysfunction.[4]

Another option for patients suffering from craniocervical pain beyond the trigeminal distribution (or also in specific cases of pain below C4 when PCC is not possible), is stereotactic mesencephalotomy. The target is the STT at the midbrain level, which carries pain and temperature fibers from the contralateral hemibody and face. The procedure is performed using standard stereotactic techniques and has been described by several authors. The target is located at the level of the red nucleus, at the anterior border of the aqueduct, 8 mm lateral from midline. The target is just a few millimeters posterior and medial than the subthalamic nucleus target used for deep brain stimulation for Parkinson's disease, and therefore should be relatively easy to accomplish for functional neurosurgeons experienced in stereotactic techniques (Figure 7.7.3).

A special consideration should be given to visceral abdominal and/or pelvic pain. Visceral pain fibers ascend through the medial tracts of the dorsal columns in the spinal cord, separate from the STT. Although limited, evidence is accumulating to suggest that targeting these fibers through a procedure called punctate midline myelotomy can result in significant relief of cancer-related visceral pain.[2] The procedure is usually performed through a single-level thoracic laminectomy and entails a small lesion of the most dorsomedial fibers about 2 mm bilaterally from the midline. Side effects are usually mild proprioceptive deficits.

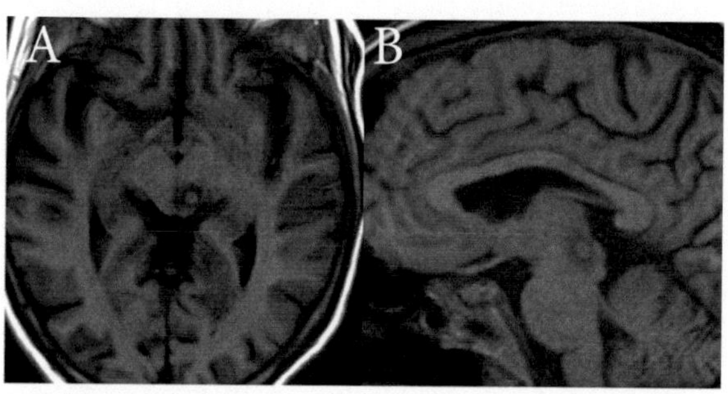

Figure 7.7.3 Axial (a) and sagittal (b) MR images acquired on post-op day 1 after stereotactic mesencephalotomy, showing a unilateral lesion in the midbrain, 7 mm lateral to the aqueduct at the level superior colliculi.

In cases of diffuse or bilateral pain, options include staged bilateral cordotomy, stereotactic cingulotomy, and hypophysectomy. Hypophysectomy is especially for pain from bony metastases.[7] Staged bilateral high cervical cordotomy has been described but carries a higher risk of respiratory complications due to bilateral damage to the reticulospinal fibers that lie just medial to the STT.

Stereotactic cingulotomy is a safe treatment option for patients suffering from diffuse pain,

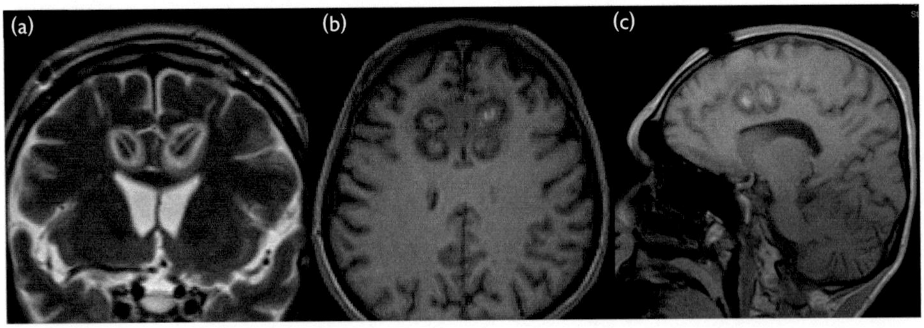

Figure 7.7.4 MR images acquired on the 1st postoperative day after stereotactic cingulotomy, showing bilateral double lesion in the dorsal anterior cingulate cortex. **a,** Coronal T2-weighted image **b,** Axial T1-weighted image, and C: Sagittal T1-weighted image.

especially if there is a significant affective component to the pain.[2] The dorsal anterior cingulate cortex (dACC) is considered part of the limbic circuit and is thought to have a major role in cognitive and emotional processing, as well as the perception of pain. The advantages of cingulotomy are that the procedure is relatively quick and can be performed under local anesthesia or mild sedation (Figure 7.7.4). It is well tolerated with minimal side effects and produces immediate relief of the suffering component of pain. Following the procedure, patients often report that they can still feel pain, however it is better tolerated, and the overall suffering associated with the perception of pain is decreased.

Palliative stereotactic radiosurgery hypophysectomy is a noninvasive treatment that has been described for diffuse refractory pain, especially due to bony metastases in patients with hormone-sensitive cancer.[7] The mechanism of pain relief is unknown, but the hypothalamo-hypophyseal axis and especially oxytocin appear to play a role in pain perception. There is currently no standard of care guideline for target selection and dosing, but there is ongoing research into the field.

References

1. WHO guidelines for the pharmacological and radiotherapeutic management of cancer pain in adults and adolescents. World Health Organization. (2019) https://www.who.int/publications/i/item/9789241550390. Accessed March 6, 2022.
2. Raslan AM, Ben-Haim S, Falowski SM, et al. Congress of Neurological Surgeons systematic review and evidence-based guideline on neuroablative procedures for patients with cancer pain. *Neurosurgery*. 2020;88(3):437–442. doi:10.1093/neuros/nyaa527
3. Purves D, Augustine GJ, Fitzpatrick D, et al., editors. Neuroscience. 2nd ed. Sunderland, MA: Sinauer Associates; 2001.
4. Salahadin S. Cordotomy for intractable cancer pain: a narrative review. *Pain Physician*. 2020 Jun;23(3):283–292. doi:10.36076/ppj.2020/23/283
5. Kanpolat Y, Ugur HC, Ayten M, Elhan AH. Computed tomography-guided percutaneous cordotomy for intractable pain in malignancy. *Neurosurgery*. 2009 Mar;64(3 Suppl):ons187–193.
6. Kanpolat Y, Ozdemir M, Al-Beyati E. CT-guided percutaneous cordotomy for intractable pain in what is more than a disease: lung malignancies. *Turk Neurosurg* 2013; 23:81–87.
7. LaRossa JT, Strong MS, Melby JC. Endocrinologically incomplete transethmoidal trans-sphenoidal hypophysectomy with relief of bone pain in breast cancer. *N Engl J Med*. 1978;298(24):1332–1335. doi:10.1056/NEJM197806152982403.

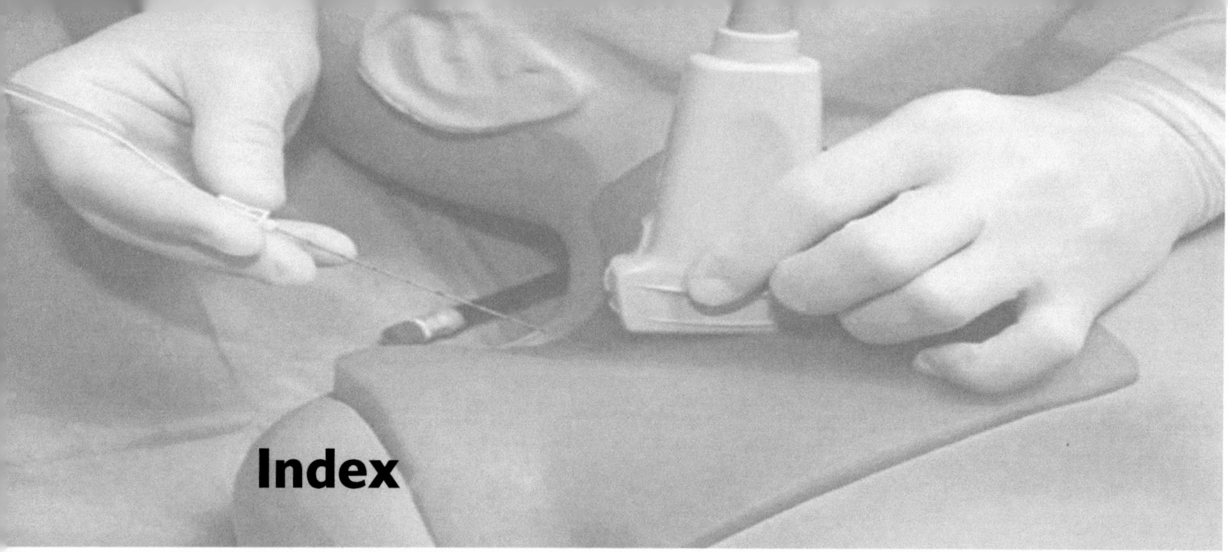

Index

For the benefit of digital users, indexed terms that span two pages (e.g., 52–53) may, on occasion, appear on only one of those pages.

Tables, figures, and boxes are indicated by an italic *t*, *f*, and *b* following the page/paragraph number.

Index

Index

Index

Index